Clinical Cases in Dental Hygiene

Clinical Cases Series

Wiley-Blackwell's Clinical Cases series is designed to recognize the centrality of clinical cases to the dental profession by providing actual cases with an academic backbone. This unique approach supports the new trend in case-based and problem-based learning. Highly illustrated in full color, the Clinical Cases series utilizes a format that fosters independent learning and prepares the reader for case-based examinations.

Clinical Cases in Endodontics
by Takashi Komabayashi
November 2017

Clinical Cases in Orofacial Pain
by Malin Ernberg, Per Alstergren
March 2017

Clinical Cases in Implant Dentistry
by Nadeem Karimbux (Editor), Hans-Peter Weber (Editor)
December 2016

Clinical Cases in Orthodontics
by Martyn T. Cobourne, Padhraig S. Fleming, Andrew T. DiBiase, Sofia Ahmad
June 2012

Clinical Cases in Pediatric Dentistry
by Amr M. Moursi (Editor), Marcio A. da Fonseca (Assistant Editor), Amy L. Truesdale (Associate Editor)
June 2012

Clinical Cases in Periodontics
by Nadeem Karimbux
December 2011

Clinical Cases in Prosthodontics
by Leila Jahangiri, Marjan Moghadam, Mijin Choi, Michael Ferguson
October 2010

Clinical Cases in Restorative and Reconstructive Dentistry
by Gregory J. Tarantola
September 2010

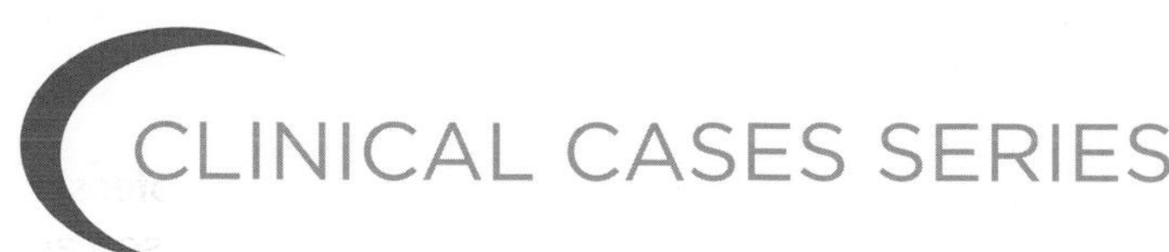

Clinical Cases in Dental Hygiene

Edited by

Cheryl M. Westphal Theile, EdD, RDH
Clinical Professor, Associate Dean for Allied Dental Programs
Director, Dental Hygiene, Dental Hygiene Programs
New York University College of Dentistry
New York, NY, USA

Mea A. Weinberg, DMD, MSD, RPh
Diplomate, American Board of Periodontology
Clinical Professor, Department of Periodontology and Implant Dentistry
New York University College of Dentistry
New York, NY, USA

Stuart L. Segelnick, DDS, MS
Diplomate, American Board of Periodontology
Diplomate, International Congress of Oral Implantologists
Adjunct Clinical Professor
Department of Periodontology and Implant Dentistry
New York University College of Dentistry
New York, NY, USA

WILEY Blackwell

This edition first published 2019

Registered Office
John Wiley & Sons, Inc., 111 River Street, Hoboken, NJ 07030, USA

Editorial Office
111 River Street, Hoboken, NJ 07030, USA

For details of our global editorial offices, customer services, and more information about Wiley products visit us at www.wiley.com.

Wiley also publishes its books in a variety of electronic formats and by print-on-demand. Some content that appears in standard print versions of this book may not be available in other formats.

Library of Congress Cataloging-in-Publication Data

Names: Theile, Cheryl M. Westphal, editor. | Weinberg, Mea A., editor. | Segelnick, Stuart L., editor.
Title: Clinical cases in dental hygiene / edited by Cheryl M. Westphal Theile, Mea A. Weinberg, Stuart L. Segelnick.
Description: Hoboken, NJ : Wiley-Blackwell, 2019. | Series: Clinical cases series | Includes bibliographical references and index. |
Identifiers: LCCN 2018027357 (print) | LCCN 2018028623 (ebook) | ISBN 9781119145035 (Adobe PDF) | ISBN 9781119145042 (ePub) | ISBN 9781119145028 (pbk.)
Subjects: | MESH: Dental Prophylaxis–methods | Dental Hygienists | Case Reports
Classification: LCC RK60.7 (ebook) | LCC RK60.7 (print) | NLM WU 113 | DDC 617.6/01–dc23
LC record available at https://lccn.loc.gov/2018027357

Cover Design: Wiley
Cover Images: (Top to Bottom) ©Marija L. Cahoon; ©Stuart L. Segelnick; ©Stuart L. Segelnick; ©Stuart L. Segelnick; ©filadendron/Getty Images; ©Hero Images/Getty Images

Set in 10/13pt Univers-Light by SPi Global, Pondicherry, India
Printed and bound in Singapore by Markono Print Media Pte Ltd

10 9 8 7 6 5 4 3 2 1

Our thanks go in general to the contributing authors, all who hold or have held affiliations with the New York University College of Dentistry Dental Hygiene, Undergraduate or Graduate programs. Without the dedication of these authors the cases could not have been developed to the expertise and application to practice they now provide. We also sincerely thank the patients and case stories reflected in these chapters as well as the permission to share the images to illustrate the content so vividly. All efforts combined to generate telling information that highlights the critical thinking and evidence-based care needed in all of our dental healthcare delivery systems.

We dedicate this book to those who quest for knowledge, seek evidence to base sound decisions, and strive to improve the quality of the care we provide.

On a personal note I wish to dedicate this book to my husband, Keith Theile, who shared many hours in this book preparation and to my three sons, James Westphal, Erik Westphal, and Jeffrey Theile, for whom I always impart that learning never stops.

Cheryl M. Westphal Theile

I dedicate this book to my family, especially my parents who gave me the desire to write.

Mea A. Weinberg

This book is dedicated to both my mother Harriet Segelnick and my father in law Milton "King" Finkelstein. They left this world way too soon, but made major impacts in my life. It would be superfluous to say without my mother I wouldn't be the dentist that I am. At this very moment, my mother is probably telling everyone in heaven of her son's accomplishments and the "King" would be just as proud.

Stuart L. Segelnick

CONTENTS

LIST OF CONTRIBUTORS

Kim Attanasi RDH, MS, PhD
Adjunct Clinical Associate Professor
Dental Hygiene Programs
New York University College of Dentistry
New York, NY, USA

Shirley S. Birenz, RDH, MS, FAADH
Clinical Assistant Professor
Dental Hygiene Programs
New York University College of Dentistry
New York, NY, USA

Marija L. Cahoon, RDH, MS
Adjunct Clinical Instructor
Dental Hygiene Programs
New York University College of Dentistry
New York, NY, USA

Stephanie E. Cruz, DMD
Former Postgraduate Student
Diplomate, American Board of Periodontology
New York University College of Dentistry
New York, NY, USA

Edgard S. El Chaar, DDS, MS
Clinical Associate Professor
Director, Advanced Education Program in Periodontics
Diplomate, American Board of Periodontology
New York University College of Dentistry
New York, NY, USA

Debra Ferraiolo, DMD, FAGD
Clinical Assistant Professor
Department of Oral and Maxillofacial Pathology, Radiology and Medicine
New York University College of Dentistry
New York, NY, USA

Winnie Furnari, MS, RDH
Adjunct Clinical Professor, Former Clinical Professor
Dental Hygiene Programs
New York University College of Dentistry
New York, NY, USA

Holly S. Harper, RDH, CDA, MEd
Faculty Chair, Dental Programs
Rio Salado College
Tempe, AZ, USA

Rosemary D. Hays, RDH, MS
Clinical Associate Professor
Coordinator, Bachelor of Science Program
Dental Hygiene Programs
New York University College of Dentistry
New York, NY, USA

Cynthia J. Howard, RDH, MS, CCRC
Adjunct Clinical Assistant Professor
Dental Hygienist
Certified Clinical Research Coordinator
Dental Hygiene Programs
New York University College of Dentistry
New York, NY, USA

Sarah Yoon Kang, RDH, MEd
Former Clinical Instructor
Dental Hygiene Programs
New York University College of Dentistry
New York, NY, USA

Analia Veitz-Keenan, DDS
Clinical Associate Professor
Department of Oral and Maxillofacial Pathology, Radiology and Medicine
New York University College of Dentistry
New York, NY, USA

Kellie R. Kennedy, RDH, MA
Clinical Assistant Professor
Dental Hygiene Programs
New York University College of Dentistry
New York, NY, USA

Lorilei Kirby, BSDHE, RDH
Clinical Assistant Professor
Dental Hygiene Programs
New York University College of Dentistry
New York, NY, USA

Judith Kreismann, RDH, MA
Adjunct Clinical Associate Professor
Former Clinical Associate Professor
Dental Hygiene Programs
New York University College of Dentistry
New York, NY, USA

Ronald J. Lehane, DDS, MS
Clinical Assistant Professor
Diplomate, American Board of Periodontology
Department of Periodontology and Implant Dentistry
New York University College of Dentistry
New York, NY, USA

Angelita L. Leon, RDH, MS
Clinical Instructor
Dental Hygiene Programs
New York University College of Dentistry
New York, NY, USA

Eva M. Lupovici, RDH, MS
Adjunct Clinical Professor
Former Clinical Associate Professor
Dental Hygiene Programs
New York University College of Dentistry
New York, NY, USA

Joan A. Phelan, DDS
Former Professor and Chair
Department of Oral and Maxillofacial Pathology, Radiology and Medicine
New York University College of Dentistry
New York, NY, USA

Miriam R. Robbins, DDS, MS, FACD
Chair, Department of Dental Medicine
New York University Winthrop Hospital
Mineola, NY, USA

Dianne L. Sefo, RDH, MEd
Clinical Associate Professor
Pre-Clinical Coordinator
Dental Hygiene Programs
New York University College of Dentistry
New York, NY, USA

Stuart L. Segelnick, DDS, MS
Diplomate, American Board of Periodontology
Diplomate, International Congress of Oral Implantologists
Adjunct Clinical Professor
Department of Periodontology and Implant Dentistry
New York University College of Dentistry
New York, NY, USA

Silvia Spivakovsky, DDS
Clinical Associate Professor
Department of Oral and Maxillofacial Pathology, Radiology and Medicine
New York University College of Dentistry
New York, NY, USA

Lisa B. Stefanou, RDH, BS, MPH
Clinical Associate Professor, Associate Director
Dental Hygiene Programs
New York University College of Dentistry
New York, NY, USA

Mea A. Weinberg, DMD, MSD, RPh
Clinical Professor
Diplomate, American Board of Periodontology
Department of Periodontology and Implant Dentistry
New York University College of Dentistry
New York, NY, USA

Cheryl M. Westphal Theile, EdD, RDH
Clinical Professor
Associate Dean for Allied Dental Programs
Director, Dental Hygiene
Dental Hygiene Programs
New York University College of Dentistry
New York, NY, USA

Stefania Moglia Willis, DMH, RDH
Clinical Associate Professor
Dental Hygiene Programs
New York University College of Dentistry
New York, NY, USA

Mark S. Wolff, DDS, PhD
Former Professor and Chair
Department of Cariology and Comprehensive Care
Former Associate Dean for Pre-Doctoral Education
New York University College of Dentistry
New York, NY, USA

Aaron E. Yancoskie, DDS
Associate Professor of Dentistry
Diplomate, American Board of Oral and Maxillofacial Pathology
Director of Pathology
Touro College of Dental Medicine at New York Medical College
Hawthorne, NY, USA

Yung Cheng Paul Yu, DDS
Clinical Assistant Professor
Department of Periodontology and Implant Dentistry
New York University College of Dentistry
New York, NY, USA

PREFACE

Clinical Cases in Dental Hygiene is the work of many established professionals affiliated in some way with New York University College of Dentistry dental and dental hygiene programs. The goal of this series published by John Wiley & Sons, Inc. is to present current dental topics in a case-based format with critical thinking and problem-based learning questions. The book is designed to provide clinical cases relating to dental hygiene practice. Included with each case are problem-based learning objectives followed by self-study questions and take-home hints that are elaborated answers of the self-study questions. This book will bring together what the dental hygiene student learned in school in a case-based format that stimulates independent thinking. This book covers all essential concepts within the scope of dental hygiene practice.

Clinical Cases in Dental Hygiene can be used as a textbook to prepare for the written boards and also as a reference book in dental hygiene practice. Group activities can focus on discussing the major points raised in the study questions or self-directed study on the major topics. The dental hygiene diagnosis and care plan are the focus of many of the cases to help guide the reader to the planned interventions and expected outcomes. Some authors have included background or additional reading resources to add to the discussion of each topic.

1

Patient Examination

Clinical Cases in Dental Hygiene, First Edition. Edited by Cheryl M. Westphal Theile, Mea A. Weinberg and Stuart L. Segelnick.

Case 1

Examination and Documentation

CASE STORY

A 55-year-old Caucasian female presented with a chief complaint of: "My mouth is always dry, and I have difficulty swallowing." She said, "I was recently diagnosed with scleroderma, and my doctor told me I should see a dentist." The vital signs were blood pressure: 159/92 mmHg; respiration: 16 breaths/min; pulse: 72 beats/min, temperature: 98°F; and nonsmoker.

PROBLEM-BASED LEARNING GOALS AND OBJECTIVES

- Discuss the role of the patient's medical, social, and dental histories (comprehensive health history) in the patient examination
- List and describe the five parts of a comprehensive clinical examination
- Differentiate between types of findings in a clinical examination including signs and symptoms, and significant and insignificant findings
- Discuss the definition, purpose, and methods of documentation
- Identify the components of care documented in the patient's permanent record

Medical History

The patient was diagnosed with scleroderma and gastroesophageal reflux disease (GERD). She is taking antacids for GERD and immunosuppressant medications and a calcium channel blocker for scleroderma.

Dental History

The patient reported that her last dental visit was one year ago. She has a history of childhood caries but has been caries free since college. Also, she has symptoms of dry mouth and difficulty opening her mouth and swallowing.

Social History

The patient is a self-described over-achieving professional concerned about her health and the appearance of her teeth. She lives with her husband in a suburb of Manhattan, has three adult children, and enjoys reading.

Review of Systems (Physical Examination)

Gastrointestinal Examination

The patient has difficulty swallowing (dysphagia) and GERD.

Cardiovascular Examination

The patient has a history of Raynaud's phenomenon and hypertension (BP: 159/92).

Cutaneous Examination

The patient stated that her fingers are extremely sensitive to the cold. The skin of her hands appeared shiny and stretched with varying degrees of pigmentation. The patient struggled to hold the pen while signing consent forms.

Head and Neck Examination

Extraoral

The patient exhibited microstomia restricting her mouth opening (<20 mm), and the lips were thin and stretched.

Intraoral

Examination of the major and minor salivary gland duct openings showed loss of quality and quantity of saliva.

Periodontal charting showed areas of bleeding on probing without CAL (clinical attachment loss).

Generalized fibrotic changes in mucosal tissues were noted with mucogingival paresthesia. Oral mucosal tissues appeared pale and tight with hardening of the soft palate. The patient's GI score was 2. Several restorations and crowns were noted. No caries present. Generalized moderate biofilm accumulation was apparent. The debris index (DI-S) and the calculus index (CI-S) were both scored as 1 (debris and calculus covered less than 1/3 of the examined tooth surfaces).

Class I: right and left sides; teeth #7 and #10 are in torso version and overlap slightly with #8 and #9.

Radiographic Examination

No significant findings.

Dental Hygiene Diagnosis

Problems	Related to Risks and Etiology
Xerostomia	Loss of quality and quantity of saliva and scleroderma Goal: The patient will experience relief from xerostomia due to scleroderma immediately upon initiation of local and systemic measures to stimulate saliva flow
Increased periodontal disease risk	Insufficient daily biofilm management, limited hand strength and mouth opening as evidenced by gingival inflammation and a high GI score Goal: The patient will reduce the GI score from 2 to <1.0 by the next visit
Increased caries risk	Low salivary flow, inadequate biofilm management and fluoride intake, an acidic environment created by GERD, and a soft, high carbohydrate diet because of dysphagia Goal: The patient will suppress potential bacterial activity by increasing caries protective factors
Blood pressure elevated above treatment goal for patients <65 years old	Blood pressure readings of 159/92 Goal: Patient will report having blood pressure evaluated by a physician before rescheduled visit

Planned Interventions

Planned Interventions (to arrest or control disease and regenerate, restore, or maintain health)		
Clinical	**Education/Counseling**	**Oral Hygiene Instruction**
BP was taken at every visit Initial exam, FMS radiographs, Adult prophylaxis In-office 5% sodium fluoride varnish Three-month continuing care interval because of scleroderma and associated medicine risks Referral to primary care physician for blood pressure evaluation Referral to occupational therapist to manage symptoms of scleroderma	Significance of management of xerostomia Determine patient's motivation to reduce plaque accumulation and oral disease risks: "What are possible benefits of removing plaque?" "On a scale of 1–10, how confident are you that you can reduce your plaque score?" Increased risk of caries because of lack of fluoride and soft, high carbohydrate diet Provide information on alternative self-care aids such as an enlarged or extended toothbrush handle, a powered toothbrush and flossing device Correlation of hypertension to general health	Use of prescribed cholinergic agonist agent Frequent use of water and saliva substitutes (Tolle 2012) Use of chlorhexidine for reduction of bacterial and gingival inflammation and prevention of Candida (Spolarich 2011) and a daily 1.1% sodium fluoride (prescription) mouthrinse for caries reduction (Featherstone 2000; Tolle 2012) Use of pump-type toothpaste dispenser and a power toothbrush with child-size brush inserts, interdental aids with elongated and enlarged handles or flosser with a toothbrush-like handle (Yuen et al. 2011)

Progress Notes

The patient arrived on time for her appointment and was treated without delay. A complete medical, social, and dental history was taken. An initial exam, FMS and adult prophylaxis were performed followed by an application of 5% sodium fluoride varnish. The patient was advised to see her physician for a BP evaluation and an occupational therapist for effects of scleroderma on daily living.

Discussion: Examination and Documentation in Patient Assessment

Patient assessment represents the most important step in the dental hygiene process of care because it provides a baseline of information, opens a dialogue between the patient and provider, and establishes trust and confidence in their relationship (Figure 1.1.1). All information collected during the assessment process is inextricably bound to each other. Information from the

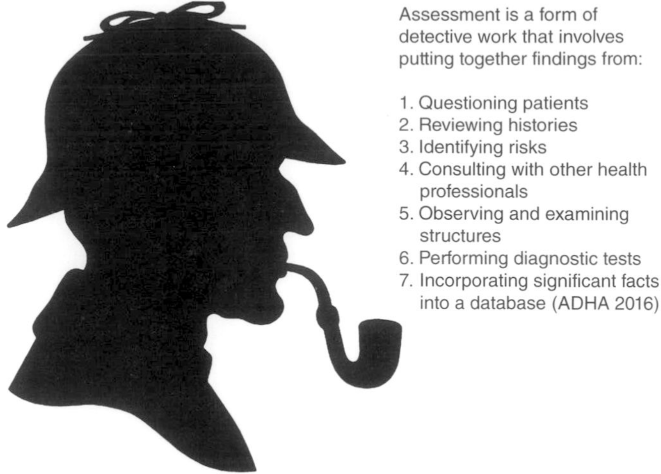

Assessment is a form of detective work that involves putting together findings from:
1. Questioning patients
2. Reviewing histories
3. Identifying risks
4. Consulting with other health professionals
5. Observing and examining structures
6. Performing diagnostic tests
7. Incorporating significant facts into a database (ADHA 2016)

Figure 1.1.1: Assessment as detective work.

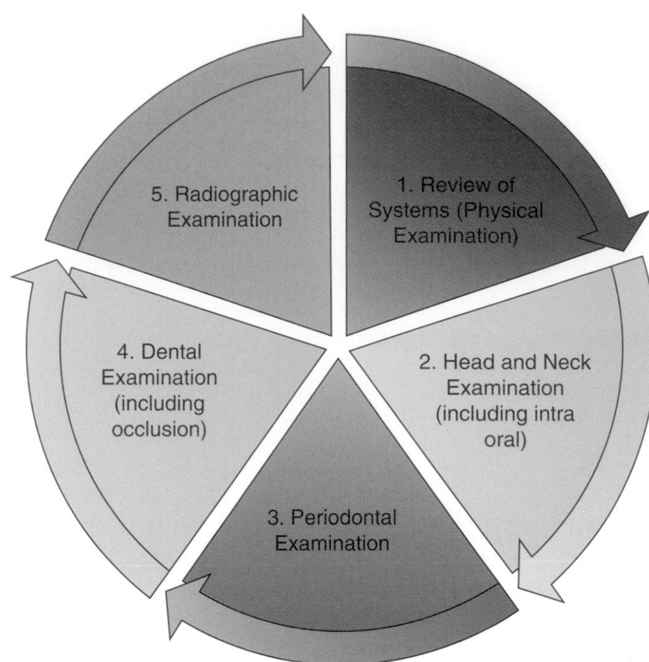

Figure 1.1.2: Five parts of the clinical examination.

patient history is used to distinguish significant from insignificant findings in a clinical examination, helps generate a list of dental hygiene diagnoses, and ultimately leads to the formation of an individualized care plan.

During an examination, the dental hygienist documents findings as signs of health or disease. On the other hand, findings revealed by the patient are referred to as symptoms of their problems. The chief complaint or concern is the primary reason that patients present for treatment and should be the first diagnostic statement in the care plan (Wilkins et al. 2017). Typically, the chief complaint is a symptom or a request and may need to be elicited by asking open-ended questions such as, "What brought you to the dental office?" or "Is there anything you hope I can do for you?" Paying close attention to a patient's chief concern(s) serves many purposes: it alerts the provider to relevant diagnostic information; it offers insight into a patient's perception regarding his or her problems; and finally, it provides insight into the patient's health literacy including their level of knowledge about dentistry.

A comprehensive clinical exam is made up of five parts (Figure 1.1.2).

1. **The Physical Exam or Review of Systems (ROS)** is a list of questions, by organ system, intended to uncover disease or dysfunction. The list is often given to patients before treatment. Along with the medical history, the ROS assists in determining a patient's MCS or ASA (methods for physical status classification). When using the ROS, clinicians must be aware of associations between noncommunicable diseases and oral disease because they share common risk factors as well as underlying infection/inflammation pathways (Jin et al. 2016).
2. **The Extraoral and Intraoral Soft Tissue Examination** evaluates head and neck structures for abnormalities or lesions. The examinations are performed systematically through a process of observation and palpation to detect variations from normal and abnormalities. Patients provide important historical context for clinical findings, such as timelines for lesions, whether the lesions are painful or tender, or can be linked to repeated exposure to sun or tobacco products.
3. **The Periodontal Examination** evaluates the patient's oral hygiene and the clinical appearance of the periodontal soft tissue. Deviations from normal healthy tissue are noted such as gingival recession, redness, suppuration, and swelling. A thorough examination requires a mouth mirror, a periodontal probe, and radiographs. A periodontal assessment provides information for long-term monitoring of a patient's periodontal disease activity (Armitage 2004).
4. **Examination of the Teeth (and Occlusion)** Before beginning the dental examination, the clinician

should review the dental history, particularly the chief complaint(s) involving the teeth. The exam is performed in conjunction with radiographs so that imaging findings can be correlated with those found clinically.

a. First note any missing teeth and type of replacement such as implants, fixed and removable partial and complete dentures. If removable prostheses are present, they are evaluated in the mouth and then removed.
b. Each tooth is evaluated visually with an excellent light source. Assess all teeth for overall condition, irregularities of color, morphology, and function.
   i. It is recommended to use the air/water syringe, with transillumination and a dull probe to detect enamel changes. However, the probe is not a better method than visual inspection alone (Newbrun 1993).
   ii. A study concluded that explorers did not improve the validity of a caries diagnosis as compared to visual detection alone (Lussi 1991); and consequently, leaders in caries research no longer support the use of a sharp explorer in caries detection (Van Dorp et al. 1988; Braga et al. 2010).
c. Document the numbers, shape, and type of existing restoration. Dental floss is used to check the integrity of interproximal contacts, and the explorer evaluates restoration margins for defects.
d. An occlusal examination is conducted by recording the intraarch and interarch relationships of adjacent teeth in the same and opposing arches. Both right and left sides are included when classifying teeth according to Angle's Classifications in the permanent dentition and when using the terminus of second primary molars.

5. **The Radiographic Examination** Radiographs are considered an essential adjunct to the visual clinical examination. They accurately detect proximal caries lesions and estimate the depth of lesion penetration into the underlying dentin (Bindra et al. 2016; Keenan and Keenan 2016). Also, radiographs are useful for monitoring the growth and development of the teeth and jaws as well as for the diagnosis and treatment of periodontal diseases and oral pathologies (American Dental Association Council on Scientific Affairs 2012).

Thorough and accurate documentation of the patient's record occurs during the assessment process and at every phase of patient care. As a result, documentation has been adopted as the sixth standard in the Standards for Clinical Dental Hygiene Practice (Figure 1.1.3) that guide practice and are designed for hygienists as a resource for providing patient-centered and evidence-based care (ADHA 2016). The patient's

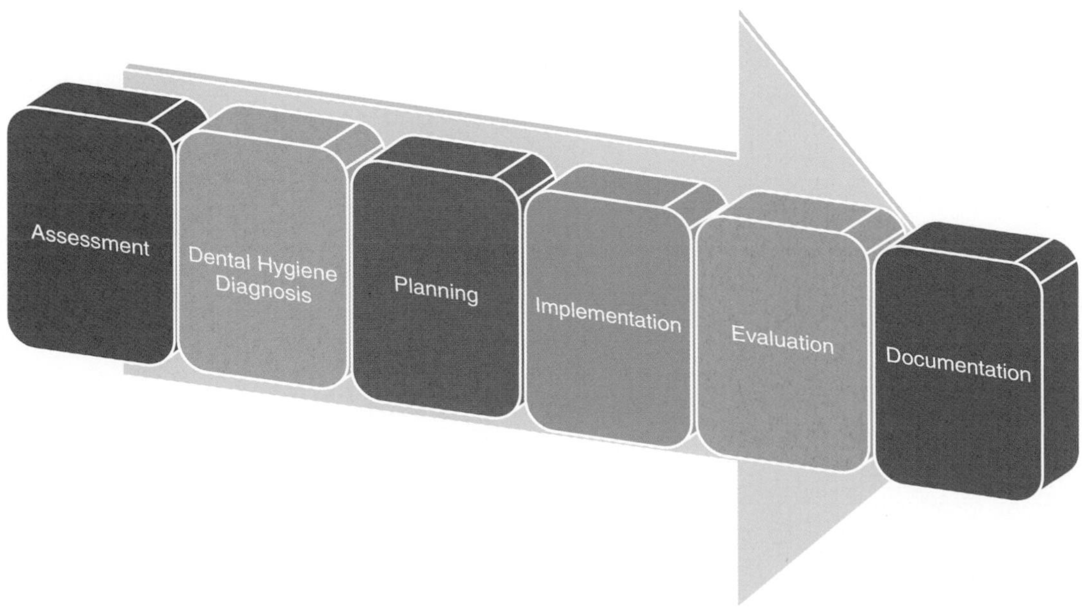

Figure 1.1.3: Standards for clinical dental hygiene practice.

record should be brief and to the point, objective (nonjudgmental) and comprehensible. Taking and documenting *all* patient data – the list of problems, planned and provided treatment, and relevant patient conversations – in a humanistic manner (with clarity, professionalism, and empathy) is an indicator of professional competence and represents the highest standard of patient care.

Using open-ended questions during a patient assessment (as opposed to direct or leading questions) results in a more nuanced examination picture (Iversen et al. 2014). Skillful clinicians elicit in-depth information about previous dental experiences and what dental care and preventive care mean to the patients. They find out how and why patients did or did not adopt prescribed preventive care, and they determine ways in which social context influences their patients' health behaviors. Humanizing the dental care experience by contextualizing clinical facts with our patients' narratives (their personal stories about general health and oral diseases) provides a bridge between evidence-based dental practice and the art of applying the knowledge to a single case (Kalitzkus and Matthiessen 2009), improves the visual exam and enriches dental hygiene practice.

Advances in technology such as imaging techniques, oral/facial photography and electronic health records (EHR) have brought improvements to the data collection and documentation processes. Proper documentation records:

- collected data from the patient interviews and clinical examination
- services planned and provided
- recommendations, and
- relevant information to the patient's case.

The process accurately and concisely records all information and interactions between the patient and provider and provides evidence that the services performed reflect the patient's specific needs. A critical part of the documentation process and a legal risk management strategy is to include the patient's acceptance or rejection of the treatment options and recommendations (after a presentation of a proposed care plan and the consequences of not receiving care by the dental hygienist) referred to as informed consent and informed refusal. After patients have agreed to and signed for treatment, errors can be corrected. However, clinicians must initial all corrections, and *any* alterations to the treatment plan require a new patient signature.

A patient's health information and clinical records are confidential and legally protected by The Health Insurance Portability and Accountability Act (https://www.hhs.gov/hipaa/for-professionals/index.html). Additionally, the ADHA Code of Ethics provides members with professional standards for ethical and moral behavior and reminds us of our professional responsibility in that regard. Hence, maintaining patient privacy when documenting information throughout the process of care and when collaborating interprofessionally on a case is critical in the application of technology to patient care.

The patient assessment process requires attention to the facts of the case but likewise, should include meaning, context (cultural and otherwise), and understanding of the patient's needs. Dental professionals conduct a patient-centered interview and examination that put the patient where she/he needs to be in the process of care, front-and-center.

Interviewing and asking questions continue throughout the patient examination to include the patient's point of view and to lend meaning to the process. The way in which questions are asked can encourage intimacy and frankness; and even though responses are typed on a computer, written on a page, or recorded, it is important to maintain eye contact with the patient, to be friendly, interested, to ask questions requiring more than a one-word response, and to reiterate for clarity and understanding.

Professionals can restore a sense of narrative into the assessment process by creating a more humanistic environment during the assessment. The patient narrative is not only a description of the facts of a case. The narrative in healthcare provides meaning, context and perspective for the patient's problem (Greenhalgh and Hurwitz 1998). Throughout the interview and examination, clinicians watch the patient's expressions, interact comfortably, engage patients verbally while simultaneously managing documentation. Consequently, patients may be more comfortable about telling their story; they may have more confidence in their provider; and they may be more willing to share in the responsibility for their health outcomes.

Health professionals cannot be detached, removed, or uncaring in what they do. Paying attention, exploring things a little bit, getting at it slowly, but carefully and thoroughly will get results throughout the entire process of care (Pirsig 1974).

Take-Home Hints

1. Assessment identifies patients' needs and oral health problems and is the first of six of the *Standards for Clinical Dental Hygiene Practice* (Figure 1.1.3).
2. The patient examination never stands alone. The clinical examination is tied to all information-gathering activities. For example, a diagnosis of scleroderma elicited during the patient interview provides historical context for changes in the patient's oral tissues.
3. The American Dental Hygienists' Association (ADHA) defines patient-centered as an approach that focuses attention on the patient and recognizes the importance of their values, beliefs, and needs in the provision of care (ADHA Standards for Clinical Dental Hygiene Practice 2016).
4. Risk assessment identifies certain behaviors, characteristics, or exposures that put our patients at risk for developing diseases. Risk factors are assessed as high, moderate, or low and are used to prevent and manage dental diseases (ADHA 2017).

Self-Study Questions

1. Findings revealed to the dental hygienist by the patient during assessment are called

A. Signs
B. Symptoms

2. Recently, a sixth standard has been added to the Standards for Clinical Dental Hygiene Practice. It is:

A. Assessment
B. Dental Hygiene Diagnosis
C. Documentation
D. Implementation

3. The six standards for Clinical Dental Hygiene Practice follow the dental hygiene process of care. The correct order of the six components is:

A. Assessment
B. Evaluation
C. Implementation
D. Dental Hygiene Diagnosis
E. Documentation
F. Planning

4. A thorough examination is made up of ________ parts. (Fill-in-the-blank).

A. Three
B. Four
C. Five
D. Six

References

ADHA Policy Manual, American Dental Hygienists' Association (2017) Glossary, [Online]. Available: https://www.adha.org/resources-docs/7614_Policy_Manual.pdf [May 30, 2018].

American Dental Association Council on Scientific Affairs (2012). The use of cone-beam computed tomography in dentistry: an advisory statement from the American dental association council on scientific affairs. *J. Am. Dent. Assoc.* 143 (8): 899–902.

American Dental Hygienists' Association (ADHA), Standards for Clinical Dental Hygiene Practice, June 2016 [Online]. Available: https://www.adha.org/resources-docs/2016-Revised-Standards-for-Clinical-Dental-Hygiene-Practice.pdf (May 15, 2018).

Armitage, G.C. (2004). The complete periodontal examination. *Periodontol.* 34 (1): 9–21.

Bindra, S., Neelkamal, Grewel, G., and Chhabra, V. (2016). Diagnosis of dental caries conventional V/S 2 recent methods. *Indian J. Dent. Sci.* [series online] 8 (1): 86–91.

Braga, M.M., Mendes, F.M., and Ekstrand, K.R. (2010). Detection activity assessment and diagnosis of dental caries lesions. *Dent. Clin. N. Am.* 54 (3): 479.

Epstein, R. and Street, R. Jr. (2011). The values and value of patient-centered care. *Ann. Fam. Med.* 9 (2): 100–103.

Featherstone, J.D. (2000). The Science and Practice of Caries Prevention. *J. Am. Dental Assoc.* 131 (7): 887–899.

Greenhalgh, T. and Hurwitz, B. (1998). Why study narrative? In: *Narrative Based Medicine: Dialogue and Discourse in Clinical Practice* (ed. T. Greenhalgh and B. Hurwitz), 3–16. London: BMJ Books.

Iversen, H.H., Bjertnaes, Ø.A., and Skudal, K.E. (2014). Health services research: patient evaluation of hospital outcomes:

an analysis of open-ended comments from extreme clusters in a national survey. *BMJ Open* 4: e004848. doi: 10.1136/bm.

Jin, L.J., Lamster, I.B., Greenspan, J.S. et al. (2016). Global Burden of Oral Diseases: Emerging Concepts, Management and Interplay with Systemic Health. *Oral Diseases* 22: 609–619.

Kalitzkus, V. and Matthiessen, P.F. (2009). Narrative-based medicine: potential, pitfalls, and practice. *Perm. J.* 13 (1): 80–86.

Keenan, J.R. and Keenan, A.V. (2016). Summary review/caries: accuracy of dental radiographs for caries detection. *Evid. Based Dent.* 17 (2): 43.

Lussi, A. (1991). Validity of diagnostic and treatment decisions of fissure caries. *Caries Res.* 25 (4): 296–303.

Newbrun, E. (1993). Problems in caries diagnosis. *Int. Dent. J.* 43 (2): 133–142.

Pirsig, R. (1974). *Paying Attention. Zen and the Art of Motorcycle Maintenance*, 291–294. William Morrow & Co.

Spolarich, A. (2011). Xerostomia and oral disease. *Dimens. Dent. Hyg.* 9 (11), Special CE Insert) Available at: http://www.dimensionsofdentalhygiene.com/2011/11_November/Features/Xerostomia_and_Oral_Disease.aspx: May 31, 2018.

Tolle, S.L. (2012). Treatment planning for patients with scleroderma. *Dimens. Dent. Hyg.* 10 (9): 50–53.

U.S. Department of Health and Human Services. (1996) H.R. 3103 — 104th Congress: Health Insurance Portability and Accountability Act of 1996 (HIPAA). HIPAA for Professionals [Online]. Available at https://www.hhs.gov/hipaa/for-professionals/index.html (May 15, 2018).

van Dorp, C.S., Exterkate, R.A., and ten Cate, J.M. (1988). The effect of dental probing on subsequent enamel demineralization. *ASDC J. Dent. Child.* 55 (5): 343.

Wilkins, E.M., Wyche, C.J., and Boyd, L.D. (eds.) (2017). *Clinical Practice of the Dental Hygienist, 12e*, Philadelphia: Lippincott Williams & Wilkins.

Yuen, H.K., Weng, J., Bandyopadhyay, D. et al. (2011). Effect of a multi-faceted intervention on gingival health among adults with systemic sclerosis. *Clin. Exp. Rheumatol.* 29 (2 Suppl 65): S26–S32.

Answers to Self-Study Questions

1. B symptoms

2. C documentation

3. Assessment, Dental Hygiene Diagnosis, Planning, Implementation, Evaluation, and Documentation (ADPIED)

4. Five. The five parts of the dental hygiene examination are

- Review of Systems
- Head and Neck exam (including intraoral exam)
- Periodontal exam
- Dental exam (including occlusion), and
- Radiographic exam

Case 2

Head and Neck Examination

CASE STORY

A 29-year-old female, recently employed as an elementary special education teacher, presented with a chief complaint of, "I am concerned about white spots on my teeth and red areas on my neck." She has been unable to see a dentist for seven years because of "a large college loan debt."

PROBLEM-BASED LEARNING GOALS AND OBJECTIVES

- Explain the steps in the head and neck exam
- State the objectives of the head and neck examination
- State the relevance of the head and neck and intraoral examinations to general health and physical wellbeing
- Identify risk factors for cancer

Medical History

Review of the patient's medical history revealed allergies to most animals, dust, and mites. The patient takes one capsule Benadryl (Diphenhydramine HCL) 25 mg every four to six hours at least four days per week for allergies. Her vital signs are within normal limits.

Dental History

The patient grew up in the Kingston, New York area without fluoride. She brushes twice daily and uses toothpaste without fluoride. The patient states she flosses once daily. Minor occlusal restorations were placed during college.

Social History

The patient teaches at a residential institution for children with emotional and academic problems. Also, she plays the violin with a local symphony orchestra. She drinks several bottles of sweetened ice tea daily and snacks on candy before, during, and after work.

Head and Neck Examination

The extraoral exam revealed hyperpigmented areas under the patient's left mandible and erythematous plaques on the left lower neck and no enlarged or palpable lymph nodes (Figure 1.2.1). The patient states that she practices violin one hour on weekdays and two hours on weekends and holds the violin against her chin and collar bone. The three lesions are slightly raised, erythematous, broad, and rough in appearance and conform to the placement position of the violin. Each lesion measures 5 × 5 mm, 3 × 7 mm, 7 × 3 mm. The patient states violinists stabilize their instrument with the sternocleidomastoid muscle (Figure 1.2.2). It is the muscle that passes diagonally across the front and side of the neck beginning at the top of the sternum and ending behind the ear. The lesions known as "fiddlers neck" are a common skin problem found on violinists (Jue et al. 2010) and conform to the performance position of the violin as described by the patient.

Intraorally, visual examination and transillumination of teeth revealed noncavitated white spot lesions on the proximal surfaces of teeth #8, #9, and #10. There is localized slight supragingival biofilm on affected tooth

(A)

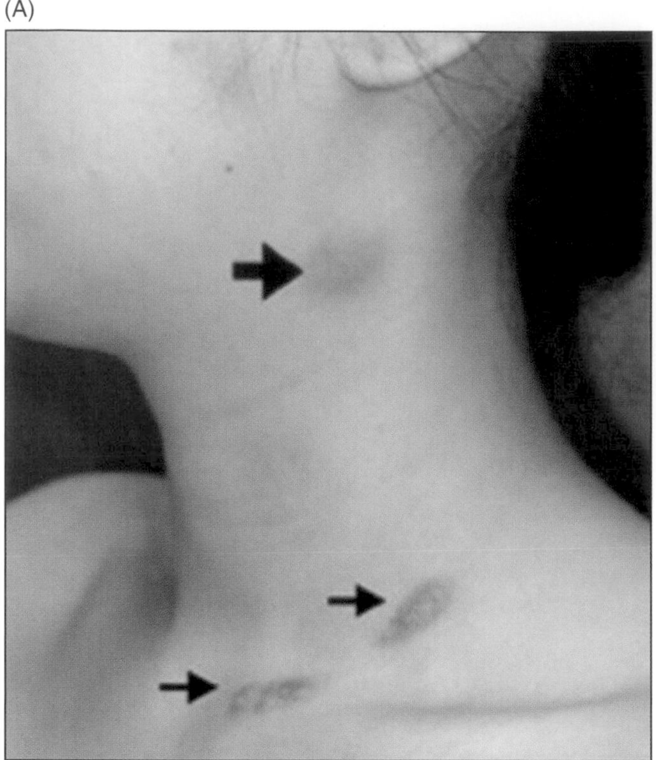

(B)

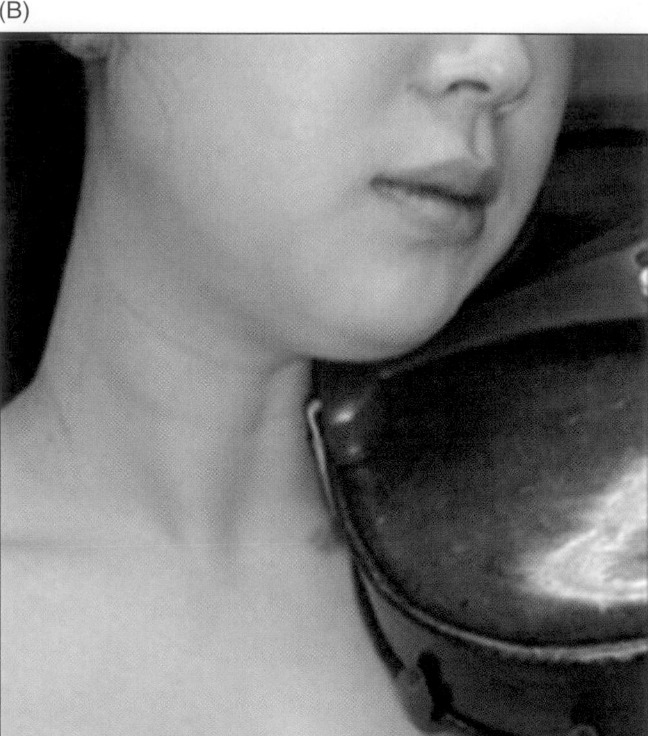

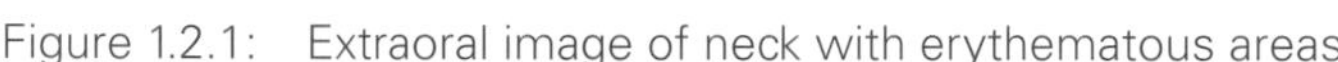

Figure 1.2.1: Extraoral image of neck with erythematous areas.

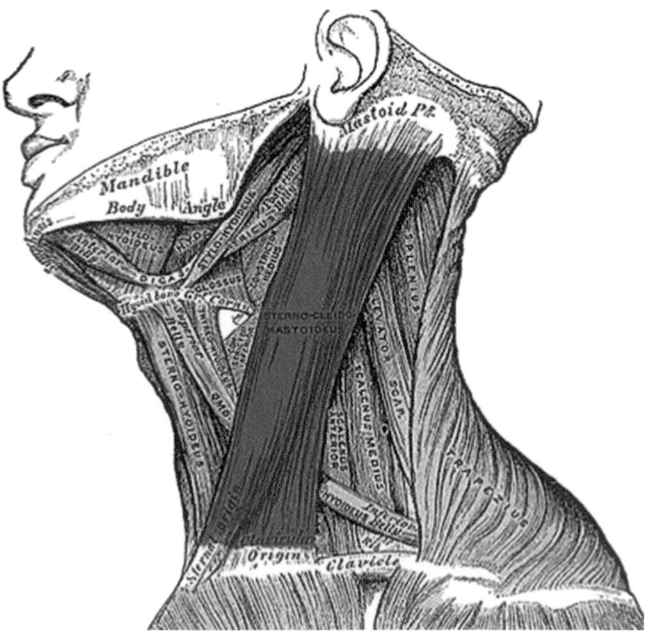

Figure 1.2.2: Sternocleidomastoid muscle.

surfaces. Supplemental oral findings indicate the patient is a mouth breather. Class I malocclusion with anterior open bite present.

Radiographic Examination

Caries lesions are visible radiographically but confined to the enamel. Partially erupted third molars are visible.

Dental Hygiene Diagnosis

Problems	Related to Risks and Etiology
Increased caries	Localized slight supragingival biofilm, frequent sugar intake, nonexistent use of fluoridated dentifrice or fluoride rinses and xerostomia (side effect of medication and mouth breathing).
Three red callus-like areas below the chin and along the neck	Violin placement, frequency of violin practice, possible allergy to varnish

Planned Interventions

Planned Interventions (to arrest or control disease and regenerate, restore, or maintain health)		
Clinical	**Education/Counseling**	**Oral Hygiene Instruction**
Initial exam, radiographs, and adult prophylaxis 5% NaF fluoride varnish with a synthetic form of colophony (to reduce risk of allergy) every 3 to 4 months Sealants Referral to dermatologist for red lesions on neck Referral to primary care physician to evaluate allergy symptoms	The importance of regular dental visits. Increased risk for caries. The role of fluoride in remineralization of noncavitated lesions. Reduction of bacterial infection through daily biofilm removal and antimicrobial therapy. Food diary for analysis of sugar exposures. Use of chamois cloth to protect exposed skin while practicing violin	Modified Bass brushing technique Recommend use of 1.1% NaF toothpaste and 0.05% NaF rinse 2X daily 10 ml 0.12% Chlorhexidine rinse one minute daily for 1 week each month for short term (evaluate at 3 months recall until risk reduced). Recommend frequent sips of water during the day and xylitol gum or candy four times daily if mouth feels dry.

Progress Notes

The patient arrived for her appointment on time. A complete medical, social, and dental history was taken. Initial exam and FMS were performed. Three atypical callus-like red lesions on the neck were noted during the head and neck exam. Noncavitated white spot lesions were charted, and bacterial infection reduction methods were explained according to patient caries risk assessment. A food diary for analysis of sugar intake was reviewed and given to the patient. The patient was instructed to return in one week for dietary analysis and counseling. The patient was advised to see a dermatologist for a differential diagnosis and treatment of neck lesions and her primary care physician for symptoms of allergies. Three to four months recall recommended for high caries risk.

Discussion: The Head and Neck Examination

Dental hygienists see patients for well-check visits more often than physicians and are at the frontline for recognizing early illness and for educating patients about their risk factors. The head and neck and intraoral examinations – often referred to as an oral cancer examination or oral cancer screening – are an important part of comprehensive dental hygiene care and can be completed in around five minutes. However, approximately half of practicing hygienists (51%) performs a head and neck exam routinely during dental visits (Forrest et al. 2001; Horowitz et al. 2002). The head and neck exam is emphasized during hygiene education as a standard of care to detect manifestations of systemic illness, early skin cancer, and lymphadenopathy. Demands on patient scheduling, working time, knowledge, and perceived risk of cancer in the United States often prevent hygienists from performing the service (Forrest et al. 2001; Horowitz et al. 2002; Cotter et al. 2011). However, failure to include this exam routinely has profound consequences such as late-stage diagnosis, more extensive surgery and therapies such as radiation and chemotherapy, and a decreased quality of life and health.

Hygienists should perform the head and neck and intraoral assessments the same way at every visit to maintain efficiency and high levels of accuracy. The head and neck exam includes checking symmetry and profile of the face, the skin, eyes, lips, lymph nodes, salivary, and thyroid glands as well as a temporomandibular joint examination (see Figure 1.2.3). If possible, clinicians visually examine each area before performing a thorough palpation. Additionally, it is important to ask permission to do the exam and to tell patients exactly what is being done and why. For example, ask your patients if you may perform an extra- and intraoral examination to look for abnormalities that affect oral and general health. Tell patients that palpation will include the clavicle area.

If a problem is identified, ask the patient about its history (onset, duration, and possible causes). As in this case, when deviations from normal are detected, patients are referred to a physician for differential diagnosis and treatment. Finally, educating patients about known risk factors for cancer such as age, genetic predisposition, sun exposure, alcohol, tobacco, viruses such as HPV and HIV, chronic inflammation and inadequate nutrition and host immunity is essential to decreasing the rate of cancer (Sciubba 2001; Neild-Gehrig 2018).

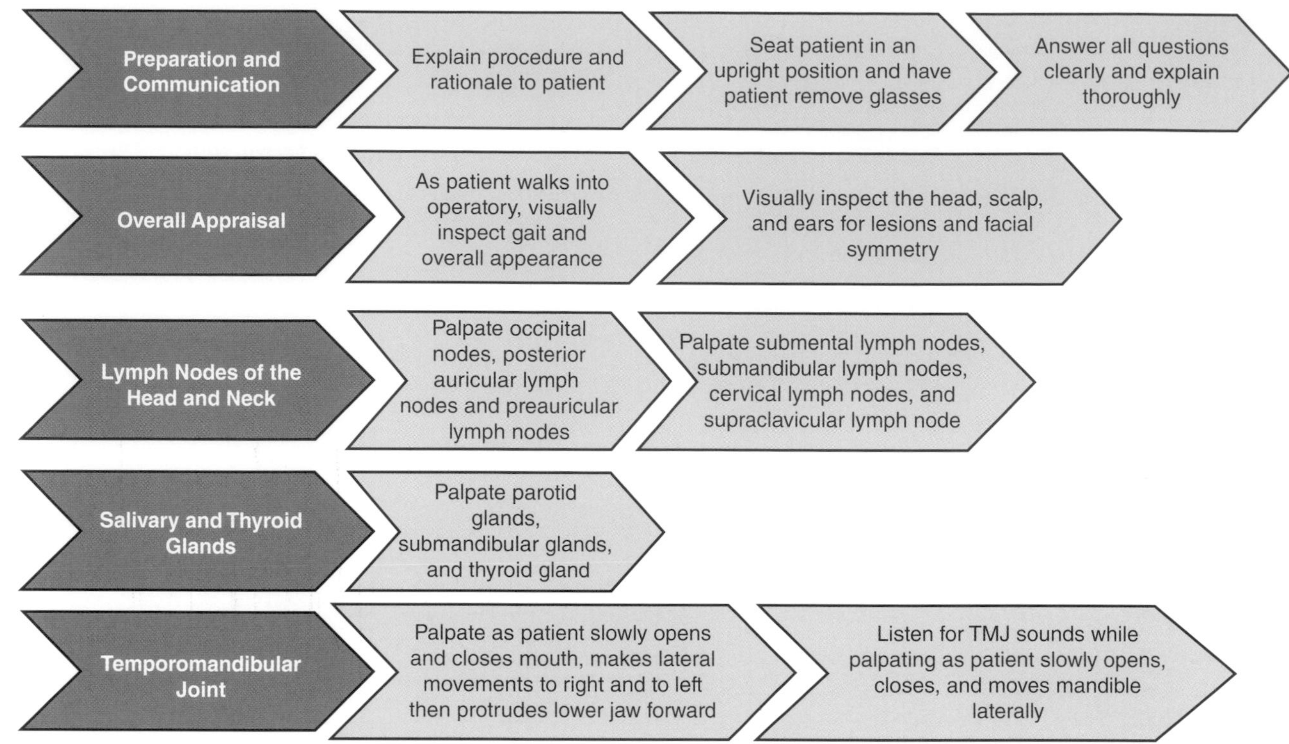

Figure 1.2.3: Steps in the head and neck examination.

Take-Home Hints

1. The American Cancer Society and the American Dental Association recommend oral cancer examinations as an essential element of routine dental examinations (Smith et al. 2013; Walsh et al. 2013).
2. The Objectives of the Head and Neck and Intraoral Exam are:
   1. To determine general wellness and ability to continue dental treatment.
   2. To provide and/or to compare to a baseline of assessment information.
   3. To determine need for additional diagnostic procedures and medical or other consultations.
   4. To enable early diagnosis of pathology.
3. Findings from the Head and Neck and Oral Examinations fall into one of three categories:
   1. Normal – found in most individuals.
   2. Atypical – a variant of normal found in some individuals but within normal limits.
   3. Pathologic– indicative of infection, trauma, neoplasms, development errors causing functional issues, inadequate nutrition and immunity, and more.
4. Include the following in your description of findings:
   1. *History* – Onset, duration, and possible causes.
   2. *Description* – Location and extent, size, surface texture, consistency, and color.
   3. *Morphology* –elevated, depressed, or flat.
5. Oral cavity and oropharyngeal cancers are considered to be the sixth most common cancers worldwide (Warnakulasurlya 2009), there will be an estimated 51,540 new cases in the United States in 2016, and an estimated 10,030 people will die of this disease (SEER Cancer Statistics 2017).
6. The most common malignancy of the head and neck, oral cavity squamous cell carcinoma (OC-SCC), is preceded often by white or red mucosal changes known as leukoplakia or erythroplakia. "Some lesions will show a combination of red and white features, termed *erythroleukoplakia*, *speckled leukoplakia*, or *speckled erythroplakia*" (Chi et al. 2015).
7. Although oral cancer is associated with aging, studies indicate a rise in the disease in adults below the age of 40 and that squamous cell carcinoma in tongues of young adults has increased sharply (Schantz and Yu 2002; Chaturvedi et al. 2011).
8. Alarmingly, cancers in younger people are more aggressive and associated with a poorer prognosis than those found in older adults (Warnakulasurlya 2009). A new study found that the human papillomavirus (HPV) may be causally linked to 70%

of oropharyngeal squamous cell carcinomas in white males in the United States, and found that by 2020 the number of oropharyngeal cancers in this population will surpass the annual number of cervical cancers (Chaturvedi et al. 2011).

9. Primary areas for the development of oral cancer in the (wet) oral tissues are:
   - Lateral borders of tongue (Figure 1.2.4)
   - Lips
   - Floor of the mouth
   - Soft tissue complex: includes "the posterior mouth such as the tonsils, tonsillar pillar and crypt, the base of the tongue, and the oropharynx" (SEER Cancer Statistics 2017).

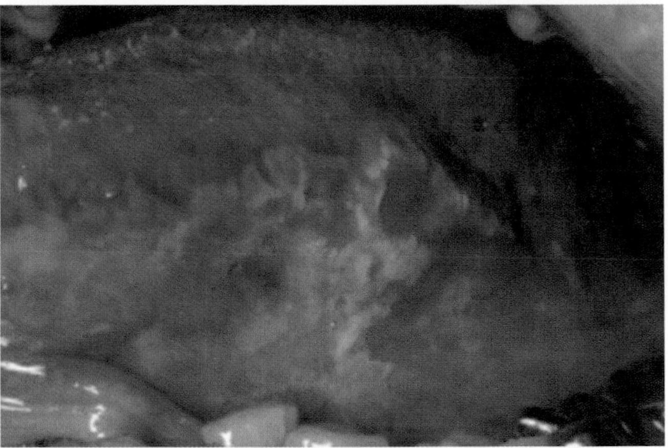

Figure 1.2.4: Lateral borders of the tongue.

Self-Study Questions

1. True or False
Clinicians should alter the sequence of the Head and Neck and Intraoral exams to keep the process from becoming routine.

2. Approximately what percent of hygienists performs a Head and Neck Examination routinely?
- **A. 100%**
- **B. 90%**
- **C. 75%**
- **D. 51%**

3. True or False?
Hygienists should only screen older adults for head, neck, and oral cancers.

4. A finding of "Atypical" means a clinical condition or lesion is:
- **A. Found in most individuals.**
- **B. Found in some individuals but within normal limits (variant of normal).**
- **C. Indicative of infection, trauma, neoplasms, development errors causing functional issues, inadequate nutrition, and immunity, and more.**
- **D. None of the above**

5. Violinists stabilize their instrument with the large strap muscle that passes diagonally across the front and side of the neck beginning at the top of the sternum and ending behind the ear. This muscle is the:
- **A. Trapezius**
- **B. Mylohyoid**
- **C. Anterior Belly of the Digastric**
- **D. Sternocleidomastoid**

References

Chaturvedi, A.K., Engels, E.A., Pfeiffer, R.M. et al. (2011). Human papillomavirus and rising oropharyngeal cancer incidence in the United States. *J. Clin. Oncol.* 29 (32): 4294–4301.

Chi, A.C., Day, T.A., and Neville, B.W. (2015). Oral cavity and oropharyngeal squamous cell carcinoma – an update. *CA Cancer J. Clin.* 65: 401–421.

Cotter, J.C., McCann, A.L., Schneiderman, E.D. et al. (2011). Factors affecting the performance of oral cancer screenings by Texas dental hygienists. *J. Dent. Hyg.* 85 (4): 326–334.

Forrest, J.L., Horowitz, A.M., and Shmuely, Y. (2001). Dental hygienists' knowledge, opinions, and practices related to oral and pharyngeal cancer risk assessment. *J. Dent. Hyg.* 75 (IV): 271–281.

Horowitz, A.M., Siriphant, P., Canto, M.T., and Child, W.L. (2002). Maryland dental hygienists' views of oral cancer prevention and early detection. *J. Dent. Hyg.* 76 (III): 186–191.

Jue, M.S., Kim, Y.S., and Ro, Y.S. (2010). Fiddler's neck accompanied by allergic contact dermatitis to nickel in a viola player. *Ann. Dermatol.* 22 (1): 88–90.

Neild-Gehrig, J.S. (2018). *Patient Assessment Tutorials: A Step-By-Step Guide for the Dental Hygienist*, 4e, 376–423. Pennsylvania: Lippincott Williams & Wilkins.

Schantz, S.P. and Yu, G.P. (2002). Head and neck cancer incidence trends in young Americans, 1973–1997, with a special analysis for tongue cancer. *Arch. Otolaryngol. Head Neck Surg.* 128 (3): 268–274.

Sciubba, J.J. (2001 Nov). Oral cancer and its detection. History-taking and the diagnostic phase of management. *J. Am. Dent. Assoc.* 132 (Suppl): 12S–18S.

SEER Cancer Statistics (2017). *Factsheets: Oral Cavity and Pharynx Cancer.* Bethesda, MD. Available at: http://seer.cancer.gov/statfacts/html/oralcav.html: National Cancer Institute (June 4, 2018).

Smith, R.A., Brooks, D., Cokkinides, V. et al. (2013). A review of current American Cancer Society guidelines, current issues in cancer screening, and new guidance on cervical cancer screening and lung cancer screening. *CA Cancer J. Clin.* 63 (2): 88–105.

Walsh, T., Liu, J.L., Brocklehurst, P. et al. (2013). Clinical assessment to screen for the detection of oral cavity cancer and potentially malignant disorders in apparently healthy adults. *Cochrane Database Syst. Rev.* 11: CD010173.

Warnakulasurlya, S. (2009). Global epidemiology of oral and oropharyngeal cancer. *Oral Oncol.* 45 (4–5): 309–316.

Additional Resources

Strings Magazine. 2018. *How to Prevent or Even Cure a Violin Hickey*, [Online]. Available at: http://stringsmagazine.com/how-to-prevent-or-even-cure-a-violin-hickey (June 4, 2018).

Answers to Self-Study Questions

1. Answer: False. The Head and Neck and Intraoral exams should be performed following the same sequence and in the same manner to ensure nothing is missed.

2. Answer: 51%. Studies indicate slightly more than half of practicing hygienists routinely performs a complete Head and Neck exam.

3. Answer: False. All patients should receive cancer screening as part of the standard of hygiene care.

4. B Answer: Atypical findings indicate the clinical condition or lesion is a variant of normal found in a portion of the population.

5. D Answer: Sternocleidomastoid.

Case 3

Radiographic Exam

Introduction

Radiographic studies provide invaluable diagnostic information to the oral health-care provider. In this section we will discuss a case of an adolescent patient who has an atypical pattern of tooth eruption, prompting the utilization of a panoramic radiograph. This case highlights the importance of identifying disease beyond caries and periodontitis by utilizing dental radiography. We will discuss how to prescribe radiographic studies, review the different types of radiographic studies commonly used in dentistry, and suggest a brief methodology for radiographic interpretation.

In this case the patient was diagnosed with Gardener syndrome (GS). GS is an autosomal dominant genetic disorder resulting from a mutation on chromosome 5 (Cristafaro et al. 2013). The oral and maxillofacial manifestations include osteomas, odontomas, supernumerary teeth, impacted teeth, and epidermoid cysts (Neville et al. 2015). Several other findings exist outside the stomatognathic region, the most important of which are colonic polyps. Patients may develop up to 2500 of these polyps, which are premalignant. Nearly 100% of patients will develop colonic carcinoma if these polyps are not addressed surgically (Cristafaro et al. 2013). It is critical that oral health-care professionals recognize the findings of GS as the clinical signs in the head and neck may manifest prior to the development of premalignant colonic polyps (Neville et al. 2015).

CASE STORY

A nine-year-old male presents to the dental clinic for an examination. This is his first visit to the dentist. Upon initial clinical examination it is noted that the patient is missing several teeth.

PROBLEM-BASED LEARNING GOALS AND OBJECTIVES

- Discuss the rationale for taking radiographs
- Describe the common radiographic studies in dentistry
- List the steps in the suggested methodology for reading images
- Describe the features of GS
- List the oral and maxillofacial findings in patients with GS
- Understand the importance of timely referrals of patients with GS to the appropriate health-care provider

Medical History

Denies.

Medications

Denies.

Review of Systems

All systems within normal limits.

Social History

Denies.

Dental History

None.

Head and Neck Exam

Extraoral Exam

Bone-hard, subcutaneous, spherical nodule present at the right mandibular angle measuring approximately 1.0 × 1.0 cm.

No other grossly visible signs of pathology are identified in the head and neck or craniofacial region. The examination is negative for clinically detectible cervical lymphadenopathy.

Intraoral Exam

Soft Tissue

All oral mucosal surfaces including upper and lower labial mucosae, gingiva, tongue, floor of mouth, bilateral buccal mucosae, bilateral maxillary and mandibular buccal vestibules, soft palate, hard palate and clinically visible oropharynx appeared healthy with no visible signs of atypical inflammation, infection, neoplasia, or other pathology.

Hard Tissue

Missing teeth C, H, #8 and #23.

Radiographic Examination

The clinical examination demonstrated missing teeth and an extraoral nodule of hard tissue consistency on the left mandibular angle. A panoramic image was prescribed in order to capture the areas of missing teeth and the angle of the mandible.

Radiographic Findings

- See Figures 1.3.1–1.3.5.
- Well-circumscribed radiopaque mass measuring approximately 1.0 × 1.0 cm located on the right mandibular angle.

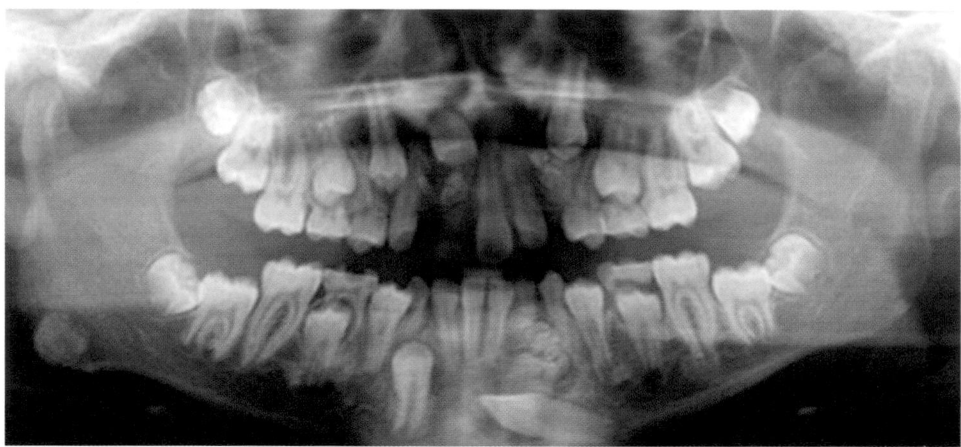

Figure 1.3.1: Panoramic radiograph demonstrating adolescent patient with a right mandibular osteoma, multiple odontomas, and impacted teeth.

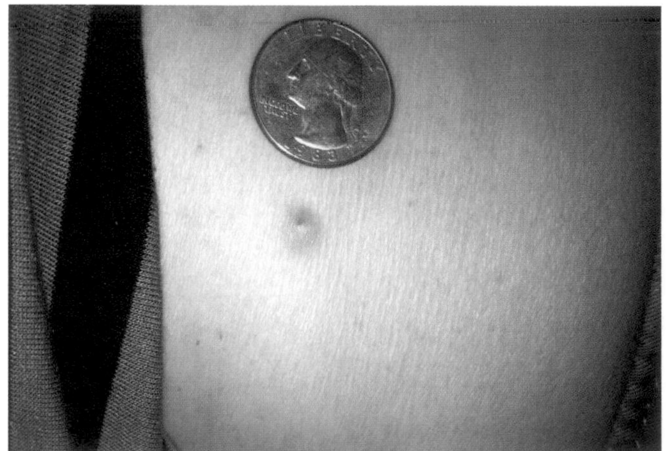

Figure 1.3.2: Clinical image of an epidermoid cyst of the skin. An elevated nodule demonstrating a darker hue compared to the adjacent skin. The nodule was doughy in consistency upon palpation.

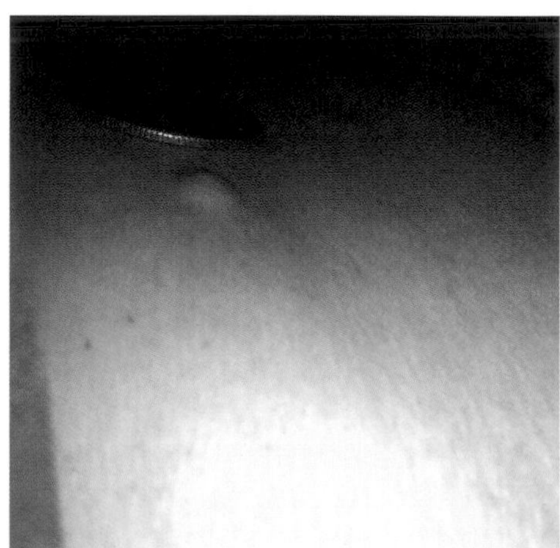

Figure 1.3.3: Clinical image of an epidermoid cyst of the skin. An elevated nodule demonstrating a darker hue compared to the adjacent skin. The nodule was doughy in consistency upon palpation.

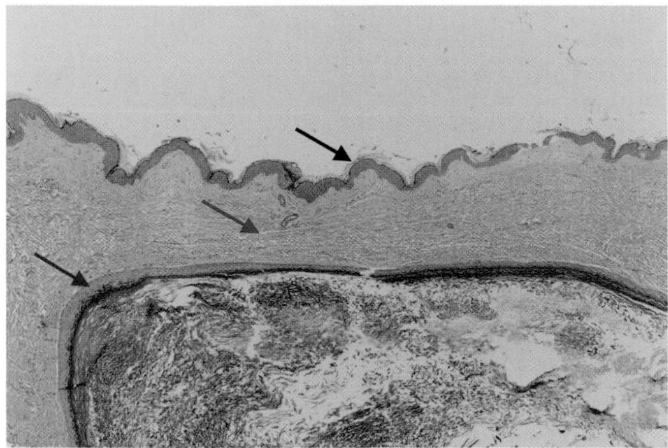

Figure 1.3.4: Low power histopathology corresponding to the epidermoid cyst of the skin seen in Figure 1.3.2 and Figure 1.3.3. The section shows an intact epidermis composed of orthokeratinized stratified squamous epithelium (black arrow), a dermis of dense fibrous connective tissue (blue arrow), a cystic structure showing orthokeratinized stratified squamous epithelium and a lumen with keratinaceous debris (red arrow).

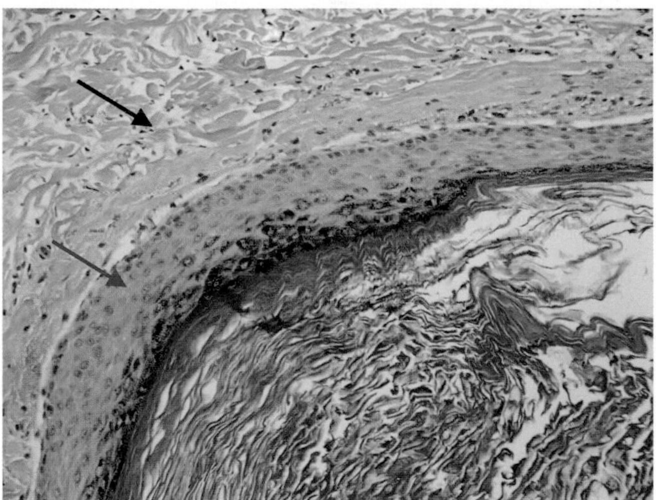

Figure 1.3.5: High power histopathology corresponding to the epidermoid cyst of the skin. The section shows the dermis comprising the cyst wall (black arrow) the cystic lining of orthokeratinized stratified squamous epithelium and a lumen with keratinaceous debris (blue arrow).

- Well-circumscribed radiopaque mass measuring approximately 0.7 × 0.5 cm located at the apex of tooth #19.
- Coalesced radiopaque masses in the anterior maxilla (areas of teeth #8 and #11) and in the anterior mandible (area of tooth #22) measuring from 1.1 × 0.9 cm to 0.8 × 0.9 cm.
- Multiple impacted teeth (# 8 and #22).
- Cystic lesion surrounding crown of impacted #22.
- Missing tooth #23.
- Multiple retained primary teeth.

Radiographic Impressions

- The well-circumscribed radiopaque masses in the right and left mandible are consistent with osteomas.
- The coalesced radiopaque masses in the anterior maxilla and anterior mandible are consistent with compound odontomas.
- The combination of findings including multiple likely osteomas and odontomas as well as multiple impacted teeth, are highly suspicious for a diagnosis of GS.

Differential Diagnosis

The combination of osteomas, odontomas, and impacted teeth place GS at the top of the differential diagnosis. It is possible that these findings could occur outside GS.

Clinical Management

- Given the high degree of suspicion for GS, the patient's parent or guardian should be questioned regarding a family history of GS and findings related to this diagnosis.
- If a diagnosis has not been established, the patient should be referred to pediatric oncology for a thorough work-up to rule out a diagnosis of GS.

Treatment Plan

Dental prophylaxis.
Referral to pediatric oncology for diagnostic work-up in consideration of findings consistent with GS.

Discussion

Radiographic examination enables the oral health-care provider to acquire essential diagnostic information for patient care that cannot be obtained by other means. Several items must be considered in deciding which studies should be performed including acquiring the necessary diagnostic information as dictated by the clinical scenario and promoting patient safety by minimizing exposure to radiation.

The radiographic studies commonly used in dental practice include the bitewing, periapical, and panoramic radiographs. Cone beam computed tomography (CBCT) is also seeing increased utilization. Bitewing radiographs allow excellent visualization of structures above the cementoenamel junction. One of the strengths of this study is diagnosis of dental caries in the posterior dentition. Periapical films enable visualization of the crown and apex of the tooth, and of the bone surrounding the apex. This is helpful in identifying inflammatory disease (periapical granulomas and cysts) as well as evaluating bone levels in patients with periodontal disease. The periapical film is also useful in diagnosing caries of the anterior dentition. The panoramic study provides a large quantity of information regarding the teeth, and bone and soft tissues of the oral and maxillofacial region. While the resolution of a panoramic radiograph renders it less sensitive to detecting periodontal disease or caries, it allows for visualization of the general condition of the oral and maxillofacial region. A CBCT scan has many uses including treatment planning for resection of gnathic pathology, implant surgery planning, and detection of crown or root fractures.

The radiographic prescription is made based on the specific clinical scenario of each patient. An initial examination is completed when the patient arrives at the dental office to decide which, if any, radiographs may be needed.

The history of recent radiographic studies must also be taken into account. Once a decision is made as to which radiographs are necessary, the clinician must inquire as to whether recent radiographic studies were performed that would provide sufficient diagnostic information. If recent studies were done and provide the necessary information, no further radiographs would be required. Attention to this principle minimizes unnecessary radiation exposure. However, exceptions do exist. For instance, if a patient presents as an emergency and the office where recent radiographic studies were performed cannot be reached, new radiographs would be necessary to aid in addressing the emergency (White and Pharoah 2009).

It is critical to assess all anatomic structures that are present within a radiographic image. Developing a systematic repeatable approach to reading radiographic images is therefore imperative. Please see Table 1.3.1 for a suggested methodology.

A descriptive clinical note should be made following the reading of the radiographic study. The mnemonic LESION (**L**ocation, **E**dge, **S**hape, **I**nternal, **O**ther structures, **N**umber) is helpful in describing any abnormalities that are identified (Dr. G's Toothpix 2016).

Location – Where is it located?
Edge – What is the degree of definition? Is it well or poorly defined or circumscribed?
Shape – What is the shape?
Internal – What is the internal character? Radiolucent, radiopaque, mixed?
Other – What other anatomic structures are involved?
Number – Is it unilocular or multilocular? Are there several components?
(Dr. G's Toothpix 2016)

Table 1.3.1: Suggested methodology for reading radiographic images.

Step	Instruction
1	Assess image radiographic artifacts and quality; if anatomic structures are clearly visible move on to step 2; if anatomic structures are not clearly visible consider retaking image
2	Assess bone for normal patterns of trabeculation and any interruptions within the pattern moving from the left to the right side of the image
3	Count the teeth if present
4	Assess lamina dura, periodontal ligament area, and apex of each tooth
5	Assess alveolar bone levels surrounding each tooth that may be indicative of periodontal bone loss
6	Assess enamel and dentin for normal degrees of thickness and uniformity (e.g., absence of fracture)
7	Assess enamel and dentin for areas of radiolucency that may be indicative of dental caries
8	Assess pulp chamber and canal of each tooth for uniformity (e.g., absence of stones)
9	Write a detailed description of any abnormalities in the patient chart and depict on a diagram if available

In this patient's case there are several radiographic abnormalities identified. These findings lead to a strong clinical suspicion of GS. GS is a rare disease resulting from a mutation on chromosome 5. Patients with this diagnosis develop up to thousands of intestinal polyps. These polyps are initially benign, but have a malignant potential, carrying a high rate of transformation into adenocarcinoma (Neville et al. 2015). Nearly 100% of patients with GS will develop colonic adenocarcinoma by middle-age if left untreated (Kumar et al. 2007). Patients are treated with prophylactic surgical removal of their colon (colectomy) to prevent development of colonic adenocarcinoma (Neville et al. 2015).

GS includes several manifestations in the oral and maxillofacial region. Hard tissue findings comprise odontomas, supernumerary teeth, impacted teeth, and dental agenesis (Cristafaro et al. 2013; Neville et al. 2015). Soft tissue abnormalities include, but are not limited to epidermoid cysts of the skin (Neville et al. 2015). Figures 1.3.2 and 1.3.3 show the typical clinical appearance of an epidermoid cyst of the skin and Figures 1.3.4 and 1.3.5 demonstrate the associated histopathology. Patients with GS are also at high risk for developing thyroid carcinoma (Neville et al. 2015).

Table 1.3.2: Findings in patients with Gardner Syndrome.

Finding	Description
Osteoma	Benign tumor of bone; most commonly identified in the skull, paranasal sinuses, and mandible
Odontomas	Benign tumor of mesenchymal and epithelial odontogenic tissue
Supernumerary teeth	Number of teeth beyond the normal complement
Impacted teeth	Tooth remaining submerged in tissue beyond normal eruption sequence
Epidermoid cysts	Cutaneous cyst
Fibromatoses	Aggressive mesenchymal tumors arising in soft tissue
Thyroid carcinoma (female patients)	Malignant tumor of the thyroid
Ocular lesions	Pigmented lesions of the fundus
Colonic polyps	Premalignant fibro-epithelial neoplasms
Small intestine polyps (less common than colonic)	Premalignant fibro-epithelial neoplasms
Stomach polyps (less common than colonic)	Premalignant fibro-epithelial neoplasms

Source: (Adapted from Neville et al. (2015) and Kumar et al. (2007)).

Please see Table 1.3.2 for a list of conditions associated with GS.

Given the serious nature of GS, it is imperative that oral health professionals are aware of the disease, its manifestations in the head and neck region, and know the next steps in ensuring the patient is referred to the correct specialist. See Table 1.3.2 for findings in patients with GS.

Take-Home Hints

1. Attention should be paid to acquiring necessary diagnostic radiographic information and minimizing patient radiation exposure.
2. Establish a systematic approach in reading radiographic studies that can be repeated.
3. Consider the LESION mnemonic in describing radiographic findings.
4. Oral and maxillofacial manifestations may be the first signs of GS and may lead to its diagnosis.
5. Consider GS in settings of multiple odontomas, impacted teeth, and osteomas.
6. Patients with GS are likely to have premalignant colonic polyps and possible gastrointestinal cancer.

Self-Study Questions

1. A patient has a large carious lesion on the occlusal surface of tooth #19. To detect periapical inflammatory disease, which would be the most appropriate radiographic study?
- **A. Cone beam computed tomography scan**
- **B. Bitewing radiograph**
- **C. Periapical radiograph**
- **D. Panoramic radiograph**
- **E. Any of the above**

2. L in the LESION mnemonic stands for:
- **A. Light energy**
- **B. Lymphatic tissue**
- **C. Location**
- **D. Laparoscopy**
- **E. Lesion**

3. Which of the following cancers are most common in patients with Gardner syndrome?
- **A. Colonic adenocarcinoma**
- **B. Thyroid carcinoma**
- **C. Oral squamous cell carcinoma**
- **D. A and B**
- **E. None of the above**

4. A combination of which of the following findings would raise the degree of suspicion for Gardner syndrome?
- **A. Odontomas**
- **B. Osteomas**
- **C. Bifid uvula**
- **D. A and B**
- **E. A and C**

5. Which of the following are considered premalignant in patients with Gardner syndrome?
- **A. Odontomas**
- **B. Osteomas**
- **C. Epidermoid cysts**
- **D. Intestinal polyps**
- **E. Supernumerary teeth**

6. The mutation in Gardner syndrome is found on chromosome:
- **A. 1**
- **B. 5**
- **C. 7**
- **D. 13**
- **E. 21**

References

Cristafaro, M.G., Giudice, A., Amantea, M. et al. (2013). Gardner's syndrome: a clinical and genetic study of a family. *Oral Surg. Oral Med. Oral Pathol. Oral Radiol.* 115 (3): e1–e6.

Dr. G's Toothpix. (2016) Describing Radiographic Lesions. [Online] Available: http://drgstoothpix.com/describing-radiographic-lesions [September 15, 2016].

Kumar, V., Kumar, V., Abbas, A.K. et al. (2007). *Robbins Basic Pathology*, 8e. Philadelphia: Saunders Elsevier.

Neville, B.W., Damm, D., Allen, C., and Chi, A.C. (2015). *Oral and Maxillofacial Pathology*, 4e. St. Louis: Saunders.

White, S.C. and Pharoah, M.J. (2009). *Oral Radiology*, 6e. St. Louis: Mosby Elsevier.

Answers to Self-Study Questions

1. C

2. C

3. D

4. D

5. D

6. B

Case 4

Occlusal Examination

CASE STORY

Miranda Hathaway is 11 years old. She is active in student government, basketball, softball, and field hockey. Miranda stated she is "being bullied and teased about her crooked teeth" and dreads going to school.

LEARNING OBJECTIVES

- Identify the parts of a thorough occlusal examination
- Differentiate between primary and permanent dentition occlusion
- Distinguish abnormal from normal interarch and intraarch relationships in a patient case

Medical History

Blood pressure: 115/70 mmHg; Pulse: 70 beats/min; Respiration: 12 breaths/min.

Review of Systems

All systems were within normal limits.

Social History

Miranda participates in school team sports five days per week. However, she reports being unhappy that members of her sixth-grade class tease her about the gaps between her teeth and her prominent incisors. The bullying impacts attendance and her ability to concentrate in class.

Dental History

The patient has an established dental home and has received comprehensive dental hygiene care under parental supervision.

Head and Neck Examination

Extraoral Exam

The temporomandibular joints and surrounding extraoral structures were within normal limits. A facial profile photograph shows a retrognathic or convex skeletal profile (Figure 1.4.1).

Intraoral Exam

There were no biofilm accumulations or calculus deposits. The patient's gingiva was pink with normal pigmentation for her ethnicity. The maxillary anterior interdental papillae were blunted due to lack of proximal

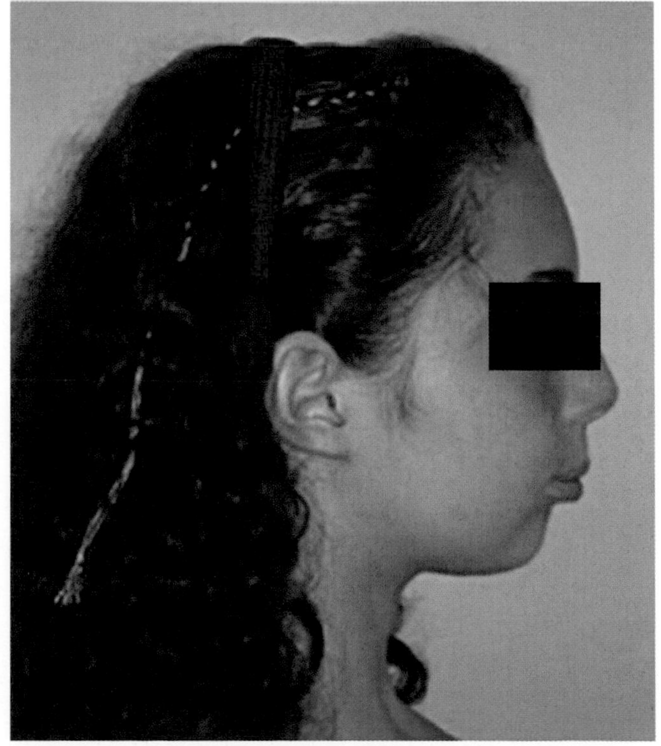

Figure 1.4.1: Patient profile image.

contacts. The gingiva exhibited normal contour and the amount of textural stippling and consistency expected in a patient in phase four of arch development (time in which the permanent canines emerge). The intraoral photographs show delayed eruption of maxillary first and second premolars (see Figures 1.4.2 and 1.4.3).

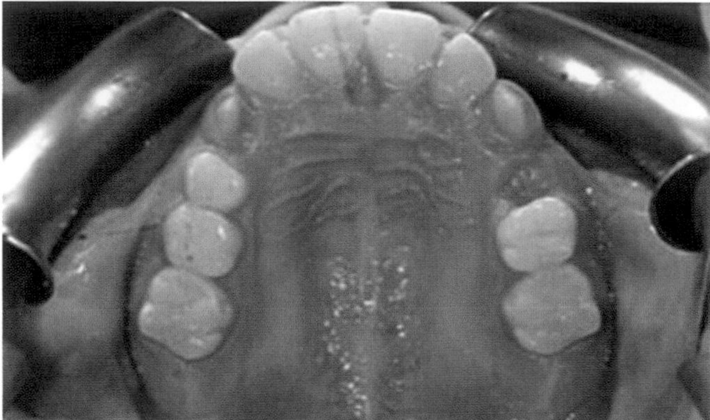

Figure 1.4.2: Patient intraoral palate.

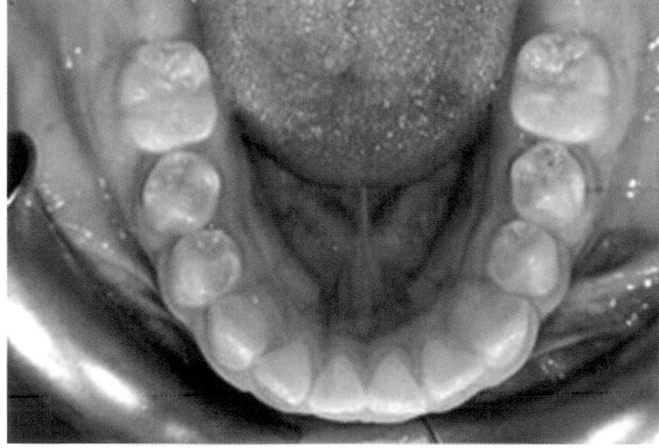

Figure 1.4.3: Patient intraoral floor of mouth.

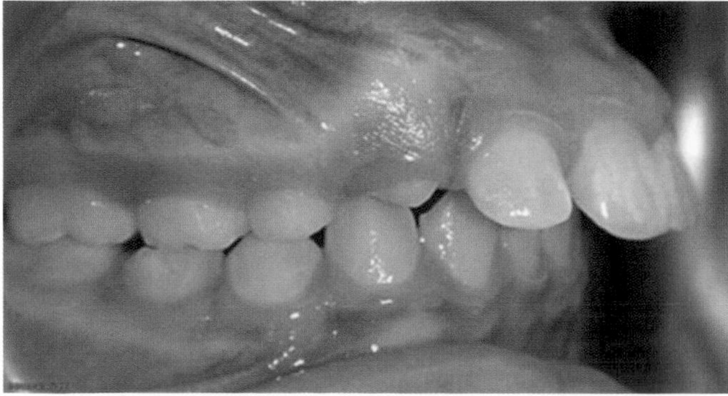

Figure 1.4.4: Malocclusion right.

Occlusion

Class II Division I malocclusion with a severe overbite and excessive overjet (9 mm) (see Figures 1.4.4–1.4.6). No occlusal habits or other parafunctional occlusal habits noted.

Radiographic Examination

Delayed eruption of maxillary first and second premolars (see Figures 1.4.7 and 1.4.8).

Dental Hygiene Diagnosis

Problems	Related to Risks and Etiology
Class II Division I malocclusion	Permanent molar and anterior teeth relationships: • mesiobuccal groove of the mandibular first molar is distal to the mesiobuccal cusp of the maxillary first molar by more than the width of a premolar • maxillary anterior teeth protrude facially with a severe overbite related to hereditary skeletal (mandibular) jaw discrepancy
Negative oral health-related Quality-of-Life (OHRQoL)	Teasing and bullying about malocclusion
Increased risk of sports-related mouth injury	Patient age and participation in sporting activities

Planned Interventions

Planned Interventions (to arrest or control disease and regenerate, restore or maintain health)

Clinical	Education/ Counseling	Oral Hygiene Instruction
Initial exam, intraoral photographs, alginate impressions, study models radiographs, and adult prophylaxis Fabrication of mouth guard Referral to an orthodontic/ orthopedic specialist Referral to primary care physician and school officials to implement appropriate services and support for bullying Six-month recall	Features of malocclusion and the importance of orthodontic intervention to OHRQoL. Proper use of a mouth guard during contact sports activities and risks of not wearing or altering protective equipment (Ranalli 2002).	OTC fluoride-containing toothpaste twice daily, after breakfast and at bedtime. Oral hygiene, flossing, and brushing. Wear mouth guard during sports activities

Progress Notes

Miranda arrived for her appointment 15 minutes late. I reminded Miranda and her mother of the office policy regarding missed and late appointments. A complete medical, social, and dental history was taken. Head and neck and dental exams including occlusal assessment were performed. Panoramic and lateral cephalogram radiographs, and alginate impressions were taken.

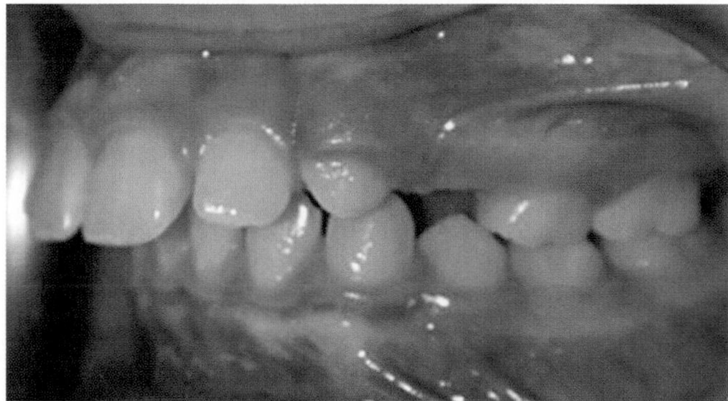

Figure 1.4.5: Malocclusion left.

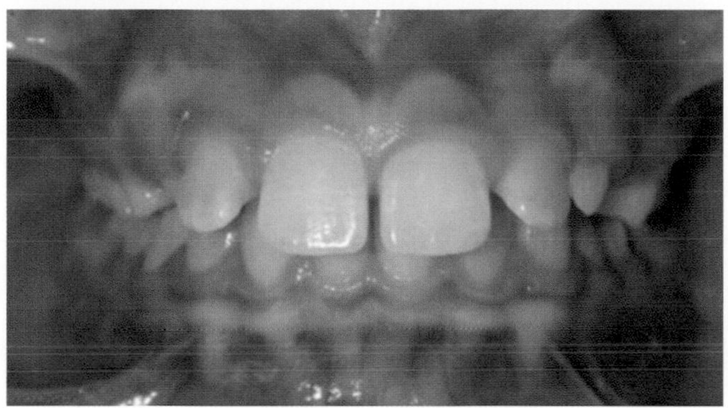

Figure 1.4.6: Malocclusion facial.

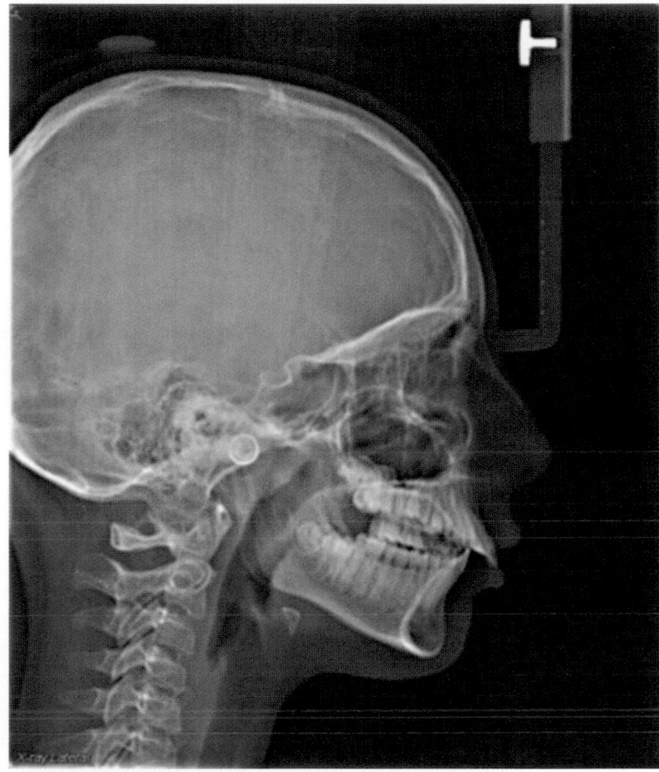

Figure 1.4.8: Relative mandibular retrognathia.

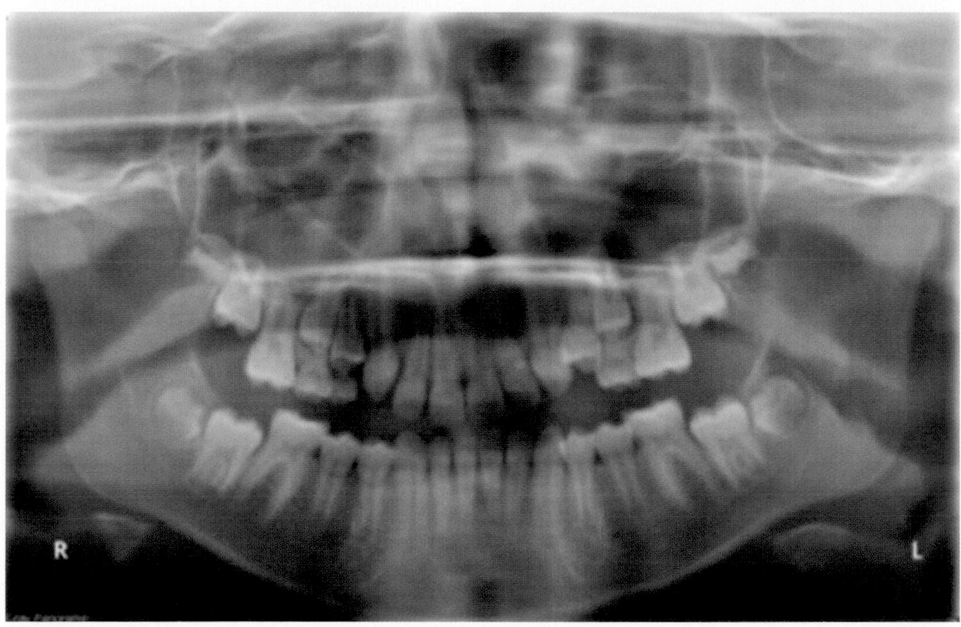

Figure 1.4.7: Radiographic image.

Study models were made for fabrication of a mouth guard. The patient had a mild to moderate gag response to the alginate impressions and was managed well by using a distraction technique: the patient was given a small puzzle to complete (For information on managing patients who gag during dental treatment, see Figures 1.4.9A and B). Oral hygiene instructions were given regarding protective factors to maintain current caries status. Correct use of mouth guard was explained to the patient. The patient was referred to an orthodontist for malocclusion and advised to speak to her guidance counselor for in-school bullying. The hygienist will make follow-up calls to Miranda's parents and her school guidance counselor regarding bullying. Six-month recall recommended.

Discussion

The occlusal examination is critical to the assessment of the patient's dentition and facial symmetry. It includes:

- Classification of occlusion,
- Identification of any teeth malrelationships,
- Examination of the temporomandibular joints, muscles of mastication and range of movements (ROM),
- Record of parafunctional habits such as bruxism and clenching.

Diagnostic records such as intraoral photographs, study casts, and panoramic radiographs and cephalograms assist in the evaluation of the patient's condition and provide a baseline growth record and database for changes during treatment. Disease development such as caries, noncaries cervical lesions (abfractions), periodontal disease and temporomandibular joint disorder (TMD) are related to occlusal disharmony. When teeth are malaligned they lose their ability to self-cleanse; also, parafunctional habit patterns (movements that are not within the normal range) may appear. Malocclusion has physical and psychological ramifications and interferes with children's Oral Health-Related Quality-of-Life (OHRQoL) regarding school attendance, performance, and psychosocial wellbeing (Jokovic et al. 2002; da Rosa et al. 2016). OHRQoL is a construct based on the World Health Organization's definition of health and is used to measure people's oral health status. OHRQoL looks at physical, mental, and social wellbeing as a determinant of oral health and not just the absence of oral disease and related ailments.

Ideal occlusion, although rare, is used as a standard for determining the need for orthodontic treatment in patients. In centric occlusion or maximum intercuspation (MI), each tooth has a particular relationship with teeth in the same arch (intraarch) and opposing arches (interarch). Centric relation (CR), the relationship of the mandible to the maxilla, should coincide with MI (when teeth are entirely interposed). When the MI and CR differ occlusal disharmony is the result. (For a list of risk factors for malocclusion, see Figure 1.4.10.)

Analysis of the permanent occlusion uses the first molars and canines to classify or confirm occlusion while the primary occlusal assessment is performed using the second molars. Analysis of the primary dentition is important because it determines the arch space required to provide room for the secondary teeth. Additionally, the identification of a distal terminal plane relationship between the primary maxillary and mandibular second molars predicts permanent molar relationships and provides valuable information for early orthodontic intervention (For an illustration of flush, mesial, and distal steps, see Figure 1.4.11).

All patients should have an orthodontic evaluation to determine the health of the masticatory system and to provide early therapy to manage the developing dentition and occlusion. The American Association of Orthodontists (AAO) recommends that an evaluation by an orthodontist should be performed no later than age seven because the first molars establish posterior occlusion and the incisors alert clinicians to crowding and poor anterior overlap relationships (American Association of Orthodontists mylifemysmile.org 2013).

Malocclusion can have an adverse effect on self-esteem, self-concept, happiness, and social development; also, it increases the risk of teasing (Seehra et al. 2011; da Rosa et al. 2016). Bullying among schoolchildren has a global prevalence rate of 5–58% and is as high as 47% in 11–12-year-old children (Al-Omari et al. 2014). The most commonly reported targets by bullies are dentofacial features; for example, children with spaces between teeth, malformed and discolored teeth, and prominent maxillary anteriors are likely to be victims of bullying (Al-Bitar et al. 2013). If a child admits to being bullied, clinicians should inform parents of the possible consequences that include psychological distress, anxiety, and depression. Also, parents should be asked to contact the school and teachers regarding the situation. The US Department of Health and Human Services website, Stopbullying.gov (U.S. Department of Health and Human Service, n.d.) provides parents, teachers, communities, and students with tools that support victims of unwanted aggressive behavior. Noting occlusal problems early, identifying possible victims of bullying, and referring patients for treatment have physical and psychosocial benefits for children with poor dentofacial features (Al-Omari et al. 2014).

(A)

Why some patients gag

Patients commonly gag during dental treatment, particularly during the taking of alginate impressions. It is interesting to note that Randall et al. found a correlation between gagging frequency and higher levels of fear related to dental care (Randall 2014).

Gagging is an involuntary defensive reaction to protect the oropharynx and upper respiratory tract from foreign objects. Some non-pharmacological and pharmacological interventions are used to manage the gag reflex (such as behavioral therapies/distraction techniques, acupuncture, local and general anesthetics, herbal remedies, and sedatives), and research has examined their effectiveness.

Effectiveness of Interventions to Manage Dental Gagging

A 2015 systematic review found weak evidence regarding the effectiveness of interventions to manage dental care related gagging and that more studies are needed (Prashanti, 2015), A recent web-based cross-sectional survey found that behavioral modification techniques such as patient distraction, relaxation, and sensory flooding are considered the most reliable methods for prevention of the gag response in 68.5% of patients (Roy 2016). This data supports previous findings that distraction techniques may temporarily divert the patient's attention and allow clinicians to perform minor dental procedures while distracting the patient from a potentially distressing situation (Krol 1963; Kovats 1971; Hoad-Reddick 1986).

Things to do

- Sit patients upright
- When taking impressions, insert the maxillary tray from posterior to anterior to direct the flow of impression material forward
- Have patients tilt their head forward
- Have patients breathe deeply through their nose
- Encourage drooling into the bib or a napkin
- Distract patients with an activity such as puzzling, (mentally) reciting the Pledge of Allegiance or conjugating the verb "to love" in Latin, talking to patients, and having your patients raise each foot until the impression material sets.
- *I find that assembling a transformer toy (Figure 1.4.9b) works with all ages, including seniors.*

(B)

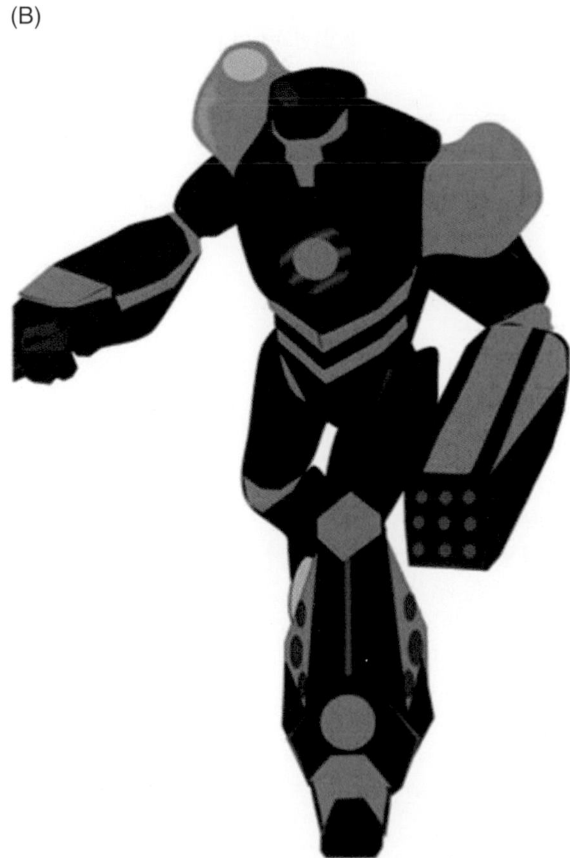

Figure 1.4.9: (A) Managing patients who gag during dental treatment. (B) Transformer puzzle toy.

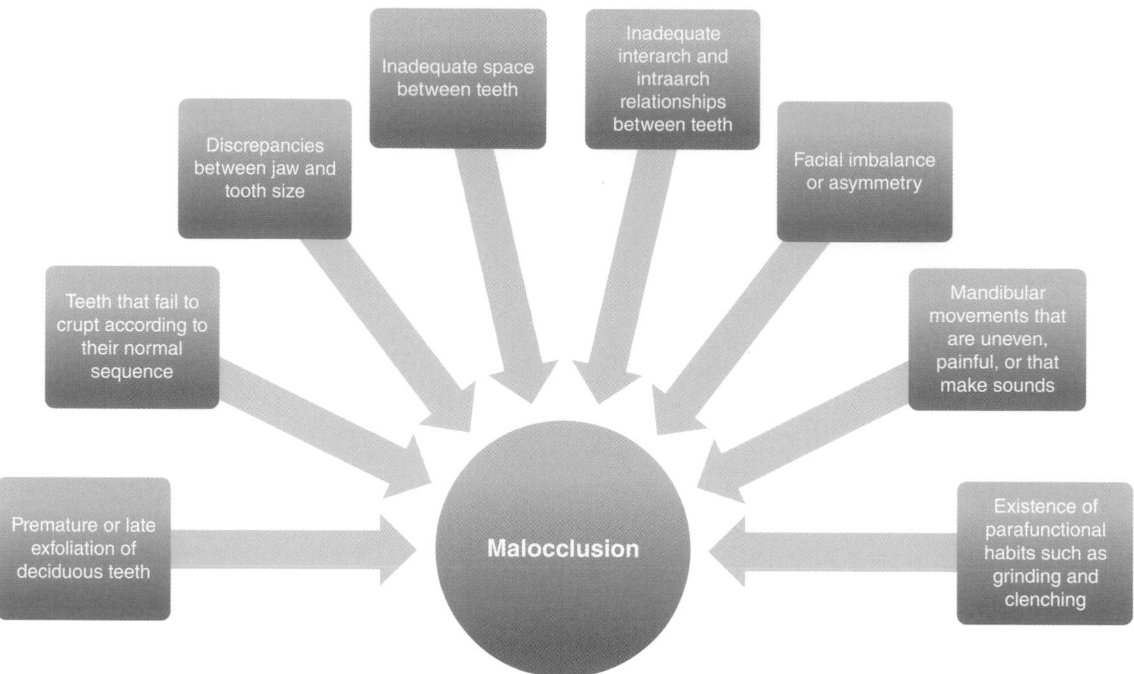

Figure 1.4.10: Risk factors for malocclusion.

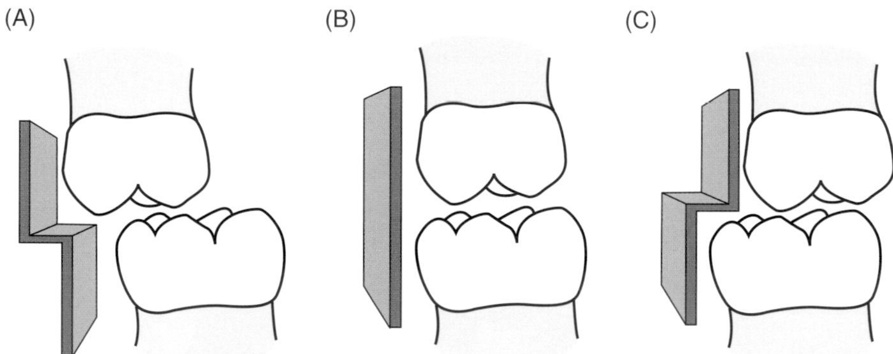

Figure 1.4.11: Distal terminal plane in determining primary occlusion. (A) mesial and (B) flush steps predict class I, (C) distal step predicts class II, extreme mesial step predicts class III.

Take-Home Hints

1. As seen in this case, the age group that is most vulnerable to sports-related injuries is children between the ages of 7 and 11 (Tesini and Soporowski 2000).
2. According Lyznicki et al. (2004) the clinician's role in bullying involves identifying the children at risk, counseling families, screening for psychiatric comorbidities, and providing preventive surgeries.
3. The dental arches go through five phases of development as the bony structures mature to accommodate the permanent teeth:
   - *Phase one* is characterized by the eruption of the permanent first molars;
   - *Phase two* is marked by the eruption of the permanent anterior teeth;
   - *Phase three* consists of the eruption of the premolars anterior to the permanent molars;
   - *Phase four* occurs when the permanent canines erupt; and finally,
   - *Phase five* occurs when the third molars erupt (Fehrenbach and Popowics 2016).
4. Flush and mesial steps in primary occlusal findings predict Class I and distal steps predict Class II in the permanent dentition. An excessive mesial step predicts Class III malocclusion (Figure 1.4.11).
5. Hygienists can reduce student bullying and its effects by collaborating with the patient's parents, school officials, and primary care physician on implementing appropriate responsive services and support.

Self-Study Questions

1. In which phase of arch development do the permanent canines erupt between lateral incisors and first premolars?

2. The following are risk factors for malocclusion EXCEPT one. Which is the EXCEPTION?

A. Premature or late exfoliation of deciduous teeth
B. Teeth that erupt according to their normal sequence
C. Discrepancies between jaw and tooth size
D. Mandibular movements that are uneven, painful or that make sounds
E. Existence of parafunctional habits such as grinding and clenching

3. Which step relationship predicts Class II malocclusion in the permanent dentition?

4. The use of which radiographs enable monitoring of tooth eruption sequence and arch development?

5. What are benefits of early identification of malocclusion in children?

References

Al-Bitar, Z.B., Al-Omari, I.K., Sonbol, N.H. et al. (2013). Bullying among Jordanian schoolchildren, its effects on school performance, and the contribution of general physical and dentofacial features. *Am. J. Orthod. Dentofac. Orthop.* 144 (6): 872–878.

Al-Omari, I.K., Al-Bitar, Z.B., Sonbol, N.H. et al. (2014). Impact of bullying due to dentofacial features on oral health-related quality of life. *Am. J. Orthod. Dentofac. Orthop.* 146 (6): 734–739.

American Association of Orthodontists mylifemysmile.org (2013) The right time for an orthodontic checkup: no later than age 7 [Online]. Available at https://www.aaoinfo.org/system/files/media/documents/Right_Time_for_Ortho-MLMS-hl.pdf (May 15, 2018).

Fehrenbach, M. and Popowics, T. (2016). *Illustrated Dental Embryology, Histology, and Anatomy*, 4e, 283–284. Missouri: Elsevier, Saunders.

Hoad-Reddick, G. (1986). Gagging: a chairside approach to control. *Br. Dent. J.* 161: 174–176.

Jokovic, A., Locker, D., Stephens, M. et al. (2002). Validity and reliability of a questionnaire for measuring child oral-health-related quality of life. *J. Dent. Res.* 81: 459–463.

Kovats, J.J. (1971). Clinical evaluation of the gagging denture patient. *J. Prosthet. Dent.* 25: 613–619.

Krol, A.J. (1963). A new approach to the gagging problem. *J. Prosthet. Dent.* 13: 611–616. 25.

Lyznicki, M.S., MCCaffree, M.A., and Robinowitz, C.B. (2004). Childhood bullying: implications for physicians. *Am. Fam. Physician* 70 (9): 1723–1728.

Prashanti, E., Sumanth, K.N., Renjith, G.P. et al. (2015). Management of gag reflex for patients undergoing dental treatment. *Cochrane Database Syst. Rev.* 1: 10.

Ranalli, D.N. (2002). A sports dentistry trauma control plan for children and adolescents. *J. Southeast Soc. Pediatr. Dent.* 8: 8–9.

Randall, C.L., Shulman, G.P., Crout, R.J., and McNeil, D.W. (2014). Gagging and its associations with dental care-related fear, fear of pain and beliefs about treatment. *J. Am. Dent. Assoc.* 145: 452–458.

da Rosa, G.N., Del Fabro, J.P., Tomazoni, F. et al. (2016). Association of malocclusion, happiness, and oral health-related quality of life (OHRQoL) in schoolchildren. *J. Public Health Dent.* 76 (2): 85–90.

Roy, S., Bhayya, D.P., Gupta, S. et al. (2016). Awareness and prevention of patient gag reflex among pedodontists in India: a web-based survey. *J. Indian Soc. Pedod. Prev. Dent.* 34: 238–243.

Seehra, J., Newton, J.T., and DiBiase, A.T. (2011). Bullying in schoolchildren-its relationship to dental appearance and psychosocial implications: an update for GDPs. *Br. Dent. J.* 210: 411–415.

Tesini, D.A. and Soporowski, N.J. (2000). Epidemiology of orofacial sports-related injuries. *Dent. Clin. N. Am.* 44 (1): 1–18.

U.S. Department of Health & Human Services (n.d.) [Online], Available at www.stopbullying.gov (May 15, 2018).

Additional Resources

American Dental Association Council on Access, Prevention, and Interprofessional Relations and Council on Scientific Affairs (2006). Using mouth guards to reduce the incidence and severity of sports-related oral injuries. *J. Am. Dent. Assoc* 137 (12): 1712–1720.

Bennadi, D. and Reddy, C. (2013). Oral health related quality of life. *J. Int. Soc. Prev. Community. Dent* 3 (1): 1–6.

American Academy of Pediatric Dentistry (2014). Clinical reference manual: guideline on adolescent oral health care Pediatr. *Dent* 36 (6): 146–153.

Dimberg, L. (2016). Oral health-related quality of life among children in Swedish dental care: the impact from malocclusions or orthodontic treatment need. *Acta Odontol. Scand.* 74: 127–133.

Answers to Self-Study Questions

1. Phase four.

2. B: Teeth that erupt according to their normal sequence.

3. Distal step predicts Class II in the permanent dentition.

4. Panoramic radiographs of the mixed dentition monitor proper growth and development of the jaws and teeth by establishing dental age and identifying eruption problems and dental anomalies/ pathologies.

5. The benefits of early identification of malocclusion in children are physical and psychosocial including an increased Oral Health-Related Quality of Life (OHRQoL).

Case 5

Gingival Examination

Introduction

The gingival exam is an aspect of the head and neck regional examination, which is a critical component of oral health care. This section will describe the gingival structures, their normal clinical appearances, disease processes that may involve the gingiva, the components of a gingival exam, and present a patient with a disease involving the gingiva.

The patient in this case has lichen planus (LP). LP is an immune-mediated disorder that can manifest in the oral cavity. Patients may be asymptomatic, have mild to moderate discomfort, or complain of intense pain. This disease has a predilection for middle-aged females, but can be seen in any segment of the population. The clinical findings in the oral cavity may include white striations, white plaques, erythematous erosions, and ulcerations anywhere on the oral soft tissues, with the buccal mucosa and the gingiva being among the most common sites (Neville et al. 2015). The diagnosis is established by combining clinical findings with histopathological examination of biopsied tissue. It is important for the oral health-care practitioner to be familiar with LP as it can clinically mimic several other oral diseases, but requires specific management. Cases of malignant transformation to oral squamous cell carcinoma are documented in the scientific literature, further necessitating knowledge of this disease entity (Cheng et al. 2016).

CASE STORY

A 32-year-old male presents to a periodontist following referral for periodontal therapy to manage moderate-to-severe chronic periodontitis. The periodontist observes atypical features (see Figures 1.5.1–1.5.3) on the gingiva of the patient.

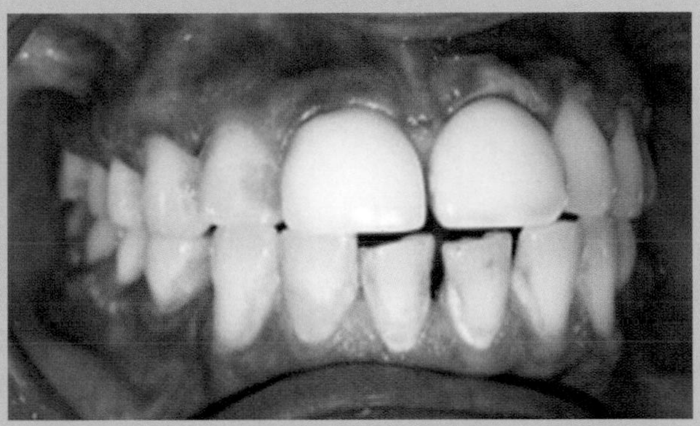

Figure 1.5.1: Clinical image of the patient from the anterior showing multiple erosions and white striated plaques of the gingiva and accumulation of plaque and calculus.

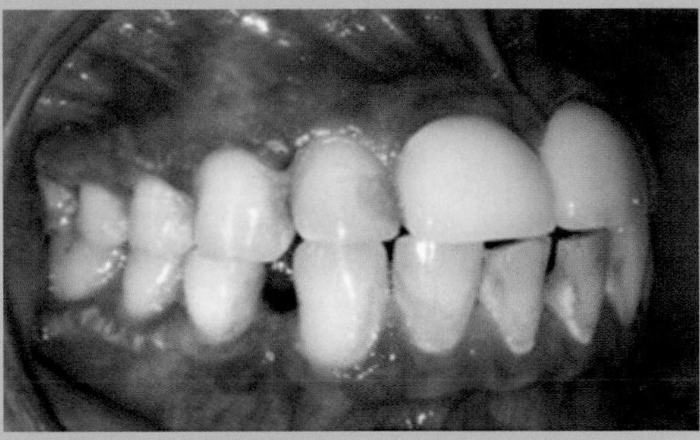

Figure 1.5.2: Clinical image of the patient from the right side showing multiple erosions and white striated plaques of the gingiva and accumulation of plaque and calculus.

The periodontist referred the patient to an oral and maxillofacial pathologist (OMP) for evaluation of the gingival findings prior to initiating periodontal therapy. The patient presents to the OMP

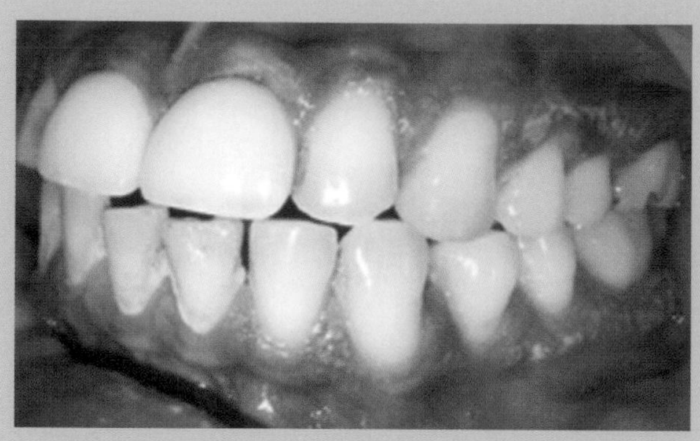

Figure 1.5.3: Clinical image of the patient from the left side showing multiple erosions and white striated plaques of the gingiva and accumulation of plaque and calculus.

requesting clearance for periodontal therapy and also mentions recent onset of sensitivity to spicy and sour foods.

PROBLEM-BASED LEARNING GOALS AND OBJECTIVES

- Describe the normal appearance of the gingiva
- List the diseases that can involve the gingiva
- Describe the components of a gingival exam
- Describe lichen planus
- Understand the importance of timely referrals for patients with LP to the appropriate provider

Medical History

Celiac disease, managed by a gluten-free diet.

Medications

Denies.

Review of Systems

All systems within normal limits.

Social History

Ten cigarettes per day for 10 years (five-pack/year smoking history).

Dental History

Regular restorative dental work.
Moderate-to-severe chronic periodontitis.
Poor oral hygiene.

Regional Head and Neck Exam

Extraoral Exam

No palpable nodules, asymmetry, or other grossly visible signs of pathology are identified in the head and neck or craniofacial region. The examination is negative for clinically detectible cervical lymphadenopathy.

Intraoral Exam

Soft Tissue

Multiple erosions on the bilateral facial and buccal aspects of the maxillary and mandibular gingiva ranging from 0.1 × 0.1 cm to 0.3 × 0.3 cm (see Figures 1.5.1–1.5.3).

Multiple white striated plaques on the bilateral facial and buccal aspects of the maxillary and mandibular gingiva ranging from 0.1 × 0.1 cm to 0.5 × 1.5 cm (see Figures 1.5.1–1.5.3).

All other oral mucosal surfaces appear healthy with no visible signs of inflammation, infection, neoplasia, or other pathology.

Hard Tissue

Multiple occlusal restorations.
Moderate plaque and calculus accumulation.

Examination Findings and Problem List

- Multiple erosions of the gingiva.
- Multiple white striated plaques on the gingiva.
- Sensitivity to spicy and acidic foods.
- Tobacco use.
- Poor oral hygiene.

Differential Diagnosis

Based on the clinical examination, patient symptoms and history, the following entities were considered as possible diagnoses:

- LP
- Epithelial dysplasia
- Squamous cell carcinoma

The color and surface texture support any of the three entities mentioned. The long history of tobacco use places the patient at an elevated risk for epithelial dysplasia and squamous cell carcinoma. The generalized involvement (bilaterality, maxillary, and mandibular locations of lesions) favored a diagnosis of oral LP.

Arrival at a definitive diagnosis required a tissue biopsy to be performed.

Treatment

Written and oral consent were obtained to biopsy the patient's gingiva. A biopsy of the gingiva adjacent to tooth #14 was performed under local anesthetic. Hemostasis was achieved within five minutes by applying local pressure with wet gauze. The specimen was submitted to an oral and maxillofacial pathology service for histopathological review.

Histopathological Description

The histopatholgical section (see Figure 1.5.4) showed a stratified squamous epithelial layer exhibiting hyperparakeratosis, saw-toothing of the rete ridges, lymphocytic infiltration, and degeneration of the basal layer. The underlying connective tissue demonstrated a band-like infiltrate of lymphocytic cells in the lamina propria. These features are characteristic of LP.

Definitive Diagnosis

Lichen planus.

Clinical Management

The patient was contacted and the diagnosis was disclosed and explained. A prescription was written for a 30-g tube 0.05% fluocinonide gel (topical cortical steroid) to be applied to the affected areas three times per day. Smoking cessation counseling was provided. A follow-up appointment was made to evaluate therapy and observe disease activity at four weeks.

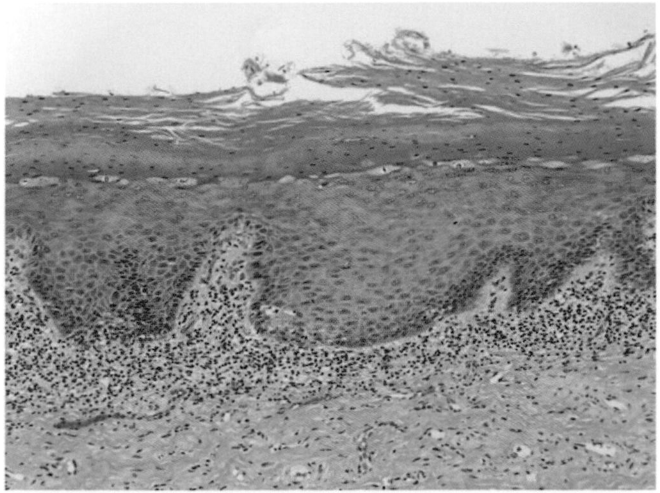

Figure 1.5.4: Histopathology of biopsied specimen demonstrating hyperparakeratosis, lymphocytic infiltration of the epithelium, degeneration of the basal layer, saw-toothing of the rete ridges and a band-like infiltrate of lymphocytes.

Discussion

The gingiva is defined as the portion of the oral mucosa that covers the alveolar bone and the cervical aspects of the teeth. It is divided into three distinct anatomic regions: the marginal gingiva, the attached gingiva, and the interdental gingiva. The marginal gingiva is the terminal end of soft tissue at the tooth and forms a collar around it. The terminating position of the marginal gingiva is at the cementoenamel junction of the tooth in health. The gingival sulcus is the shallow space between the tooth and the marginal gingiva. The attached gingiva extends from the marginal gingiva to the mucogingival junction and is tightly bound to the underlying alveolar bone. The interdental gingiva is comprised of the mucosa occupying the embrasure space between adjacent teeth (Newman et al. 2012).

Healthy gingiva is of a firm consistency upon palpation. The surface texture of the attached gingiva bears multiple small depressions. This characteristic is termed stippling and is similar to the peel of an orange. Stippling is best viewed by drying the gingiva (Newman et al. 2012). A "salmon-pink color" has often been included in the classical description of a healthy gingiva. In actuality the color of the gingiva in health can vary significantly from individual to individual. This variation depends on several factors. For instance, patients with darker skin often have a darker hue to their gingiva, or may have areas of scattered hyperpigmentation, known as physiologic or racial pigmentation (Neville et al. 2015).

The list of diseases that may involve the gingiva is extensive. The general categories include reactive, inflammatory and immune-mediated, infectious, nutritional and metabolic, and neoplastic (benign and malignant). Please see Table 1.5.1 for examples of these categories of disorders.

Many gingival diseases include a degree of inflammation. Inflammation of the gingiva is termed gingivitis. It is characterized by bright erythema (redness), swelling and loss of stippling. The swelling may be edematous or fibrotic. Inflamed gingival tissues may bleed with minimal provocation (e.g., palpation, brushing). Hence, in disease the clinical appearance of the gingival tissues change from those associated with health. Forms of gingivitis include plaque-related, necrotizing ulcerative gingivitis, medication-influenced, allergic, specific infection related, and dermatosis-related gingivitis. There are also several systemic factors that are associated with gingivitis, including hormonal changes, stress, poor nutrition, and substance abuse (Neville et al. 2015).

Examination of the gingiva should be performed in a systematic, thorough, and repeatable manner. Attention

Table 1.5.1: Examples of disease processes involving the gingiva.

Category	Disease	Etiology	Clinical Features	Clinical Management
Reactive	Frictional hyperkeratosis	Repetitive mechanical habit	Homogenous white patch	• Determine origin • Clinical observation
	Hematoma	Trauma and subsequent extravasation of blood under mucosa	Dark red to purple, fluctuant nodule	• Determine origin • Clinical observation
Inflammatory and Immune-Mediated	Plaque –induced gingivitis	• Local reaction to presence of bacteria in intimate association with the tissues • Process influenced by several factors including, but not limited to hormonal levels, medications and local factors such as crowding of the dentition.	Erythematous, swollen tissue with absence of stippling	• Oral hygiene instruction • Plaque removal • Addressing of local mechanical factors (e.g. orthodontics for dental crowding)
	Pyogenic Granuloma	Local reaction to accumulation of plaque and calculus	Pedunculated or sessile, nodule; color may be that of mucosa or more erythematous with or without ulceration	• Excisional biopsy
	Peripheral Ossifying Fibroma	Local reaction to accumulation of plaque and calculus	Pedunculated or sessile, nodule; color may be that of mucosa or more erythematous with or without ulceration	• Excisional biopsy
	Peripheral Giant Cell Granuloma	Local reaction to accumulation of plaque and calculus	Pedunculated or sessile, nodule; color may be that of mucosa or more erythematous with or without ulceration and occasionally exhibit a purple hue	• Excisional biopsy
	Fibroma	Trauma	Pedunculated or sessile, nodule; color may be that of mucosa, paler or more erythematous with or without ulceration	
	Lichen Planus	• Unknown • Primarily mediated by T lymphocytes	White striations, erythema, erosions and ulcerations	• Biopsy to establish diagnosis • Multiple therapies are available, topical cortical steroids being the most common
	Mucous Membrane Pemphigoid	Autoantibodies directed at components of the basement membrane-epithelial junction	Erythema, erosions and ulcerations with occasional identification of bullae	• Biopsy to establish diagnosis (often direct immunofluorescence studies are required) • Multiple therapies are available, cortical steroids are often utilized

Infectious	Primary Herpetic Gingivostomatitis	Infection by herpes simplex virus	Erythema, edema, absence of stippling, purulence from the gingival sulcus and occasional vesicle formation (frequently accompanied by malaise, fever and lymphadenopathy)	• Establish diagnosis (e.g., mucosal smear, serum titers, etc....) • Antiviral medications and supportive care including hydration, rest and analgesics
Nutritional	Ascorbic Gingivitis (Scurvy)	Vitamin C deficiency	Swelling, ulceration and hemorrhage	• Establish diagnosis • Administration of Vitamin C and nutritional counseling
Neoplastic- Benign	Peripheral odontogenic tumors (e.g., peripheral ameloblastoma, peripheral odontoma, peripheral odontogenic fibroma)	Genetic mutations in some cases and unknown etiology in others	Mucosa-colored, smooth surfaced nodule	• Biopsy to establish diagnosis • Complete excision
Neoplasti- Premalignant	Epithelial Dysplasia	Genetic mutations in epithelial cells	Leukoplakia, erythroleukoplakia, erythroplakia	• Biopsy to establish diagnosis • Complete excision in most cases
Neoplastic- Malignant	Squamous Cell Carcinoma	Genetic mutations in epithelial cells	Leukoplakia, erythroleukoplakia, erythroplakia, ulcerations and ulcerative masses	• Biopsy to establish diagnosis • Referral to head and neck oncology
	Lymphoma	Genetic mutations in lymphocytic cells	Mucosa-colored or erythematous broad based mass, often compressible	• Biopsy to establish diagnosis • Referral to head and neck oncology
	Leukemia	Genetic mutations in white blood cells	Generalized enlargement or broad based mass with compressible consistency and a range of color from that of mucosa to erythematous to dark green; may bleed with minimal provocation	• Biopsy to establish diagnosis • Referral to head and neck oncology
	Melanoma	Genetic mutations in melanocytic cells	Darkly pigmented nodule or mass that may exhibit ulceration	• Biopsy to establish diagnosis • Referral to head and neck oncology
	Metastatic Tumor	Genetic mutations in primary tumor	Often an ulcerative mass; great variety of appearance that may fit description of any of the above	• Biopsy to establish diagnosis • Referral to head and neck oncology

must be paid to any changes in color, surface architecture, size, position of the gingiva on the teeth, or any other abnormality. Please see Table 1.5.2 for a suggested stepwise methodology in performing a gingival exam.

Reviewing Figures 1.5.1–1.5.3 and applying the steps of the gingival exam in Table 1.5.2 to the patient in this case, one can rapidly identify features in this patient not associated with gingival health. These would include the atypical white striations, deeply erythematous areas of erosion, and an absence of stippling. Furthermore, application of moderate pressure through digital palpation would induce bleeding. Once these features are noted, the clinician would formulate a differential diagnosis and recommend biopsy. As noted above, the definitive diagnosis was LP based on the clinical and histopathological data.

Oral LP has an estimated worldwide prevalence of 2.2% (Cheng et al. 2016) with a 3:2 female-to-male ratio with most cases occurring in middle-aged patients. The disease is considered to be an immune disorder with damage to the tissues primarily mediated by T lymphocytes (Kurago 2016).

The disease can take many forms in the oral cavity including white striations, white plaques, erythematous erosions, and ulcerations. Any surface of the oral mucosa may be involved in the disease process. Common locations include the buccal mucosa, gingiva, lateral tongue, palate, and labial mucosa and vermilion (Neville et al. 2015). Patients occasionally present with oral and cutaneous lesions. While LP may be completely asymptomatic, common symptoms include mild sensitivity to spicy or acidic foods. Certain patients may even report intense pain with minimal tissue manipulation.

Several diseases may have a similar clinical appearance to oral LP. Diseases that mimic oral LP include plaque-induced gingivitis, lupus, epithelial dysplasia, mucous membrane pemphigoid, and pemphigus vulgaris (Cheng et al. 2016). A definitive diagnosis is made based on histopathological review of biopsied material.

Oral LP is an immune-mediated disorder, therefore plaque control and attention to oral hygiene alone is not sufficient to manage the disease process. Several treatments are available, the most common of which include cortical steroid derivatives. While medications can help to manage the disease, and some patients experience spontaneous resolution, there is no known cure for oral LP.

There are several documented cases in the scientific literature of oral LP transforming to oral squamous cell carcinoma. Therefore it is imperative that oral health-care providers become familiar with the clinical findings of this disease in order to make appropriate referrals to ensure adequate patient management and follow-up.

Table 1.5.2: Suggested stepwise methodology for performing a gingival exam.

Step	Instruction
1	Retract the right buccal mucosa to allow visualization of the facial aspect of the upper right quadrant (URQ)
2	Beginning from the distal aspect of the most distal tooth, run the tip of your second digit along the surface of the gingiva applying moderate pressure
3	Dry the gingiva of the facial aspect of the upper right quadrant (URQ) with an air syringe or cotton tip applicator
4	Beginning from the distal aspect of the most distal tooth visualize the facial gingival surface; follow the above steps for the facial aspect of the upper left quadrant (ULQ)
5	Complete the above steps for the palatal surface of the ULQ and URQ, using indirect vision with a dental mirror as necessary; complete the above steps for the mandibular arch, retracting the tongue as necessary
6	Write a detailed description of any abnormalities in the patient chart and depict on a diagram if available

Take-Home Hints

1. Develop a systematic approach to examining the gingiva.
2. The list of diseases that can involve the gingiva is extensive and ranges from minimally symptomatic to life threatening.
3. LP has several clinical manifestations and may appear similar to other oral diseases.
4. Patients with LP must receive timely referrals to ensure appropriate clinical management of disease and long-term follow-up.

Self-Study Questions

1. Healthy gingiva has a firm texture upon palpation and demonstrates stippling. Healthy gingiva is always characterized by a salmon-pink color.
- **A. Both statements are true**
- **B. Both statements are false**
- **C. The first statement is true and the second statement is false**
- **D. The first statement is false and the second statement is true**

2. Which of the following are recommended practices when examining the gingiva?
- **A. Retraction of soft tissues (e.g. buccal mucosa and tongue) to allow visualization**
- **B. Air-drying the tissues prior to visual examination**
- **C. Utilizing a mirror for indirect vision as necessary**
- **D. Noting all abnormalities in the patient chart**
- **E. All the above**

3. Which of the following are locations in the oral cavity where lichen planus may occur?
- **A. Buccal mucosa**
- **B. Lateral tongue**
- **C. Labial mucosa**
- **D. Palate**
- **E. All of the above**

4. What type of cancer occurs in cases where oral lichen planus transforms into a malignancy?
- **A. Basal cell carcinoma**
- **B. Oral squamous cell carcinoma**
- **C. Adenoidcycstic carcinoma**
- **D. Mucoepidermoid carcinoma**
- **E. Osteosarcoma**

5. Which cells are most likely responsible for the damage to the mucosa in oral lichen planus?
- **A. Osteocytes**
- **B. T lymphocytes**
- **C. Neutrophils**
- **D. Eosinophils**
- **E. Langerhans cells**

6. Oral lichen planus most often occurs in middle-aged adults. This statement is:
- **A. True**
- **B. False**

7. Clinical findings in oral LP may include:
- **A. White plaques**
- **B. White reticulations**
- **C. Erosions**
- **D. Ulcerations**
- **E. All of the above**

References

Cheng, Y.S.L., Gould, A., Kurago, Z. et al. (2016). Diagnosis of oral lichen planus: a position paper of the American Academy of oral and maxillofacial pathology. Oral Surg. Oral Med. Oral Pathol. Oral Radiol. 1–23.

Kurago, Z.B. (2016). Etiology and pathogenesis of oral lichen planus: an overview. *Oral Surg. Oral Med. Oral Pathol. Oral Radiol.* 122 (1): 72–80.

Neville, B.W., Damm, D., Allen, C., and Chi, A. (2015). *Oral and Maxillofacial Pathology*, 4e. St. Louis: Saunders.

Newman, M.G., Takei, H., Fermin, K. et al. (2012). *Carranza's Clinical Periodontology*, 11e. St. Louis: Saunders.

Answers to Self-Study Questions

1. C

2. E

3. E

4. B

5. B

6. A

7. E

Case 6

Periodontal Exam

Introduction

The periodontium comprises the gingiva, periodontal ligament, alveolar bone, and the cementum. It provides support to the teeth, keeping them anchored in the maxilla and mandible. While the stability of the teeth is directly affected by the health of the periodontium, it may be involved with several other diseases processes. There are at least two types of relationships the periodontium may have with other diseases: diseases that directly involve the periodontium and those diseases that are indirectly impacted by its relative state of health or disease. Examples of the former include the patient presented in this case, and other infectious and neoplastic diseases. An example of the latter is diabetes mellitus (DM). The periodontal exam is therefore a critical aspect of oral health care as it functions to assess the health of the periodontal structures that are related not only to the health of the teeth in isolation, but to overall health.

In this section we will review the basic structures of the periodontitium, discuss the components of the periodontal exam and review a case of a patient with periodontal bone loss. The patient in this case has Langerhans cell histiocytosis (LCH). LCH is characterized by a proliferation of histiocyte-like cells that infiltrate and destroy various tissues of the body including the hard and soft tissues of the oral and maxillofacial region (Badalian-Very et al. 2011; Neville et al. 2015). Disease may be solitary or multifocal involving several anatomic sites. LCH occurs in a wide range of patients, but has a predilection for the pediatric population (Neville et al. 2015). The diagnosis of LCH is confirmed by histopathological review of biopsied tissue. Treatment of this disease ranges from simple curettage to radiation and chemotherapy. The prognosis depends on the extent of involvement and the specific tissues affected by disease (Badalian-Very et al. 2011; Neville et al. 2015).

CASE STORY

A 42-year-old male presents to the dental clinic for evaluation of vague pain and loose teeth. Teeth #17, #18, and #19 were extracted at a different dental office two weeks prior due to severe mobility.

PROBLEM-BASED LEARNING GOALS AND OBJECTIVES

- List the components of the periodontitium
- Describe the importance of the periodontitium in terms of oral and overall health
- List the components of the periodontal exam
- Describe chronic and aggressive periodontitis and their variants
- Be able to describe the clinical aspects of LCH
- Understand the importance of timely referrals of patients with LCH to the appropriate healthcare provider

Medical History

Hypertension.

Medications

Hydrochlorothiazide 25 mg.

Review of Systems

All systems within normal limits.

- Vital Signs
  - Blood pressure: 126/88 mmHg
  - Respiration: 16 breaths/min
  - Pulse: 80 beats/min

Social History

Denies.

Dental History

Regular dental recall.
Restorative treatment.
Maxillary third molars (#1 and #16) extracted 22 years prior.
Extraction of teeth #17, #18, and #19 two weeks prior due to severe mobility.

Head and Neck Examination

Extraoral Exam

No palpable nodules, asymmetry, or other grossly visible signs of pathology are identified in the head and neck or craniofacial region. The examination is negative for clinically detectible cervical lymphadenopathy.

Intraoral Exam

Soft Tissue

Gingival tissues of teeth #s 2–6, 20, and #s 29–32 demonstrate marked erythema and enlargement.
Extraction sockets of teeth #s 17–19 demonstrate marked erythema and redundant soft tissue.
Generalized gingival recession.
All other oral mucosal surfaces appear healthy with no visible signs of inflammation, infection, neoplasia, or other pathology.

Hard Tissue

See Figure 1.6.1 panoramic radiograph and Figure 1.6.2 Periodontal Chart.

Minimal plaque and calculus accumulation.

Radiographic Findings and Problem List

- Well-circumscribed radiolucency in the left posterior mandible extending from the ascending ramus to tooth #20 and involving the inferior alveolar nerve canal.
- Well-circumscribed radiolucency in the right posterior mandible extending from the apices of tooth #32 to the interproximal bone between teeth #28 and #29.

Clinical Impressions

1. Multiple, large bony defects of this type can often be identified in certain populations including adults with advanced chronic severe periodontitis, young adults with a history of aggressive periodontitis, and patients with syndromes predisposing them to rapid periodontal bone such as Down or Papillon-Lefevre syndrome. This pattern of bone loss, in a patient of this age and health status is uncommon. Furthermore, the loss of attachment pattern and the patient age of do not fit well for either variant of aggressive periodontitis or chronic periodontitis. The differential diagnosis would include both infectious and neoplastic processes. The initial examination should focus on identifying any source of pulpal necrosis of the involved teeth that could be responsible for the defect, such as a fractured tooth or gross carious lesion. Once a pulpal etiology has been ruled out, the remaining entities on the differential diagnosis may include aggressive periodontitis, a benign neoplastic process such as ameloblastoma, and a malignant neoplastic process such as lymphoma. A biopsy is appropriate to arrive at a definitive diagnosis in this clinical scenario.

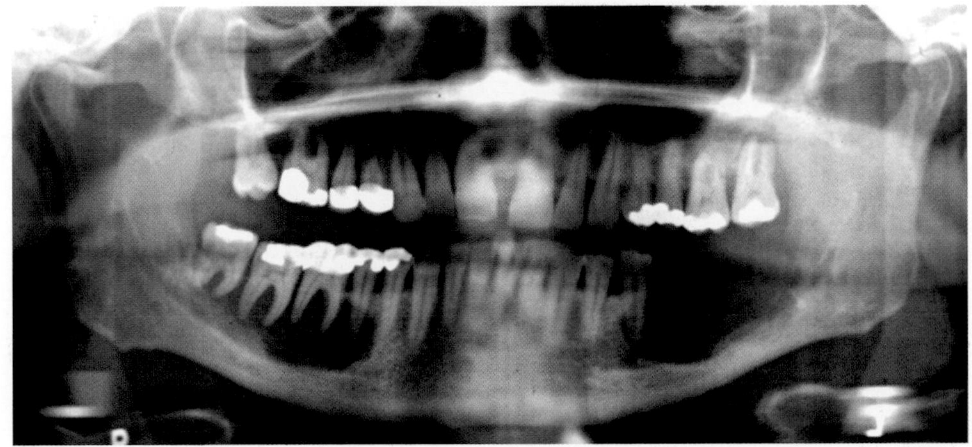

Figure 1.6.1: Panoramic radiograph demonstrating multiple large, unilocular radiolucencies. *Source:* White et al. (2009).

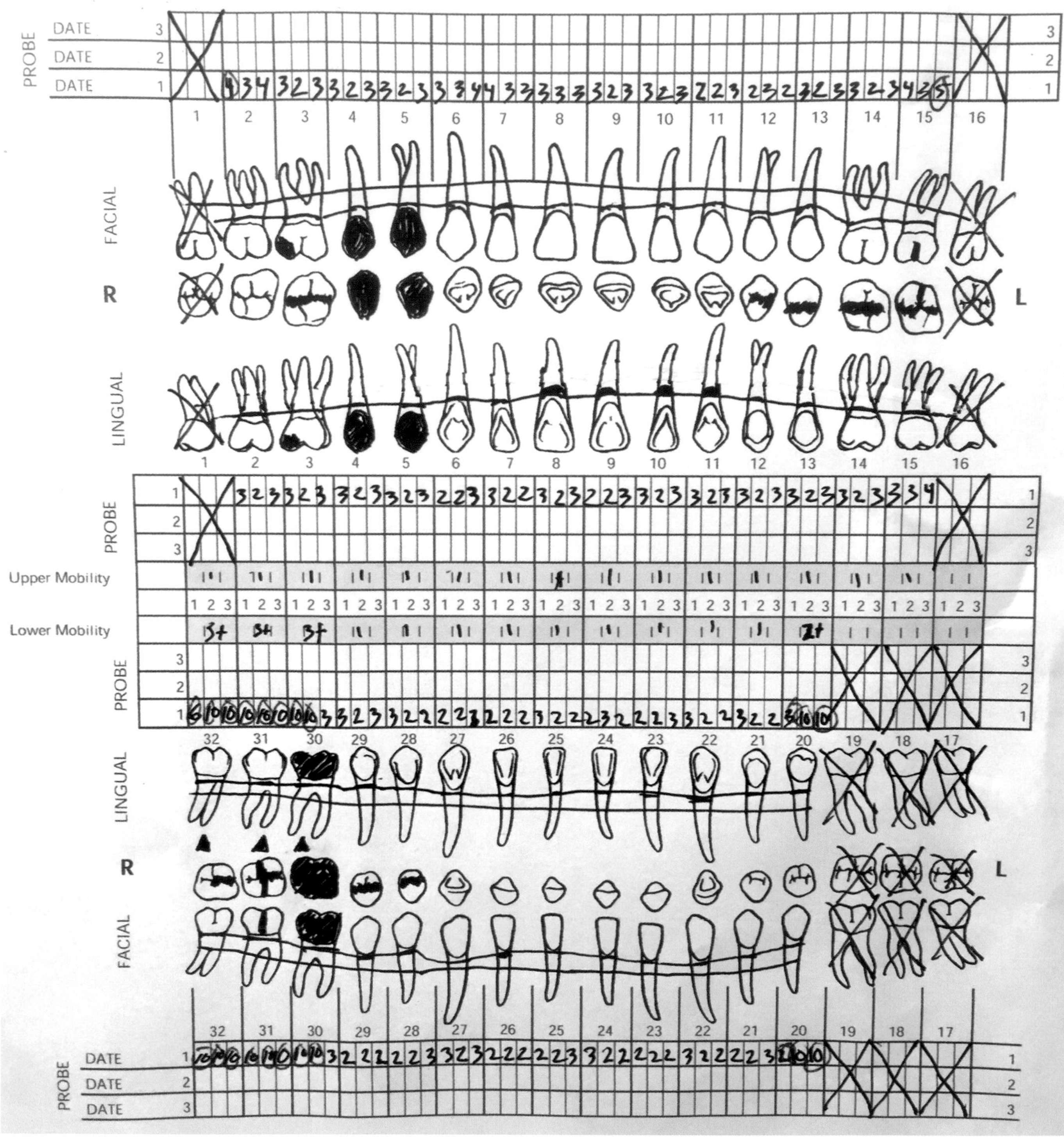

Figure 1.6.2: Periodontal charting.

Treatment Plan

- Referral to oral and maxillofacial surgery for an incisional biopsy of the tissue involved with the radiolucencies.

Discussion

The gingiva, periodontal ligament, cementum, and alveolar bone are the four components that comprise the periodontium. These components work together providing structural support to the dentition. Assessment of periodontal health depends on the periodontal exam. This exam includes four parts: the medical history, the dental history, radiographic exam, and clinical exam (Newman et al. 2012). The medical history may reveal critical information related to periodontal health. For instance, DM has been strongly correlated with periodontal health in the scientific literature (Chapple et al. 2013). Identification of a history of DM is likely to impact the periodontal status of the patient. The dental history is important for determining the patient's past and ongoing treatment, current oral hygiene regimen, and general attitude toward oral health (Newman et al. 2012). Following the medical and dental history, a radiographic exam is usually required. For details concerning the radiographic exam, please see Case 3 of this chapter, Radiographic Examination.

With the medical and dental history obtained and radiographic studies completed, the clinical examination of the periodontium can commence. This exam consists of several steps. As emphasized thus far in the text, deciding on a systematic, repeatable method for performing this task is foundational. Critical elements of any methodology should contain at least the following steps: assessment of mobility, sensitivity to percussion, plaque, and calculus accumulation, a gingival examination, inspection of all dental restorations, assessment of periodontal pocketing and furcation involvement, and detailed notation of all findings. Please see Table 1.6.1 for a suggested methodology.

Periodontal attachment loss is most commonly related to chronic periodontitis. The American Academy of Periodontology (AAP) classifies slight to moderate loss of periodontal support as periodontal pockets up to 6 mm and clinical attachment loss of up to 4 mm. Advanced loss of periodontal support is classified as pocketing greater 6 mm and clinical attachment loss greater than 4 mm (American Academy of Periodontology 2000a). While loss of periodontal

Table 1.6.1: Periodontal examination: a suggested methodology.

Step Number	Procedure	Additional Information
1	Study the mobility of each tooth placing a fingertip on the lingual/palatal surface and the blunt end of an explorer on the buccal/facial surface	Mobility Grading: • Normal • Grade I: Slight • Grade II: Moderate • Grade III: Severe with displacement in the horizontal and vertical planes
2	Sensitivity to percussion	Test any teeth reported to be symptomatic by the patient for sensitivity to percussion by gentle tapping with the blunt end of a dental explorer
3	Inspection of existing dental restorations	Identification of defective dental restorations that may negatively impact the health of the periodontium (e.g., restorations with overhanging margins, over-contoured crowns)
4	Assessment of plaque and calculus	Utilization of one of several indices
5	Gingival exam	Please see Chapter 1 Case 5: Gingival Exam for a detailed description of this component of the periodontal exam.
6	Assessment of periodontal pocketing	Probing of all surfaces of the teeth with notation of fluids expressed including blood and purulence; areas of pocketing may be indicated by areas of bone loss seen on radiographs
7	Assessment of furcation involvement on posterior teeth	A Nabers probe is used to assess furcation involvement of posterior teeth that demonstrate pocketing on probing; classification is based on one of several grading systems
8	Charting of all the above findings	Charting is typically entered simultaneously by an assistant as the clinician performs the exam

Source: Adapted from *Carranzas Clinical Periodontology*, 11th Edition and "Parameter on Comprehensive Periodontal Examination," American Academy of Periodontology.

support is most often mediated by chronic periodontitis, aggressive periodontitis (AP), although less common, can result in similar clinical outcomes. AP progresses more rapidly than the chronic variant and generally occurs in patients who are healthy and have a level of plaque and calculus that do not seem to correspond to the level of attachment loss. Two variants of AP exist; a localized variant, commonly occurring around adolescence, and a generalized variant with a predilection for those under 30 years of age. Localized AP typically affects the permanent incisors and first molars; generalized AP involves three permanent teeth besides the incisors and first molars (American Academy of Periodontology 2000b).

A cursory review of the panoramic radiograph and periodontal charting of the patient in this case may appear as some form of severe periodontitis. However, a closer study of this patient reveals a pattern that does not correspond to either chronic or aggressive periodontitis. The severe loss of attachment is isolated to the posterior lower right and left quadrants. The loss of attachment would be more generalized to fit a diagnosis of generalized AP or chronic periodontitis. A diagnosis of localized AP is questionable as the central incisors are not involved and the patient is outside the age group where this disease is typically identified. It is critical to consider other disease processes when a clinical pattern does not fit into the diagnostic parameters of the common variants of periodontitis. These considerations should prompt the clinician to refer the patient to an oral and maxillofacial surgeon for an incisional biopsy. The definitive diagnosis in this case was LCH.

LCH is characterized by a destructive proliferation of histiocyte-like cells (Badalian-Very et al. 2011; Neville et al. 2015). The first designation given to this disease was "histiocytosis X." The term used more commonly today, LCH, points to the phenotypic characteristics shared by the disease and the Langerhans cells of epidermal and mucosal surfaces. In the past it was believed that disease cells originated from the Langerhans cells. Recent research indicates that this may not be the case with the most likely origin of the cells being a myeloid-derived precursor (Badalian-Very et al. 2011).

The presentation of this disease may take several forms. The disease may be solitary, or multifocal involving various anatomic sites including skin, mucosa, bone, lymph nodes, soft tissue, and organs. In the past the terms Hand-Schuller-Christian disease and Letterer-Siwe disease were used to describe chronic and acute disseminated LCH, respectively. These eponyms have largely been set aside and replaced with a description of the focus of disease and sites of involvement (Neville et al. 2015; Badalian-Very et al. 2011).

LCH is diagnosed in patients over a wide age range. However, over 50% of cases are diagnosed in those younger than 15 years. The disease demonstrates an equal distribution between the sexes (Neville et al. 2015).

LCH is capable of destroying hard tissue and results in radiolucent lesions on radiography. Destruction of tooth-supporting bone can produce a similar radiographic pattern to that seen in severe periodontitis (Neville et al. 2015). It is important to keep LCH on one's differential diagnosis in cases of atypical periodontal bone loss, particularly in pediatric patients. Lesions involving bone may present with symptoms of tenderness or dull pain (Neville et al. 2015). When lesions are diagnosed in the oral soft tissues they often present initially as an ulcerative mass (Neville et al. 2015).

Diagnosis of LCH is based on histopathological review of biopsied specimens coupled with immunohistochemical evaluation (Neville et al. 2015). Treatment depends upon the extent of disease involvement. Mainstays of therapy have included curettage, local steroid injection and radiation for isolated, single focus disease (Neville et al. 2015; Badalian-Very et al. 2011). Disseminated disease is often treated by a combination of systemic steroids and chemotherapeutics (Neville et al. 2015; Badalian-Very et al. 2011). The discovery of the $BRAF^{V600E}$ mutation in 38–69% of LCH cases has opened the possibility of molecular-targeted therapy (Badalian-Very et al. 2011; Haroche et al. 2013). The prognosis varies from patient to patient and depends upon several factors including age at the time of diagnosis, the degree of dissemination as well as the specific organs involved in the disease process (Neville et al. 2015). Some cases of LCH have exhibited spontaneous resolution, while others will lead to the patient's demise.

It is critical that oral health-care providers become familiar with the presenting signs of LCH as the oral and maxillofacial region is not an uncommon site of involvement. Identification of the disease and a timely referral is likely to have a positive impact on the patient's long-term prognosis.

Take-Home Hints

1. The variants of periodontitis follow demographic and clinical parameters.
2. It is critical to consider other disease processes when a clinical pattern does not fit into diagnostic parameters of the common variants of periodontitis.
3. LCH and other neoplastic processes can mimic periodontitis clinically and radiographically.

Self-Study Questions

1. Which of the following are components of the periodontitium?
 A. Gingiva
 B. Alveolar bone
 C. Periodontal ligament
 D. Cementum
 E. All of the above

2. In which age group is localized aggressive periodontitis typically identified?
 A. Elderly adults
 B. Middle-aged adults
 C. Adolescents
 D. Children
 E. None of the above

3. What is the most likely radiographic presentation of LCH?
 A. Radiolucency
 B. Radiopacity
 C. Mixed radiolucency-radiopacity
 D. A and B
 E. All of the above

4. Which of the following therapeutic modalities may be utilized in the treatment of LCH?
 A. Curettage
 B. Local steroid injection
 C. Radiation
 D. Chemotherapy
 E. All of the above

5. The radiographic presentation of LCH may appear similar to severe periodontitis. The preceding statement is:
 A. True
 B. False

References

Badalian-Very, G., Vergilio, J.A., Degar, B.A. et al. (2011). Recent advances in the understanding of Langerhan cell histiocytosis. *Br. J. Haematol.Br J Haematol* 156 (2): 163–172.

Chapple, I.L.C., Genco, R., and working group 2 of the joint EFP/AAP workshop (2013). Diabetes and periodontal diseases: consensus report of the joint EFP/AAP workshop on periodontitis and systemic diseases'. *J. Clin. Periodontol.* 40 (Suppl. 14): S106–S112.

Haroche, J., Cohen-Aubart, F., Emile, J.F. et al. (2013). Dramatic efficacy of vemurafenib in both multisystemic and refractory Erdheim-Chester disease and Langerhans cell histiocytosis harboring the *BRAF* V600E mutation. *Blood* 121 (9): 1495–1500.

Neville, B.W., Damm, D., Allen, C., and Chi, A. (2015). *Oral and Maxillofacial Pathology*, 4e. St. Louis: Saunders.

Newman, M.G., Takei, H., Fermin, K. et al. (2012). *Carranza's Clinical Periodontology*, 11e. St. Louis: Saunders.

The American Academy of Periodontology (2000a). Parameter on chronic periodontitis with advanced loss of periodontal support. *J. Periodontal.* 71 (Suppl): 856–858.

The American Academy of Periodontology (2000b). Parameter on aggressive periodontitis. *J. Periodontal.* 71 (Suppl): 867–869.

White, SC, et al. (2009) *Oral Radiology*, 6e. Mosby Elsevier, St. Louis.

Answers to Self-Study Questions

1. E

2. C

3. A

4. E

5. A

2

Dental Hygiene Diagnosis

Clinical Cases in Dental Hygiene, First Edition. Edited by Cheryl M. Westphal Theile, Mea A. Weinberg and Stuart L. Segelnick.

Case 1

Plaque-Induced Gingivitis

CASE STORY

A 20-year-old Caucasian male presents for treatment. His chief complaint is "My gums bleed when I brush and it hurts to floss." He has not been to the dentist for three years. He lives at home, works full time, and is a part time student.

PROBLEM-BASED LEARNING GOALS AND OBJECTIVES

- Differentiate between a dental hygiene diagnosis and a dental diagnosis for gingival diseases
- Identify signs/symptoms and causes of plaque-induced gingival disease
- Identify health promotion strategies or interventions for gingival diseases
- Develop a problem list and/or unmet human need for a dental hygiene diagnosis

Medical History

The patient's medical history revealed a car accident five years ago resulted in a broken collarbone. He does not take any medications and is not under the care of a physician. The patient does not smoke and his vital signs were within normal limits.

Dental History

The patient has not had a dental exam or prophylaxis in three years. He has no restorations. He has had orthodontia and his third molars removed. The patient brushes once a day in the morning and flosses occasionally.

Social History

Patient works full time at an automotive parts store and is studying automobile mechanics part time in the evenings at a community college to earn his certifications. He does his own and his friends' automotive repairs on weekends. He lives at home and eats out at

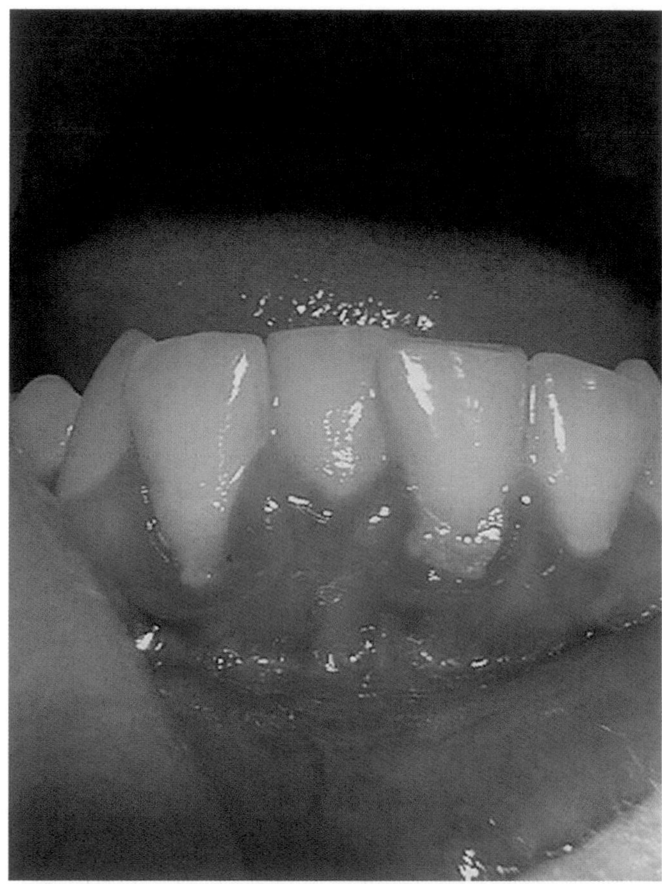

Figure 2.1.1: Note the plaque accumulation around the gingival margin and associated inflammation. *Source:* Photo courtesy of Rio Salado College.

lunch and sometimes dinner. Occasionally he will have dinner with his parents.

Head and Neck Examination

Extraoral/Intraoral Examination

Nonremarkable

Periodontal Assessment

Gingival Statement: Generalized moderate marginal and papillary redness with rolled margins and edematous papilla, localized severe redness facial of maxillary anterior #6–#11 and mandibular anterior #22–#26 (see Figure 2.1.1)

Generalized 4 mm pocket depths, no recession present, no furcations or mobility

Sulcular bleeding index (SBI) 65%

Plaque control record (PCR) 90% (see Figure 2.1.2)

Calculus classification: light to moderate supragingival and subgingival deposits

Dental Charting

Occlusion: Class I right/left with a mandibular lingual bar from #22 to #27

Sealants on teeth #3, #14, #19, and #30

Missing teeth: #1, #16, #17, and #32

Radiographic Findings

No radiographic loss of crestal bone

Risk Assessments

Caries: low risk

Periodontal: low risk

Cancer: low risk

Problem List

Gingival inflammation and bleeding

Probing depths of 4 mm

High plaque score

Dental Hygiene Diagnosis

Unmet human need	Evidenced (caused) by	Signs/Symptoms
Integrity of the skin and mucous membrane due to plaque accumulation	Biofilm accumulation 90% PCR	Bleeding on probing
Responsibility for oral health	Last dental visit 3 years Lack of brushing	90% PCR

Planned Interventions

Interventions	Goals	Evaluation
Oral Hygiene Instructions (OHI) toothbrushing instruction	Patient will demonstrate the proper brushing method	Immediate + next visit by reduction of PCR
	Reduce PCR to 50%	Next visit
	Patient will understand the disease process and the importance of routine dental visits	Patient will schedule appointment for follow up and 6-month recare
Biofilm reduction	Patient will leave office plaque free	End of appointment

Appointment Schedule

First appointment

Assessments with dental examination and radiographs

Oral Hygiene Instructions

Adjunct chemotherapeutics as needed

Full-mouth debridement or prophylaxis

Second appointment if necessary

Re-evaluation

Prophylaxis as needed

Selective polishing and fluoride as needed

Discussion

Assessments should include a medical and dental history, social and cultural factors, activities of daily living, extraoral and intraoral examinations, gingival statement, periodontal assessment, plaque and bleeding indices, risk assessments, and radiographs. Through the interview process the clinician can discuss the stresses this patient might be having and how it may relate to his oral conditions. A nutritional assessment would also benefit the patient in his overall health and in the healing of gingival tissues.

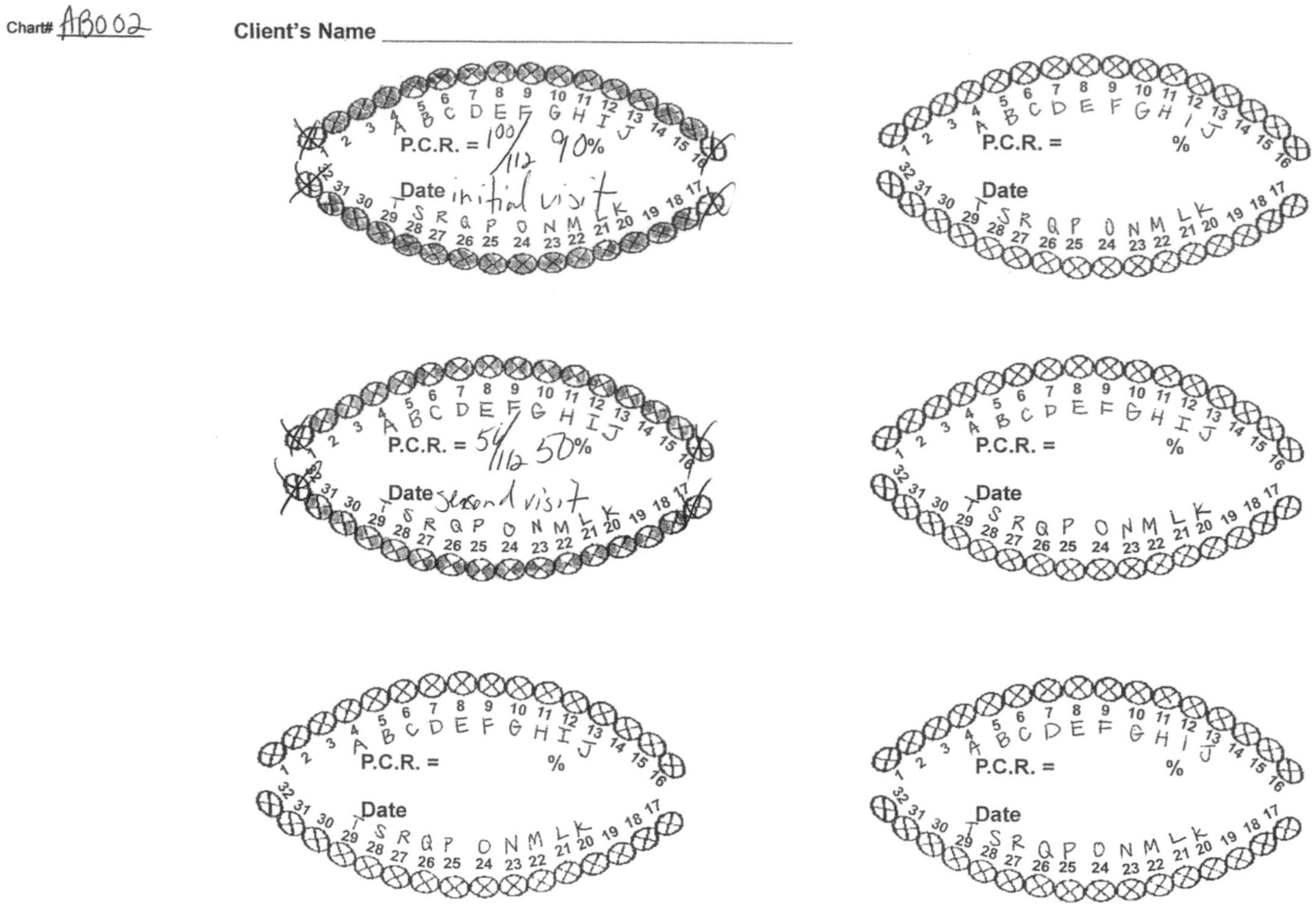

Chart# AB002 Client's Name ______________________

P.C.R. = 100/112 90%
Date initial visit

P.C.R. = 54/112 50%
Date second visit

Figure 2.1.2: Plaque control record for initial and second appointments note the decrease in PCR score from the initial appointment.

A dental diagnosis of plaque-induced gingivitis is defined as inflammation of the gingiva in the absence of clinical attachment loss (perio.org 2016). A dental diagnosis is based on clinical findings that may include: redness, edema, bleeding, and changes in gingival contour and consistency. It is a disease process that begins where plaque or biofilm is present. Clinical signs can be seen as early as four to seven days following plaque accumulation. In Figure 2.1.1 note the inflammation around the gingival margin and the associated plaque control record shown in Figure 2.1.2. This is consistent with a dental diagnosis of plaque-induced gingivitis. Treatment considerations may include many of the same interventions as a dental hygiene diagnosis, but can also include surgical interventions.

It is important for the dental hygienist to recognize that a dental hygiene diagnosis is a part of the process of care. A dental hygiene diagnosis will include a problem list determined from the assessment data collected. The problem list may include some of the same clinical signs as a dental diagnosis. These findings may be redness, edema, bleeding, changes in gingival contour and consistency, and plaque accumulation. At this stage disruption of the plaque accumulation through patient self-care and the host's immune response can reverse the disease process and prevent further progression. Further interviews with the patient can determine his chief complaint and oral hygiene habits to determine an appropriate dental hygiene diagnosis based on the individual's needs.

A dental hygiene diagnosis is key to successful prevention efforts. Why not just perform an oral prophylaxis without ascertaining a dental hygiene diagnosis, dismissal of the patient, and a six-month recare appointment? What prevents this patient from returning in six months with the same condition or a progression of the current condition? What if the patient is not properly educated and does not return for another three years or perhaps a longer span?

From the assessments and patient interview the dental hygienist can develop a diagnosis that focuses on the problems, causes, and prevention rather than a disease entity. The dental hygiene diagnoses for this patient can include several unmet human needs; goals for care and planned interventions. For this particular patient one of the unmet human needs chosen was skin and mucous membrane integrity of the head and neck as evidenced by biofilm accumulation and bleeding on probing. An intact and functioning mucosal membrane and periodontium defend against harmful microbes. Bleeding is a key indicator of inflammation and a determinant of the human need deficit (Darby and Walsh 2015). Interventions such as detailed oral hygiene instructions, patient education so that the patient understands the need for a sound mucosal membrane and the progression of disease play a role in prevention. In Figure 2.1.1 note the inflammation around the gingival margin and the associated plaque control record. The goal to reduce the plaque puts the onus of care on the patient and not on the dental hygienist.

The second unmet human need identified was responsibility for oral health due to the patient's high plaque control score. Utilizing the unmet human needs model and incorporating preventative interventions and goals will hopefully prevent disease progression. It is important to include the patient in the development of goals for their care. Education and oral hygiene for the promotion of health is a clear goal for plaque-induced gingivitis to prevent its progression and to reverse the disease process. Studies have been conducted regarding self-care, self-efficacy, and self-monitoring as playing roles in lasting behavioral modifications. Taking the time to develop the patient's confidence in their ability to perform oral hygiene properly increases the likelihood they will be compliant with self-care behaviors (Schwarzer et al. 2015).

Including a combination of therapies such as oral prophylaxis, debridement, chemotherapeutic agents, and patient education will improve expected outcomes. Assisting the patient with goals and educating the patient can eliminate gingivitis and improve the patient's health for years to come. Scolding the patient for noncompliance with brushing will lead to a lack of understanding on the patient's part and possible future oral health disease.

Take-Home Hints

1. Keep the patient involved in development of goals.
2. Relate the dental hygiene care to the dental hygiene diagnosis.
3. Interventions can include a variety of procedures, education, and oral hygiene instructions.

Self-Study Questions

1. A dental diagnosis for plaque-induced gingivitis is based on clinical findings, which may include all of the following except one. Which one is the exception?

A. Color of gingiva
B. Self-care habits
C. Probing depths
D. Bleeding

2. A dental hygiene diagnosis is based on a disease process that identifies conditions that a dental hygienist is licensed to treat.

A. Both statements are true.
B. Both statements are false.
C. The first statement is true; and the second statement is false.
D. The first statement is false; and the second statement is true.

3. Patient education should include all of the following except one, which is the exception?

A. Smoking cessation
B. Brushing technique
C. Relationship of plaque to bleeding gums
D. Nutritional counseling

4. Signs and Symptoms for integrity of the skin and mucous membrane may include:

A. Bleeding
B. Pain
C. Lack of care and inadequate plaque control
D. Missing teeth and defective restorations

References

Darby, M. and Walsh, M. (2015). *Dental Hygiene Theory and Practice*. St Louis: Evolve Elsevier.

Schwarzer, R., Antoniuk, A., and Gholami, M. (2015). *A brief intervention changing oral self-care, self-efficacy, and self-monitoring. British Journal of Health Psychology* 20: 56–67. doi: 10.1111/bjhp.12091.

Answers to Self-Study Questions

1. B

2. D

3. A

4. D

Case 2

Non-Plaque-Induced Gingivitis

CASE STORY

A 25-year-old Caucasian female presents for treatment. Her chief complaint is "My gums bleed all the time." She goes to the dentist every six months.

PROBLEM-BASED LEARNING GOALS AND OBJECTIVES

- Differentiate between a dental hygiene diagnosis and a dental diagnosis for gingival diseases
- Identify unmet human needs that may pertain to gingival diseases
- Identify signs/symptoms and causes of non-plaque-induced gingival disease
- Identify health promotion strategies or interventions for gingival diseases

Medical History

The patient's medical history revealed she is 14 weeks pregnant and is taking prenatal vitamins. She is under the care of an obstetrician-gynecologist (OB-GYN) for prenatal visits. Her obstetrician recommended a dental check-up. The patient does not smoke and her vital signs were within normal limits.

Dental History

Patient has had routine dental exams and prophylaxis every six months since she can remember. She has had a few occlusal restorations when she was younger. The patient brushes twice a day in the morning and the evening with a fluoridated toothpaste. She flosses about three to four times per week. She has questions about her gums bleeding and her baby's teeth development.

Social History

The patient works full time as an administrative assistant. She is recently married. She is very excited about her pregnancy and has been reading pregnancy and parenting books. She likes to cook and frequently has dinner parties with friends.

Assessments

Extraoral/Intraoral Examination

Nonremarkable

Periodontal Assessment

Gingival Statement: Generalized moderate marginal and papillary redness with edematous papilla; localized severe edematous papilla between tooth #29 and #30 (see Figure 2.2.1)

Generalized 4 mm pocket depths with localized 5 mm between #'s 29 and 30, no recession present, no furcations or mobility

SBI 75% (see Figures 2.2.2A and B)

PCR 15% (see Figure 2.2.3)

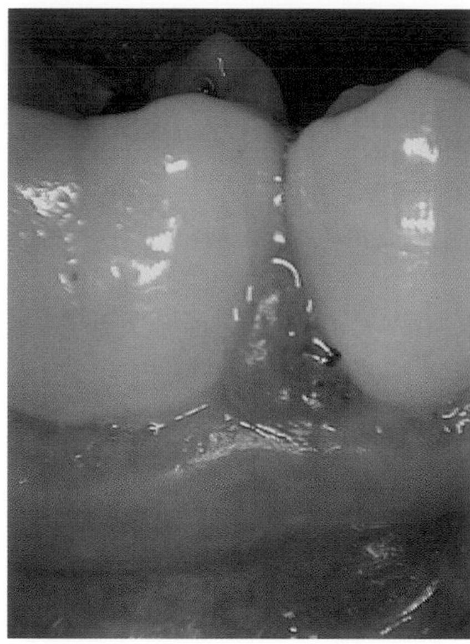

Figure 2.2.1: Note the edematous papilla between teeth #29 and #30 indicative of a pyogenic granuloma. *Source:* Photo courtesy of Rio Salado College.

Calculus classification: light supragingival and no subgingival deposits

Dental Charting Assessment

Occlusion: Class I right/left
Composite restorations on #3, #14, #19, and #30
Missing teeth: #1, #5, #12, #16, #17, #21, #28, and #32

Radiographic Findings

No radiographic loss of crestal bone

Risk Assessments

Caries: low risk
Periodontal: low risk
Cancer: low risk

Problem List

Bleeding
Edematous papilla

(A)

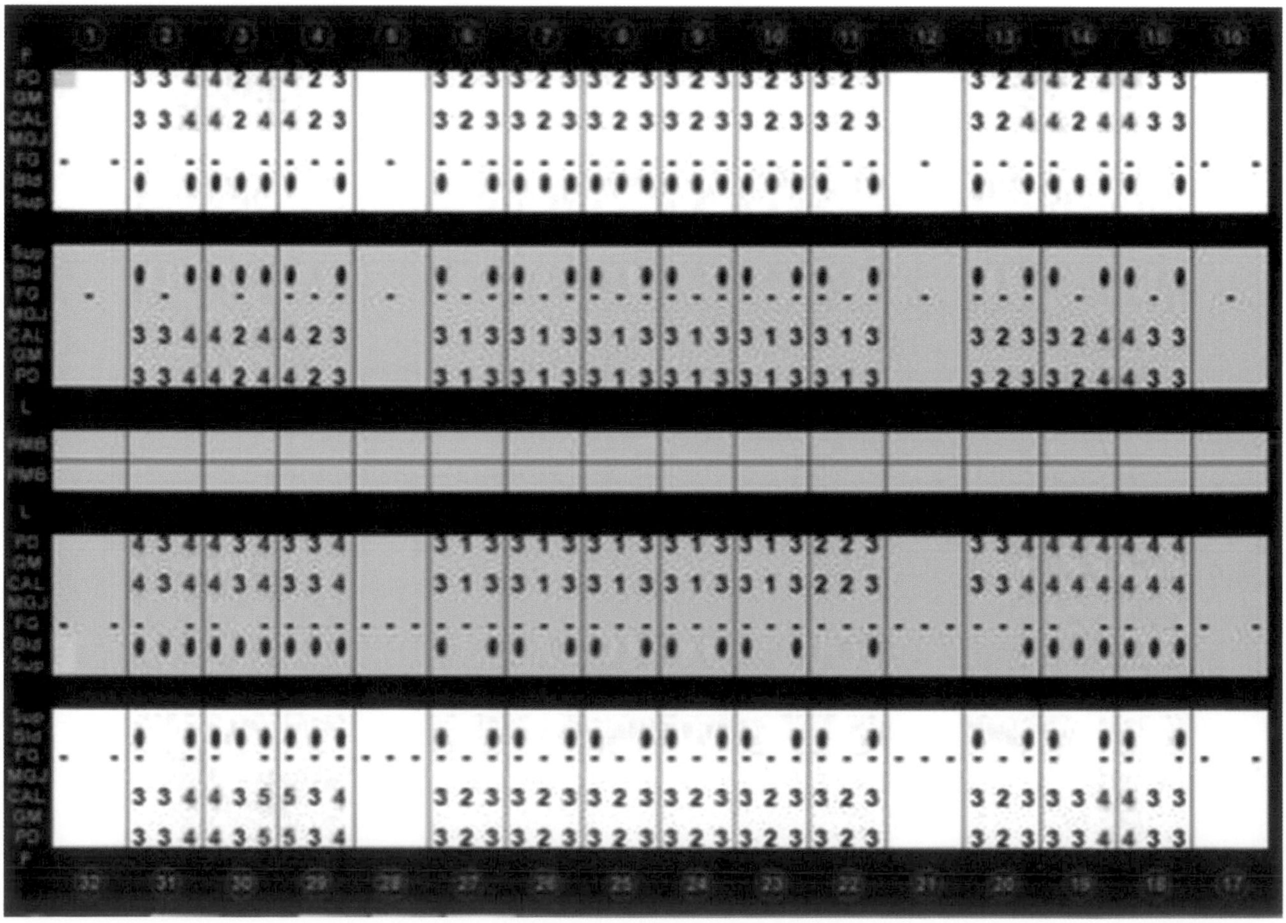

	1	2	3	4	5	6	7	8	9	10	11	12	13	14	15	16
PD		3 3 4	4 2 4	4 2 3		3 2 3	3 2 3	3 2 3	3 2 3	3 2 3	3 2 3		3 2 4	4 2 4	4 3 3	
CAL		3 3 4	4 2 4	4 2 3		3 2 3	3 2 3	3 2 3	3 2 3	3 2 3	3 2 3		3 2 4	4 2 4	4 3 3	
CAL		3 3 4	4 2 4	4 2 3		3 1 3	3 1 3	3 1 3	3 1 3	3 1 3	3 1 3		3 2 3	3 2 4	4 3 3	
PD		3 3 4	4 2 4	4 2 3		3 1 3	3 1 3	3 1 3	3 1 3	3 1 3	3 1 3		3 2 3	3 2 4	4 3 3	

	32	31	30	29	28	27	26	25	24	23	22	21	20	19	18	17
PD		4 3 4	4 3 4	3 3 4		3 1 3	3 1 3	3 1 3	3 1 3	3 1 3	2 2 3		3 3 4	4 4 4	4 4 4	
CAL		4 3 4	4 3 4	3 3 4		3 1 3	3 1 3	3 1 3	3 1 3	3 1 3	2 2 3		3 3 4	4 4 4	4 4 4	
CAL		3 3 4	4 3 5	5 3 4		3 2 3	3 2 3	3 2 3	3 2 3	3 2 3	3 2 3		3 2 3	3 3 4	4 3 3	
PD		3 3 4	4 3 5	5 3 4		3 2 3	3 2 3	3 2 3	3 2 3	3 2 3	3 2 3		3 2 3	3 3 4	4 3 3	

Figure 2.2.2: (A) Periodontal charting for non-plaque-induced gingivitis. (B) Periodontal charting summary for a patient with non-plaque-induced gingivitis – note the total sites and the bleeding sites compare with the plaque control record in Figure 2.2.3.

(B)

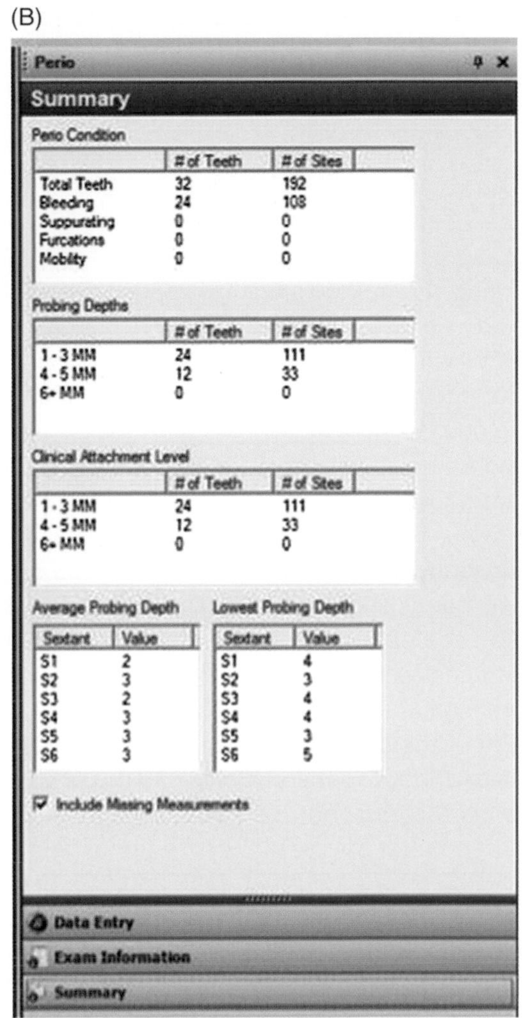

Perio

Summary

Perio Condition

	# of Teeth	# of Sites
Total Teeth	32	192
Bleeding	24	108
Suppurating	0	0
Furcations	0	0
Mobility	0	0

Probing Depths

	# of Teeth	# of Sites
1-3 MM	24	111
4-5 MM	12	33
6+ MM	0	0

Clinical Attachment Level

	# of Teeth	# of Sites
1-3 MM	24	111
4-5 MM	12	33
6+ MM	0	0

Average Probing Depth

Sextant	Value
S1	2
S2	3
S3	2
S4	3
S5	3
S6	3

Lowest Probing Depth

Sextant	Value
S1	4
S2	3
S3	4
S4	4
S5	3
S6	5

☑ Include Missing Measurements

Data Entry

Exam Information

Summary

Figure 2.2.2: (Continued)

Client's Name ______________________

P.C.R. = 14/96 15%

Date 7-2-16

P.C.R. = %

Date

P.C.R. = %

Date

Figure 2.2.3: Plaque control record for a patient with non-plaque-induced gingivitis – note the low plaque score and compare with the bleeding points in Figures 2.2.2A and B.

Dental Hygiene Diagnosis

Unmet human need	Evidenced (caused) by	Signs/Symptoms
Protection from health risks	Inadequate control of a systemic condition – pregnancy	Evidence on the medical history and patient interview
Integrity of the skin and mucous membrane	Inadequate control of a systemic condition – pregnancy	Bleeding on probing
Conceptualization and problem solving	Knowledge deficit	Patient asking questions regarding bleeding gums and baby's development

Planned Interventions

Interventions	Goals	Evaluation
Address safety factors with patient	Referral to medical doctor	Patient consult with primary care provider
OHI tooth brushing instruction	Patient will demonstrate the proper brushing method	Immediate
Teach patient about systemic conditions and oral health	Patient will understand the relationship between pregnancy and gingival conditions	End of appointment
Biofilm reduction and calculus removal with ultrasonic	Patient will leave office plaque free	End of appointment

Appointment Schedule

First appointment
Assessments with dental examination and radiographs as needed
OHI – includes education on the relationship between oral health and pregnancy
Prophylaxis
Second appointment if necessary
Re-evaluation – determination of increasing the frequency for recare appointments

Discussion

Assessments should include a medical and dental history, social and cultural factors, and activities of daily living, extraoral and intraoral examinations, gingival statement, periodontal assessment, plaque and bleeding indices, risk assessments, and radiographs. Through the interview process the clinician can discuss the patient's pregnancy and relationship with gingival conditions. A discussion of the nutritional needs during pregnancy and reinforcing the obstetrician's recommendations would benefit the patient. Educating the expectant mother on fetal oral health and when the development and calcification of teeth occurs is an important function of the dental visit (Darby and Walsh 2015).

A dental diagnosis of non-plaque-induced gingivitis is defined as inflammation of the gingiva caused by factors other than plaque. These may include allergic reactions, bacterial associated infections, viral associated infections, foreign body response, or physical trauma (perio.org 2016). Pregnancy and other conditions can also be associated with non-plaque-induced gingivitis. As in plaque-induced gingivitis a dental diagnosis is based on clinical findings, which may include: redness, edema, bleeding, and changes in gingival contour and consistency. Treatment considerations with a dental diagnosis may include surgical interventions.

The unmet human need of protection from health risks addresses the potential intervention of a medical referral to the patient's OB-GYN if necessary. In the case of pregnancy-associated gingivitis this may or may not be required, dependent on the patient's individual health concerns. It is addressed here as other conditions that relate to non-plaque-induced gingivitis may require a medical consult.

A dental hygiene diagnosis addressing the bleeding gingiva and the patient's questions regarding oral health and pregnancy will engage and involve her in dental hygiene care and the care of her developing fetus.

An unmet human need chosen was skin and mucous membrane integrity of the head and neck. This is a common unmet human for a dental hygiene diagnosis related to gingival and periodontal problems. An intact and functioning oral mucous membranes and periodontium defends against harmful microbes. Bleeding and inflammation relate to problems associated with gingival and periodontal conditions (Darby and Walsh 2015). Figure 2.2.1 shows the associated enlarged papilla between teeth s #29 and #30. This area serves as a pathway for bacteria to enter the blood stream and body. Refer to the patient's periodontal charting and bleeding points. The sulcular bleeding index is high and unrelated to the accumulation of plaque as in Case 1 in this chapter.

Conceptualization and problem solving was identified as evidenced by the patient's knowledge deficit shown by her asking questions. The definition conceptualization and problem solving is the need to grasp ideas and abstractions to make sound decisions about one's oral health (Darby and Walsh 2015). Teaching and education of the patient will address this unmet human need. Educational factors to consider are oral hygiene instructions, nutritional counseling, and education on fetal oral health. While the patient has a relatively low plaque control record and previously did not have bleeding issues, oral hygiene instructions are important to incorporate the importance of biofilm accumulation and the host response. Basic nutritional counseling to include both gingival health and fetal development may begin to address the patient's questions and educate her regarding oral health and nutrition.

Including a combination of therapies such as oral prophylaxis and patient education may contribute to the expected outcomes. The need for a medical referral may be necessary to improve the final outcome of care. All three unmet human needs maybe met with the same interventions. Patient education and understanding is key. Monitoring the status of the patient may include increased frequency for dental hygiene care and consideration of the gestational period.

Take-Home Hints

1. Relate the dental hygiene care to the dental hygiene diagnosis.
2. Interventions can include a variety of procedures, education, oral hygiene instructions, and will take into account medical conditions that may require a referral.

Self-Study Questions

1. A dental diagnosis for non-plaque-induced gingivitis is based on factors other than plaque. These may include all of the following except one. Which one is the exception?
- **A. Pregnancy**
- **B. Diabetes**
- **C. Probing depths**
- **D. Allergic reactions**

2. The need to grasp ideas to make sound decisions is related to which one of the dental hygiene diagnoses?
- **A. Responsibility for oral health**
- **B. Freedom from pain**
- **C. Biologically sound and functional dentition**
- **D. Conceptualization and problem solving**

3. The dental hygiene diagnosis addresses the condition (problem) of bleeding, which is related to which contributing factor?
- **A. Pregnancy**
- **B. Plaque**
- **C. Trauma – floss cut**
- **D. Prenatal vitamins**

References

American Academy of Periodontology. (2016). Parameter on Nonplaque-Induced Gingivitis [Online]. Available: http://www.joponline.org/doi/pdf/10.1902/jop.2000.71.5-S.851 (July 2, 2016).

Darby, M. and Walsh, M. (2015). *Dental Hygiene Theory and Practice*. St Louis: Evolve Elsevier.

Answers to Self-Study Questions

1. C

2. D

3. A

Case 3

Drug-Induced Gingivitis

CASE STORY

There are multiple cases in which drug-induced gingivitis may occur. According to the American Academy of Periodontology there are an increasing number of medications that can be associated with gingival enlargement (*Journal of Periodontology* 2004). Three primary drug classifications associated with gingival enlargement are anticonvulsants, calcium channel blockers, and immunosuppressants.

PROBLEM-BASED LEARNING GOALS AND OBJECTIVES

- Differentiate between a dental hygiene diagnosis and a dental diagnosis for gingival diseases.
- Identify signs/symptoms and causes of drug plaque-induced gingival disease.
- Identify health-promotion strategies or interventions for gingival diseases.
- Identify drugs that may cause gingival enlargement

Medical History

A medical history related to calcium channel blocker medication would be a patient with hypertension taking medication such as nifedipine commonly known as Procardia.

A medical history related to anticonvulsant medication would be a patient who suffers from seizures or diagnosed with epilepsy. The most common drug taken for this condition is phenytoin also known as Dilantin.

A medical history related to immunosuppressants would be a patient who has received an organ transplant. A commonly used medication to prevent organ rejection is cyclosporine. Brand names for cyclosporine are Gengraf, Meoral, and Sandimmune (Lexicomp 2016).

Immunosuppressant medications may be prescribed for autoimmune conditions such as rheumatoid arthritis, Crohn's disease, lupus, and immune thrombocytopenia (Lexicomp 2016). Immunosuppressant medications for these conditions include methotrexate or azathioprine.

Dental History

There are various dental histories depending upon the patient's history. These may include restorations, missing teeth, and or broken teeth, orthodontia, and lack of care due to the patient's medical condition. Medications that cause drug-induced gingivitis may also cause xerostomia. Xerostomia can precipitate dental conditions such as dental caries. A thorough review of the patient's dental history will be necessary for accurate caries and periodontal risk assessments.

Assessments

Periodontal Assessment

Gingival Statement: Gingival descriptors for drug-induced gingival enlargement will vary depending upon the oral condition and may include generalized gingival enlargement; localized papillary enlargement; fibrotic, firm, and stippled gingiva. If associated with plaque accumulation the gingival descriptors may include the above gingival enlargement with marginal or papillary redness, edema, and bleeding.

Pocket depths will vary according to the patient's conditions. Pockets associated with drug-induced gingival enlargement may be pseudo pockets if there is no clinical attachment loss. An indication of this would be that the junctional epithelium attachment is at the level of the cementoenamel junction, the probe tip is on the enamel and the gingival growth is covering the enamel and tooth crown. A periodontal pocket would indicate the probe tip is on the cementum or dentinal surface and is associated with clinical attachment loss and bone loss.

Radiographic Findings

Bone loss would be dependent upon the individual patient's condition and can range from none to severe.

Risk Assessments

Caries – dependent upon findings, history, modifiable, and non-modifiable factors
Periodontal – dependent upon findings, history, modifiable, and non-modifiable factors

Problem List

Gingival enlargement (see Figure 2.3.1)
Probing depths

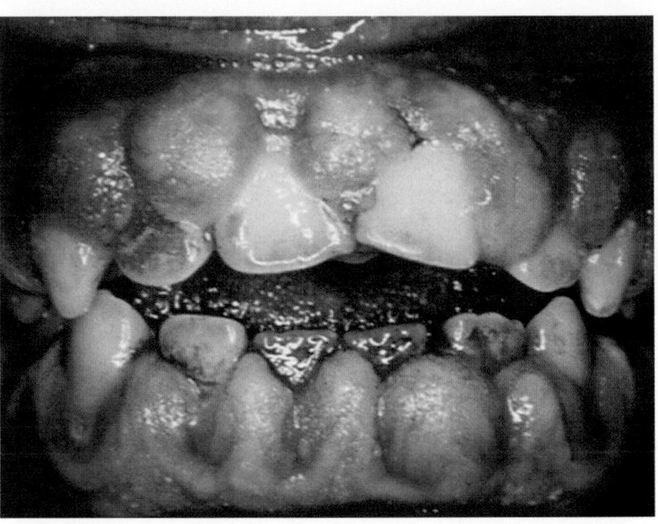

Figure 2.3.1: Phenytoin-induced gingival enlargement (Darby and Walsh 2015, p. 882).

Bleeding
Dental findings may include: missing or broken teeth, caries, crowding

Dental Hygiene Diagnosis

Unmet human need	Evidenced (caused) by	Signs/Symptoms
Freedom from health risks	Medications/health condition requiring medical consult	Need for prophylactic antibiotics Uncontrolled hypertension
Biologically sound and functioning dentition	Risk factors for dental disease	Teeth with signs of disease Broken teeth
Skin and mucous membrane integrity	Risk factors for periodontal disease Presence of plaque accumulation Medication	Probing depths Bleeding Enlarged gingiva

Planned Interventions

Interventions	Goals	Evaluation
Medical consult	The patient will return to primary health-care provider for evaluation of condition	Continuation of planned care Consultation on medications – dependent on outcomes
Education	Patient will understand the disease condition and relationship to medication	Patient will schedule appointment for follow up with medical personnel
Intraoral photos and risk assessments, caries prevention (xylitol, fluoride, amorphous calcium phosphate [ACP] interventions), Education on prevention for broken teeth	Schedule appointment with dentist for exam and treatment plan Schedule appointment with hygienist for care planned	Appointment scheduled
OHI toothbrushing instruction	Patient will demonstrate the proper brushing method	Immediate + next visit by reduction of PCR 6–8 weeks re-evaluation or 3–4-month recare visits
Prophylaxis or non-surgical periodontal therapy	Patient will schedule appointment for care planned Reduction of pocket depths, gingival enlargement	Appointments scheduled 6–8 weeks re-evaluation or 3–4-month recare visits

Appointment Schedule

The appointment sequence may vary depending upon the necessity for a medical consult. Inclusion of the medical and dental team for planning the patient's care may increase overall outcomes of the care provided.

Discussion

Assessments should start with a thorough review of the patient's medical history. Patients with a complex medical history may be taking multiple medications and as such drug interactions should be noted. Oral side effects and side effects related to dental treatment will assist the practitioner in developing an appropriate dental hygiene diagnosis and care plan based on the patient's need. It is good practice to review all medications patients are taking. An example of a medication summary form is Table 2.3.1. When looking at the side effect for medications one can see that all the medications listed cause gingival hyperplasia. See Table 2.3.1 to review the medications discussed in the case (Lexicomp 2016).

Assessments should include a medical and dental history, social, and cultural factors, activities of daily living, extraoral and intraoral examinations, gingival statement, periodontal assessment, plaque and bleeding indices, risk assessments, and radiographs. Through the interview process the clinician can assess risk for developing caries and periodontal diseases and structure planned interventions related to these risks.

Clinical findings for drug-induced gingivitis may include: interdental papilla gingival overgrowth predominantly on the facial surfaces, fibrotic lobulations, and dependent upon plaque accumulation, gingivitis. See Figure 2.3.1 for an example of the lobulations associated with phenytoin induced gingival enlargement.

For this particular patient group focusing on a primary unmet human need would be freedom from health risks. Darby and Walsh define this as the need to avoid medical contraindications to dental hygiene care (Darby and Walsh 2015). Protecting the patient's health is central to our code of ethics. Nonharming or do no harm is an obligation of every health-care provider. Keeping this as the primary dental hygiene diagnosis will ensure the patient's safety.

Protection from health risks for the patient taking antirejection medications may include a medical consult prior to any dental hygiene care. Organ transplant patients can be immunocompromised and require antibiotic prophylactic coverage prior to any care. They are most likely on multiple medications with various side effects and considerations prior to dental treatment will eliminate complications or medical emergencies. Consultation with medical providers will assist the dental hygienist with developing interventions related to the patient such as the oral effects of multiple medications and the effects that dental hygiene care may have on the patient that is immunocompromised.

For patients taking medication for hypertension, the dental hygienist will need to establish through the patient interview and taking the patients vital signs if the condition is controlled. Uncontrolled hypertension can lead to emergencies in the dental office. Other protection considerations during the dental hygiene appointment are sitting the patient up slowly and having them sit for a few minutes after care will help prevent orthostatic hypertension. Recommendations such as changing hypertensive medication or structuring more frequent dental hygiene care visits are possibilities when evaluating outcomes.

For patients taking Dilantin, knowing triggers for a seizure and the date of their last seizure to determine if they are controlled or not will help to protect the patient during their dental hygiene appointment and help prevent or prepare for any likely emergencies that may occur.

A thorough review of the patient's history and any medical consultations can decrease the incidence of these emergencies. Focusing on patient-centered care and protecting the patient from health risks related to dental hygiene care is essential. Communication with the patient is important. Keeping them informed regarding why and how this affects their health will have a positive impact on the patient and their treatment.

The next dental hygiene diagnosis chosen was biologically sound and functioning dentition. Darby and Walsh describe this as the need to have intact teeth and restorations. Dentition that functions properly aids in chewing and digestion. Preventing the progression of dental disease can result in the prevention of pain and another dental hygiene diagnosis. Broken teeth as a result of a seizure can also be considered in this dental hygiene diagnosis. Another diagnosis for broken teeth would be change in the facial image if they were located in the anterior region and prevented the patient from smiling or feeling confident.

Planned interventions for biologically sound and functioning dentition would involve the patient

Table 2.3.1: A medication summary form for reviewing patients medications and summarizing drugs reactions, side effects, and dental considerations to be used in formulating a dental hygiene care plan.

Date	Medication and Dosage	Prescribed for	Side Effects/Adverse Reactions	Drug Effects of Concern to Dentistry	Dental Considerations
02/16/15	Sandimmune (cyclosporine) 1–3 mg day^{-1}	Antirejection organ transplant	Hypertension, headaches, susceptible to infection, gingival hyperplasia	Mouth sores, swallowing difficulty, gingivitis, gingival hyperplasia, xerostomia, abnormal taste, tongue disorder, and gingival bleeding	Caries, bleeding with procedures, no special precautions with local anesthetic/vasoconstrictors, gingival overgrowth
2/16/15	Procadia (nifedipine) 30 or 60 mg day^{-1}	High blood pressure	Flushing, dizziness/ lightheaded	Gingival hyperplasia	Orthostatic hypertension – sit up slowly, no special precautions with local anesthetic/vasoconstrictors, gingival overgrowth
2/16/15	Dilantin (phenytoin	Epilepsy	Cardiac arrhythmias, cerebral dysfunction, dermatitis	Gingival hyperplasia	No special precautions with local anesthetic/vasoconstrictors, no information available on bleeding that require special precautions

Source: Lexicomp (2016).

scheduling with the dentist. The level of destruction or pain involved would determine the sequence for appointment scheduling. At this point the dental hygienist would provide appropriate patient education and interventions for prevention such as fluoride and home-care procedures. Evaluation includes following up to reinforce the need for dental care.

The last dental hygiene diagnosis of skin and mucous membrane integrity of the head and neck may or may not be evidenced by plaque accumulation. The determination of plaque accumulation as related to gingivitis and gingival enlargement will determine the interventions needed. Gingival enlargement may be ameliorated by removal of local factors, frequent maintenance, and meticulous self-care but these interventions will not completely eliminate the condition. Establishing realistic goals and evaluation timelines is important.

Interventions will be dependent upon the problem list, signs and symptoms, and causes. Aligning the diagnosis with interventions and outcomes or goals will ensure comprehensive care for the patient and can include: detailed oral hygiene instructions, patient education on the relationship of medication and gingival enlargement, and specific rationale for planned treatment. Interventions may range from a prophylaxis to nonsurgical periodontal therapy. Many of the gingival conditions may not be reduced after dental hygiene care or oral hygiene interventions and incorporating referrals in the care plan should be considered. A referral to a periodontist for evaluation of gingival and periodontal conditions beyond the scope of a dental hygienist may be required. Referrals to the primary care provider and discussions of conditions as they relate to the patient may help improve outcomes.

Beginning with the dental hygiene diagnosis of freedom from health risks will eliminate any risks related to care and reduce the incidence of medical emergencies. Having the ability to proceed safely will allow the health-care provider to focus on subsequent dental hygiene diagnoses and planned care.

Take-Home Hints

- Remember dental professionals are health-care providers, keep the patient's other health-care providers informed of your findings.
- An intra- and interdisciplinary approach is in the best interest of the patient.
- Interventions can include a variety of procedures, education, and oral hygiene instructions dependent on the problem list, signs and symptoms, and evidence.

Self-Study Questions

1. The three primary medications related to drug-induced gingival enlargement include all of the following except one. Which is the exception?
- **A. Sandimmune**
- **B. Metformin**
- **C. Procardia**
- **D. Methetraxate**

2. Protection from health risks is defined in the dental hygienists code of ethics; the dental hygiene code of ethics includes nonmaleficence and means doing no harm.
- **A. Both statements are true**
- **B. Both statements are false**
- **C. The first statement is true; and the second statement is false**
- **D. The first statement is false; and the second statement is true**

3. Assessments include medical history; part of the medical history should include a pharmacologic summary.
- **A. True**
- **B. False**

4. Signs and symptoms for freedom from health risks may include:
- **A. Bleeding**
- **B. Probing depths**
- **C. Uncontrolled hypertension**
- **D. Missing teeth and defective restorations**

References

Darby, M. and Walsh, M. (2015). *Dental Hygiene Theory and Practice*. St Louis: Evolve Elsevier.

Journal of Periodontology (2004). *Informational paper: drug-associated gingival enlargement. Journal of Periodontology* 75 (10): 119–122 [Online]. Accessed at: http://www.joponline.org/doi/pdf/10.1902/jop.2004.75.10.1424. (May 28, 2018).

Lexicomp (2016). [online] Accessed at: http://www.online.lexi.com/lco/action/doc/retrieve/docid/dental_f/2074477 (subscribers only).

Answers to Self-Study Questions

1. B
2. D
3. A
4. C

Case 4

Chronic Periodontitis

CASE STORY

A 48-year-old Caucasian male presents for treatment. His chief complaint is "My teeth are rotted out at the bottom." He has experienced bleeding and sore gums. He has not been to the dentist for eight years. He is currently between jobs.

PROBLEM-BASED LEARNING GOALS AND OBJECTIVES

- Differentiate between a dental hygiene diagnosis and a dental diagnosis for periodontal diseases
- Identify signs/symptoms and causes of chronic periodontal disease
- Identify health-promotion strategies or interventions for periodontal diseases

Medical History

The patient's medical history states he is in good health. He currently does not take any medications and is not under the care of a physician. The patient does not smoke and his vital signs were within normal limits.

Dental History

Patient has not had a dental exam or prophylaxis in eight years. He has amalgam and composite restorations, carious lesions, and is missing teeth #3, #14, #18, and #19. The patient brushes using fluoridated toothpaste twice a day and flosses twice a day.

Social History

Patient is between jobs. He is divorced. He does not smoke or drink. He likes to ride bikes and watch sports.

Assessments

Extraoral/intraoral examination – bilateral linea alba, white-coated tongue, fistula present on the facial attached gingiva around tooth #25.

Periodontal Assessment

Gingival Statement: Generalized moderate marginal and papillary redness with rolled margins and edematous papilla, localized severe redness facial of lower anterior #22–#26

Calculus classification: moderate to heavy supragingival and subgingival deposits (see Figure 2.4.2)

Generalized 4–9 mm pocket depths, recession present, furcation on #30 or mobility (see Figure 2.4.3 for periodontal charting).

SBI 36%

PCR 44%

Dental Charting Assessment

Occlusion: Class II left / Class I on the right

Amalgam and composite restorations

Carious lesions: #14, #15

Generalized

Missing teeth: #3, #14, #18, and #19

All third molars are present

Radiographic Findings

Horizontal bone loss – 30%

Risk Assessments

Caries: high risk

Periodontal: high risk
Cancer: low risk

Problem List

Gingival inflammation and bleeding
Probing depths of 4–9 mm
Plaque accumulation
Bone loss
Missing teeth
Furcation
Abfractions
Carious lesions

Dental Hygiene Diagnosis

Unmet Human Need	Evidenced (caused) by	Signs/Symptoms
Freedom from head and neck pain	Untreated dental condition (abfractions and recession) / plaque accumulation / calculus	Sensitivity to cold / sore gums / bleeding
Integrity of the skin and mucous membrane	Microbial infection and host response	Bleeding/plaque accumulation
Responsibility for oral health	Inadequate dental care	Last dental visit 8 years

Planned Interventions

Interventions	Goals	Evaluation
Fluoride/desensitization	Patient will return for desensitization treatment Patient will see dentist for evaluation of caries and abfractions	Patient scheduled an appointment
OHI tooth brushing instruction	Patient will demonstrate the proper brushing method Patient will reduce PCR score by 10%	Immediate + next visit by reduction of PCR
Oral Hygiene Education	Patient will understand the disease process	Patient will schedule appointments for care
Removal of calculus deposits and biofilm accumulation	Patient will understand the disease process and the importance of dental visits	Patient will schedule appointment for treatment and follow up with a periodontist
Biofilm reduction with ultrasonic	Patient will leave office plaque free	End of appointment

Appointment Schedule

First appointment
Assessments
OHI
Full mouth debridement (D4355) / oral prophylaxis
Desensitization as needed
Second appointment
OHI
Nonsurgical periodontal therapy (D4341) URQ
Local anesthetic or pain control
Chemotherapeutic as needed
Desensitization as needed
Third appointment
OHI
Nonsurgical periodontal therapy (D4341) LRQ
Local anesthetic or pain control
Chemotherapeutic as needed
Desensitization as needed
Fourth appointment
OHI
Nonsurgical periodontal therapy (D4341) ULQ
Local anesthetic or pain control
Chemotherapeutic as needed
Desensitization as needed
Fifth appointment
OHI
Nonsurgical periodontal therapy (D4341) LLQ
Local anesthetic or pain control
Chemotherapeutic as needed
Desensitization as needed
Sixth appointment
OHI
Four to six week re-evaluation – referral to periodontist
Chemotherapeutic as needed
Desensitization as needed

Discussion

A dental diagnosis of chronic periodontitis is defined as inflammation of the gingiva extending into the adjacent attachment apparatus. Clinical features include edema, redness, bleeding, and suppuration (*American Academy of Periodontology* 2000). Chronic periodontitis is further divided into slight to moderate loss of support and advanced loss of support. Treatment considerations for both include much of the same interventions as for the dental hygiene diagnosis. It is important in both diagnosis to include contributing factors, systemic conditions, and the host's response.

Choosing freedom from head and neck pain addresses the patient's chief complaint regarding sore gums. Evidence to support this would be plaque accumulation and calculus deposits. Addressing any pain is key to gaining the trust and cooperation of the patient. Interventions to address this would be the nonsurgical periodontal therapy for the plaque and calculus accumulation. Desensitization to address any tooth sensitivity due to the abfractions and recession could be included in the implementation of care. Figure 2.4.1 shows generalized recession and severity of the abfractions. Setting a patient goal of seeing the dentist to address these areas and his concerns is a priority. The patient stated in his chief complaint of "My teeth are rotted out at the bottom." According to Maslow's hierarchy of needs one does not move into upper tiers of human needs until the needs at each lower level are met (Jackson et al. 2014). Freedom from pain is on the physiological first-tier level and must be met first.

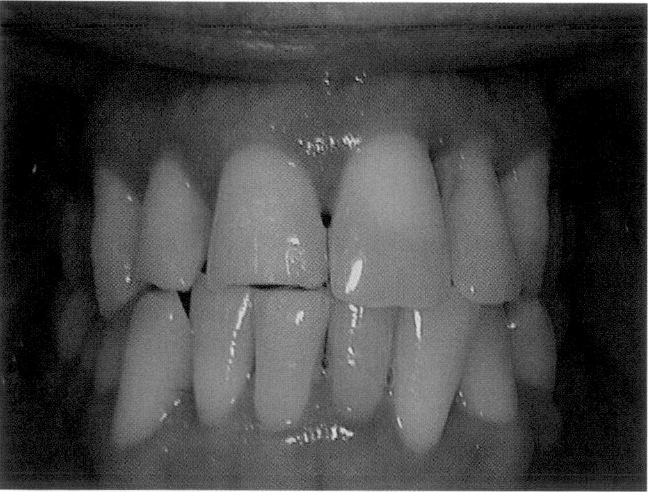

Figure 2.4.1: Generalized recession and abfractions causing tooth sensitivity. *Source:* Photo courtesy of Rio Salado College.

Secondly using the dental hygiene diagnosis of human need for integrity of the skin and mucous the dental hygienist will be able to provide services they are licensed to treat. Interventions include nonsurgical periodontal therapy, chemotherapeutics, pain control as needed, desensitization as needed, and most importantly oral hygiene education. Addressing the need for therapeutic services such as scaling and debridement will eliminate contributing factors such as calculus and biofilm. Figure 2.4.2 shows calculus accumulation on the lingual of the mandibular anterior teeth. Removal of the calculus can establish a clean environment for healing. Figure 2.4.3 shows the patients periodontal charting with probing depths, bleeding points, and attachment loss all contributing to integrity of the mucosal membrane.

The disease process for chronic periodontitis includes the host's response. The host response may

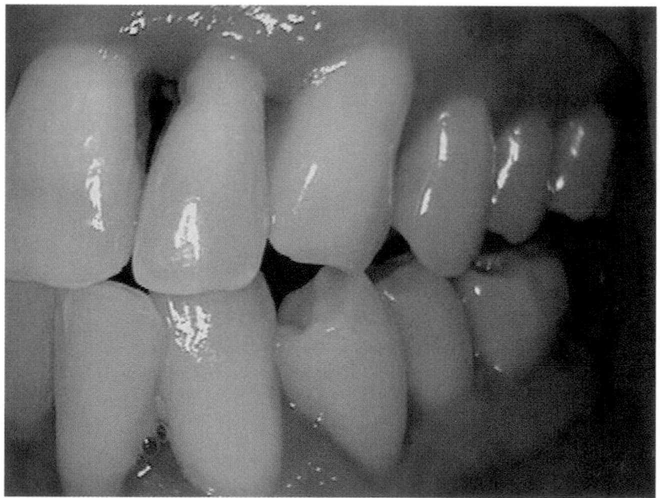

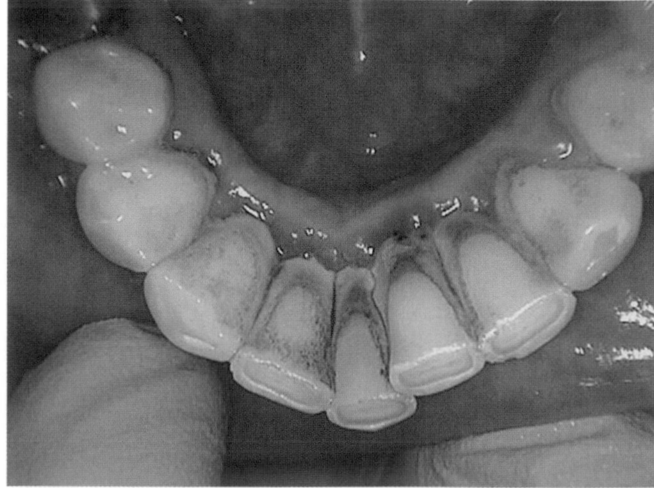

Figure 2.4.2: Calculus accumulation on the mandibular anterior teeth. *Source:* Photo courtesy of Rio Salado College.

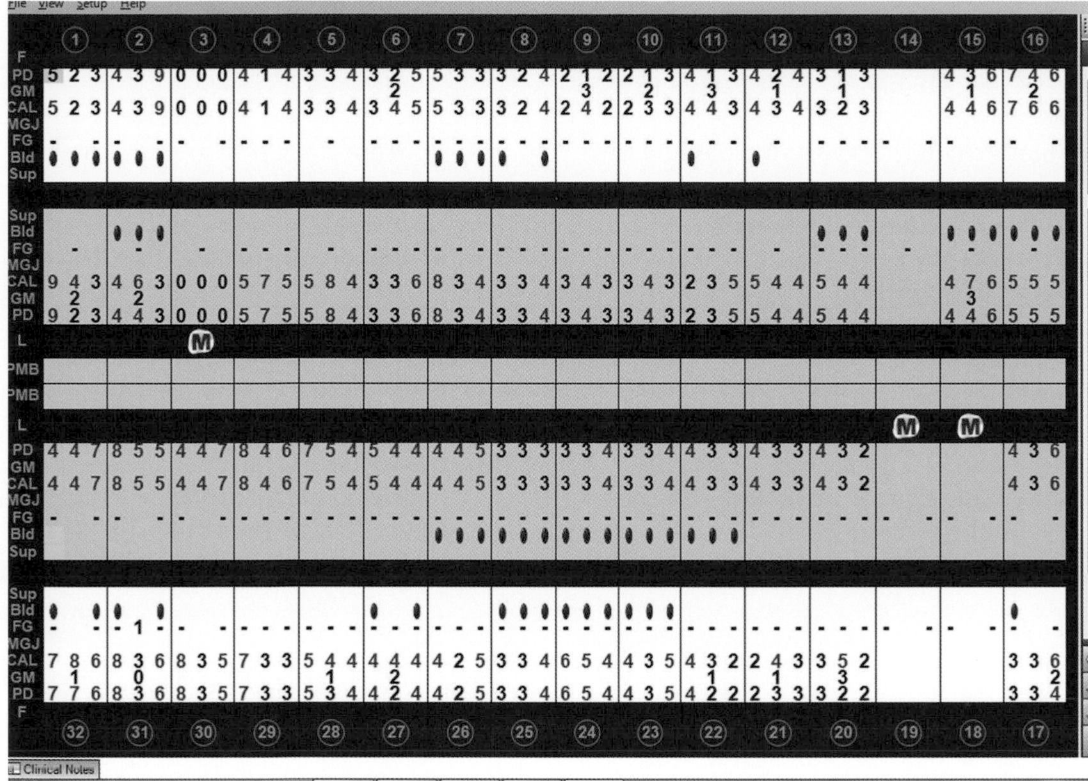

Figure 2.4.3: Periodontal charting note probing depths and bleeding points on the posterior teeth associated with deeper pockets.

trigger the patient's own immune system to destroy tissue and resorb bone (Nield-Gehrig and Willmann 2016). Addressing all the factors to establish health, including calculus removal, biofilm disruption, and chemotherapeutics to assist the host's immune response, increase outcomes for care.

Lastly, including responsibility for oral health establishes the patient's accountability for their health. It takes the burden off the health-care professional. Is the patient motivated to improve their health? Are they interested in keeping their teeth? Are they physically and financial capable? Incorporating these questions and establishing interventions to address this human need will assist the dental hygienist to transfer ownership of the patient's health from the clinician to the patient. Education and setting goals can assist with patient's acceptance and follow through with treatment.

Including a combination of therapies such as debridement, chemotherapeutic agents, and patient education, dental referrals will improve expected outcomes. Assisting the patient with goals and education can improve the patient's health for years to come and hopefully save teeth in the future. Providing the traditional scaling and root planing and scolding the patient for noncompliance with brushing will not support the patient, coming in for care, to improve his health.

Take-Home Hints

- Considerations of Maslow's hierarchy when addressing the problem list.
- Keep the patient involved in the development of goals.
- Relate the dental hygiene care to the dental hygiene diagnosis.
- Interventions can include a variety of procedures, education, and oral hygiene instructions.
  Include dental referrals from the problem list.

Self-Study Questions

1. In Maslow's hierarchy it is important to address the patient's lower level of need, this patient's lower need is freedom from head and neck pain.

A. Both statements are true.
B. Both statements are false.
C. The first statement is true and the second statement is false.
D. The first statement is false and the second statement is true.

2. Which dental hygiene diagnosis places accountability for health on the patient?

A. Conceptualization and problem solving
B. Integrity of the skin and mucous membrane of the head and neck
C. Responsibility for oral health
D. Freedom from head and neck pain

3. Clinical signs of chronic periodontitis include all of the following EXCEPT one; which one is the exception?

A. Edema
B. Halitosis
C. Loss of bone support
D. Loss of attachment

References

American Academy of Periodontology (2000). Parameter on Plaque-Induced Gingivitis [Online], Available: http://www.joponline.org/doi/pdf/10.1902/jop.2000.71.5-S.851 (June 3, 2018).

Darby, M. and Walsh, M. (2015). *Dental Hygiene Theory and Practice*. St Louis: Evolve Elsevier.

Jackson, J.C., Santoro, M.A., Ely, T.M. et al. (2014). Improving patient care through the prism of psychology: application of Maslow's hierarchy to sedation, delirium, and early mobility in the intensive care unit. *Journal of Critical Care* 29: 438–444.

Nield-Gehrig, J.S. and Willmann, D.E. (2016). *Foundations of Periodontics for the Dental Hygienist*, 4e. Philadelphia: Wolters Kluwar.

Answers to Self-Study Questions

1. A

2. C

3. B

Case 5

Aggressive Periodontics

CASE STORY

A 53-year-old Caucasian female presents for treatment. Her chief complaint is "sensitive teeth." She has experienced bleeding and sore gums. She has not been to the dentist in the last two years. She is currently a homemaker, works part time and has three adult children.

LEARNING GOALS AND OBJECTIVES

- Differentiate between a dental hygiene diagnosis and a dental diagnosis for periodontal diseases
- Identify signs/symptoms and causes of aggressive periodontal disease
- Identify health promotion strategies or interventions for periodontal diseases

Medical History

The patient's medical history states she is in good health. She reported a hospital visit for a broken rib in 2014. She currently takes multivitamins and is not under the care of a physician. The patient does not smoke and her vital signs were within normal limits.

Dental History

The patient has not had a dental visit in the past two years. She has single surface amalgam restorations and a broken tooth #3. Missing teeth are #1, #7, #10, #16, #17, and #32. The patient brushes using toothpaste for sensitive teeth or multiple benefit toothpaste twice a day and flosses once a day. She is concerned about yellowing, crowding, and spacing.

Social History

She has been a full-time mother and housekeeper. She has recently entered the work force part time as an aide at an elementary school. She is very active in her local church and volunteers.

Assessments

Extraoral/intraoral examination – large, firm thyroid gland, popping and clicking on the left TMJ, lower labial mucosa magenta and reddened, tonsils have been removed, reddened area bilateral anterior tonsillar pillars.

Periodontal Assessment

- Gingival Statement: Generalized moderate marginal and papillary redness with rolled margins and edematous papilla; localized area lingual teeth #12–#14 deeper blue color with frayed margins (see Figure 2.5.1)

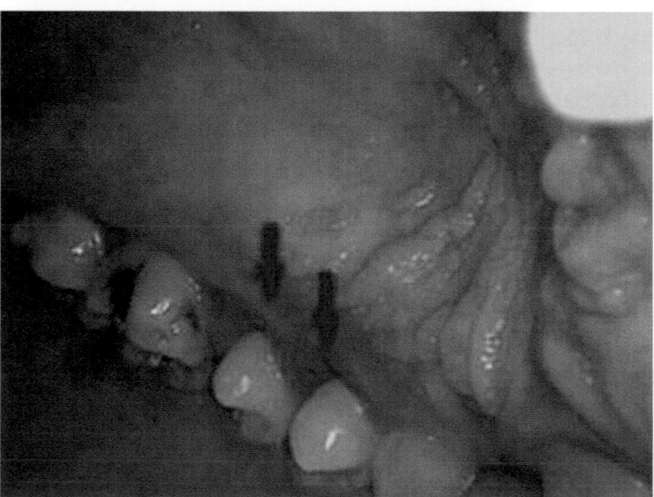

Figure 2.5.1: During the visual examination of the gingiva the dental hygienist would interpret the gingival changes and further conduct a thorough periodontal examination. *Source:* Photo courtesy of Rio Salado College.

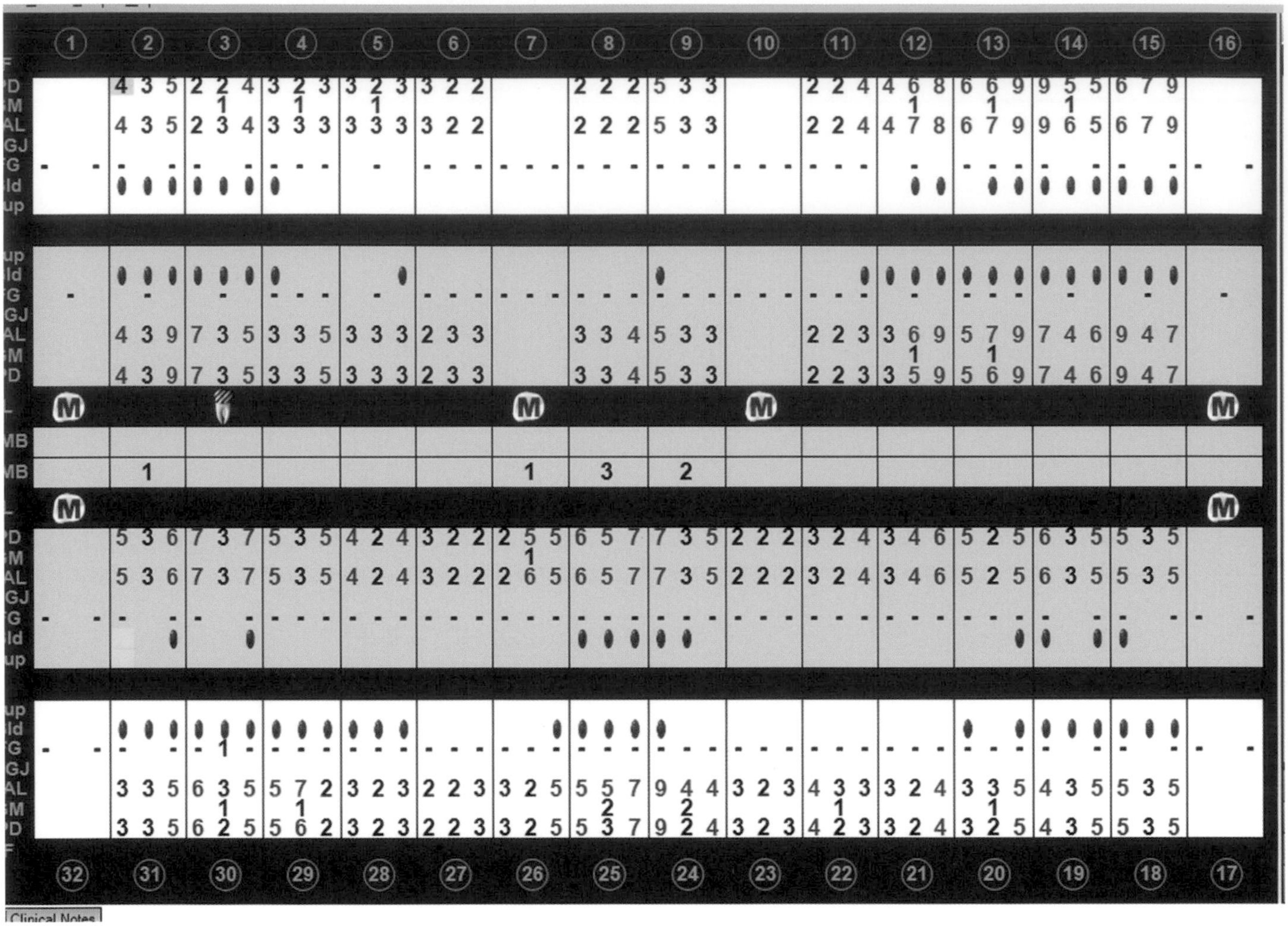

	1	2	3	4	5	6	7	8	9	10	11	12	13	14	15	16
PD		4 3 5	2 2 4	3 2 3	3 2 3	3 2 2		2 2 2	5 3 3		2 2 4	4 6 8	6 6 9	9 5 5	6 7 9	
GM			1	1	1							1	1	1		
AL		4 3 5	2 3 4	3 3 3	3 3 3	3 2 2		2 2 2	5 3 3		2 2 4	4 7 8	6 7 9	9 6 5	6 7 9	
AL		4 3 9	7 3 5	3 3 5	3 3 3	2 3 3		3 3 4	5 3 3		2 2 3	3 6 9	5 7 9	7 4 6	9 4 7	
GM												1	1			
PD		4 3 9	7 3 5	3 3 5	3 3 3	2 3 3		3 3 4	5 3 3		2 2 3	3 5 9	5 6 9	7 4 6	9 4 7	
MB		1					1	3	2							

	32	31	30	29	28	27	26	25	24	23	22	21	20	19	18	17
PD		5 3 6	7 3 7	5 3 5	4 2 4	3 2 2	2 5 5	6 5 7	7 3 5	2 2 2	3 2 4	3 4 6	5 2 5	6 3 5	5 3 5	
GM							1									
AL		5 3 6	7 3 7	5 3 5	4 2 4	3 2 2	2 6 5	6 5 7	7 3 5	2 2 2	3 2 4	3 4 6	5 2 5	6 3 5	5 3 5	
FG			1													
AL		3 3 5	6 3 5	5 7 2	3 2 3	2 2 3	3 2 5	5 5 7	9 4 4	3 2 3	4 3 3	3 2 4	3 3 5	4 3 5	5 3 5	
GM			1	1				2	2		1		1			
PD		3 3 5	6 2 5	5 6 2	3 2 3	2 2 3	3 2 5	5 3 7	9 2 4	3 2 3	4 2 3	3 2 4	3 2 5	4 3 5	5 3 5	

Clinical Notes

Figure 2.5.2: Periodontal charting for patient with aggressive periodontitis. Note the deep pockets and multiple bleeding sites.

- Generalized 4–9 mm pocket depths, recession present, furcation on #30 and mobility (see Figure 2.5.2)
- SBI 44%
- PCR 14%
- Calculus classification: moderate to heavy supragingival and subgingival deposits

Dental Charting Assessment

- Occlusion: Class I right and left
- Amalgam restorations
- Broken tooth: #3
- Missing teeth: #1, #7, #10, #16, #17, #32

Radiographic Findings

Severe bone loss both vertical and horizontal (see Figure 2.5.3)

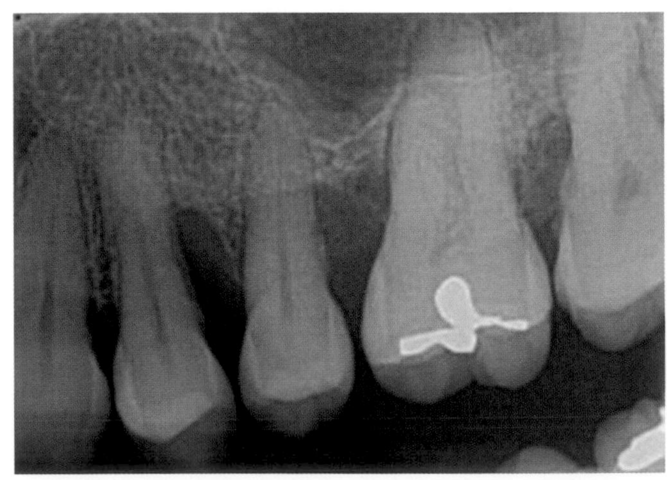

Figure 2.5.3: Periapical image of the maxillary left premolars. Note both vertical and horizontal bone loss.

Risk Assessments

Caries: low risk
Periodontal: high risk
Cancer: low risk

Problem List

Gingival inflammation and bleeding
Probing depths of 4–12 mm
Severe bone loss both vertical and horizontal (see Figure 2.5.3)
Missing teeth
Broken tooth #3
Mobility
Furcation

Dental Hygiene Diagnosis

Unmet human need	Evidenced (caused) by	Signs/Symptoms
Conceptualization and problem solving	Lack of exposure to information	Patient has lack of knowledge about advanced periodontal diseases
Integrity of the skin and mucous membrane	Microbial infection and host response	Bleeding/severe bone loss
Biologically sound and functional dentition	Inadequate dental care	Missing teeth and broken tooth

Planned Interventions

Interventions	Goals	Evaluation
Oral Health Education	Patient will understand the disease process	Patient will schedule appointments for care and follow up with periodontist
Removal of calculus deposits and biofilm accumulation	Patient will understand the disease process and the importance of dental visits	Patient will be as plaque and calculus free as possible
Periodontal referral	Patient will make an appointment with the periodontist for evaluation and consultation	Patient will schedule appointment for treatment and follow up with a periodontist
Dental treatment	Patient will make an appointment with the dentist for consultation on missing teeth (permanent replacements) and broken tooth	After dental hygiene care and periodontal referral

Appointment Schedule

First appointment
Assessments
OHI
Full mouth debridement (D4355) / oral prophylaxis
Chemotherapeutic
Second appointment
OHI
Nonsurgical periodontal therapy (D4341) URQ
Local anesthetic or pain control
Chemotherapeutic as needed
Third appointment
OHI
Nonsurgical periodontal therapy (D4341) LRQ
Local anesthetic or pain control
Chemotherapeutic as needed
Fourth appointment
OHI
Nonsurgical periodontal therapy (D4341) ULQ
Local anesthetic or pain control
Chemotherapeutic as needed
Fifth appointment
OHI
Nonsurgical periodontal therapy (D4341) LLQ
Local anesthetic or pain control
Chemotherapeutic as needed
Sixth appointment
OHI
Four to six week re-evaluation – referral to periodontist
Chemotherapeutic as needed

Discussion

According to the American Academy of Periodontology (2000), aggressive periodontitis encompasses distinct types of periodontitis that affect people who, in most cases, otherwise appear healthy. This patient has no systemic considerations for the advanced state of bone loss in areas. Aggressive periodontitis tends to have a rapid rate of disease progression and can occur in generalized or localized forms. It typically is seen in patients aged under 30, but can occur in older adults. Clinical features may include the same as chronic periodontitis such as edema, redness, bleeding, and suppuration (American Academy of Periodontology 2000).

It is important for the patient to understand the aggressive form of this type of periodontal disease. Conceptualization and problem solving as a dental hygiene diagnosis will allow the dental hygienist to prioritize the patient's education. Educating the patient on the progression and prognosis of the disease can initiate them to act. Discussing the bacteria associated with the disease and the host immune response may increase the patient's willingness to help control the disease. The long-term outcome may depend on the patient's compliance and the host response (American Academy of Periodontology 2000).

To determine a dental hygiene diagnosis, the clinician must be able to critically analyze and interpret the assessment data. For example, during the assessment phase noted on the extra- and intraoral examination were popping and clicking TMJ and enlarged thyroid. The dental hygienist needs to interpret this data to determine if a problem exists that a dental hygienist is licensed to treat, formulate a dental hygiene diagnosis, and determine interventions for care. A thorough review of all the assessment data such as the gingiva, periodontal charting, and radiographs will help the dental hygienist to determine a dental hygiene diagnosis and direct patient care. During the patient's gingival assessment (Figure 2.5.1) the arrows point to friable gingival margins and a diffuse magenta color during the observation, the dental hygienist would need to further assess the periodontal findings. The periodontal charting (Figure 2.5.2) indicates deep periodontal pocketing and further review of the radiograph on the upper left (Figure 2.5.3) shows both vertical and horizontal bone loss with calculus deposits on the root surfaces. Putting all the assessment data together (Figure 2.5.4) the dental hygienist is able to synthesize and interpret the information to produce a diagnosis.

Using the dental hygiene diagnosis of human need for integrity of the skin and mucous with the sign and symptom of pocket depths and bone loss as shown in Figure 2.5.2 and Figure 2.5.3 the dental hygienist will be able to provide services they are licensed to treat. Basic initial interventions include nonsurgical periodontal therapy, chemotherapeutics, pain control as needed, desensitization as needed, and most importantly oral hygiene education. In addition to these, more forms of chemotherapeutics such as antibiotic therapy, genetic testing, and microbiological identification may be needed. Initial therapy may prove to be ineffective with aggressive periodontitis (*American Academy of Periodontology*, 2000). Establishing an oral environment as free from periodontal pathogens as possible to provide an environment for healing is a first step. With aggressive forms of periodontitis, referral to a periodontitis should always be a planned intervention.

Including biologically sound and functioning dentition will address the patient's broken and missing teeth and potential tooth loss due to the aggressive nature of the

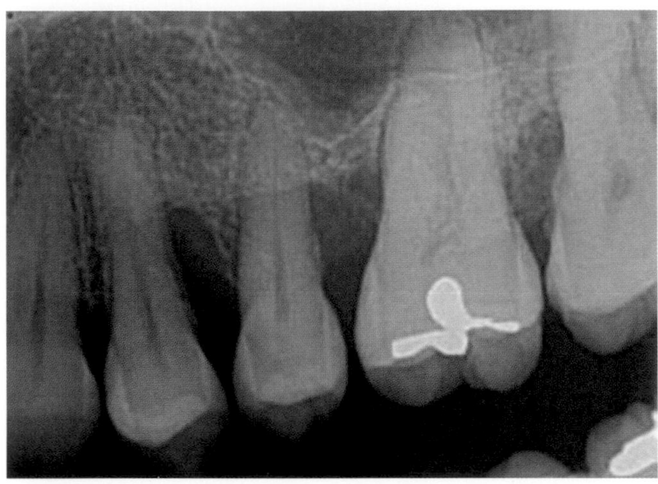

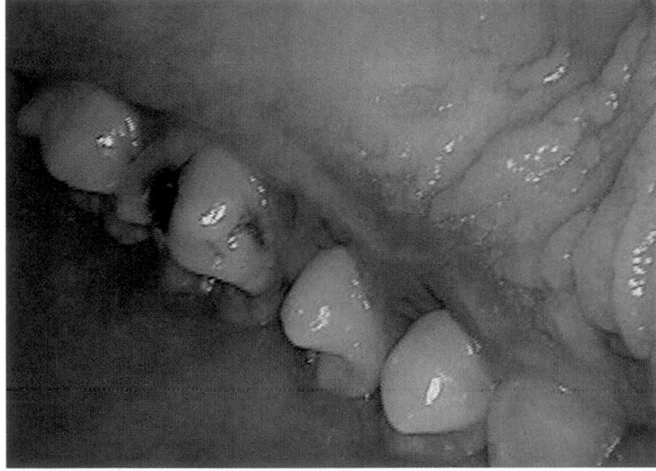

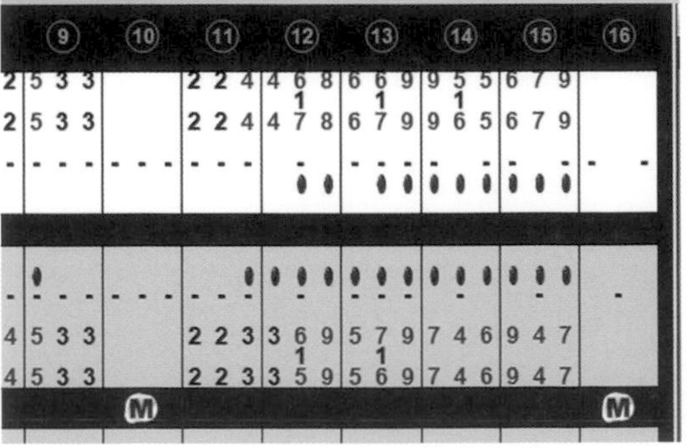

Figure 2.5.4: Amalgamated assessment data allow the dental hygienist to analyze and interpret the information to provide a diagnosis.

disease. Dental and periodontal referrals need to be included in the care plan and overall treatment plan for the patient with aggressive periodontitis. The human need for functioning dentition is a part of creating a healthy oral environment.

Take-Home Hints

1. Consideration of advanced disease state.
2. Education of the patient.
3. Relate the dental hygiene care to the dental hygiene diagnosis.
4. Include dental referrals from the problem list.

Self-Study Questions

1. A rapid rate of destruction characterizes aggressive periodontitis, and occurs mainly in adults under 30.
- **A. Both statements are true**
- **B. Both statements are false**
- **C. The first statement is true and the second statement is false**
- **D. The first statement is false and the second statement is true**

2. Which dental hygiene diagnosis addresses the broken tooth?
- **A. Conceptualization and problem solving**
- **B. Integrity of the skin and mucous membrane of the head and neck**
- **C. Responsibility for oral health**
- **D. Biologically sound and functioning dentition**

3. An etiology for conceptualization and problem solving would be:
- **A. Lack of adequate dental care**
- **B. Lack of adequate self-care**
- **C. Lack of exposure to information**
- **D. Lack of biofilm removal**

References

American Academy of Periodontology (2000). Parameter on Aggressive Periodontitis [Online], Available at: http://www.joponline.org/doi/pdf/10.1902/jop.2000.71.5-S.851 (July 2, 2016).

Darby, M. and Walsh, M. (2015). *Dental Hygiene Theory and Practice*. St Louis: Evolve Elsevier.

Nield-Gehrig, J.S. and Willmann, D.E. (2016). *Foundations of Periodontics for the Dental Hygienist*, 4e. Philadelphia: Wolters Kluwar.

Answers to Self-Study Questions

1. A

2. D

3. C

Case 6

Local Contributing Factors

CASE STORY

As with drug-induced gingivitis, there are many cases in which local contributing factors play a role in the development of gingival and periodontal diseases. They may be found in most patients that a dental professional would see on a daily basis. Depending upon the patient's risk assessment and immune response local contributing factors may or may not play a role in the development of the gingival or periodontal disease. Patients may present with restorations that have poor, open, or over hanging margins. The patient may also have crowns, crown and bridge, or removable partials among other dental restorations. Calculus build-up is also a contributing factor and should be considered. There are many other local factors that play a role in developing or contributing to an already existing gingival or periodontal condition.

PROBLEM-BASED LEARNING GOALS AND OBJECTIVES

- Identify local contributing factors.
- Identify how local contributing factors increase the risk for developing a periodontal disease.
- Identify health-promotion strategies or interventions for local contributing factors in periodontal diseases.

Medical History

The patient's medical history can vary and range from the adolescent to the geriatric populations.

Dental History

The patient's dental history may include a lack of dental care or below-standard care resulting in a large formation of calculus deposits or poor broken-down restorations.

Social History

The patient's social history would be dependent upon the age and values of the individual.

Assessments

Extraoral/intraoral examination

Dependent upon the individual.

Periodontal Assessment

Gingival Statement: Consideration for a generalized gingival statement as well as significant attention to localized gingival inflammation. Gingival inflammation can range from mild to severe. It can involve all areas of the gingiva including marginal, attached, and mucogingiva.
Pocket depths: Vary
SBI: Vary but would be high around local contributing factor
PCR: Vary but most likely would be high around local contributing factor
Calculus classification: Vary but most likely would be heavy if calculus is a local contributing factor

Dental Charting Assessment

Occlusion: Dependent upon individual but may include: crowding; open contacts; and lingual, buccal, and torsoversions
Restorations: Vary but consideration for Class II and Class V restorations, crowns and bridges, partials
Broken teeth: Dependent upon individual
Missing teeth: Dependent upon individual

Radiographic Findings

Bone loss will vary: Slight to severe

Risk Assessments

Vary depending upon the patient's modifiable and nonmodifiable factors

Problem List

Gingival inflammation and bleeding
Probing depths
Bone loss
Missing or broken teeth
Malocclusion that may include: lingual, buccal, and torsoversions; and crowding

Dental Hygiene Diagnosis

Unmet Human Need	Evidenced (caused) by	Signs/Symptoms
Integrity of the skin and mucous membrane	Plaque and calculus accumulation	Bleeding, inflamed gingiva
Biologically sound and functional dentition	Inadequate dental care Malocclusion-crowding, malpositioned teeth	Ill contoured restorations Bleeding, inflamed gingiva, bone loss, mucogingival involvement

Planned Interventions

Interventions	Goals	Evaluation
Oral Health Education	Patient will understand the disease process and contributing factors associated with the periodontal condition	Patient will schedule appointments for care and follow up with periodontist
Removal of calculus deposits and biofilm accumulation	Patient will understand the disease process and the importance of dental visits	Patient will schedule appointment for treatment and follow up with a periodontist
Dental treatment	Patient will make an appointment with the dentist for consultation on missing teeth (permanent replacements) and broken tooth Patient will make an appointment with a periodontist Patient will make an appointment with an orthodontist	After dental hygiene care and periodontal referral

Discussion

The appointment schedule would be dependent upon the level of periodontal involvement and the local contributing factor(s). It could range from a simple prophylaxis to nonsurgical periodontal therapy. Referrals for dental, periodontal, and orthodontia care must also be considered to remove the local contributing factors.

Local contributing factors play a role by increasing the risk for developing a periodontal condition or increase the severity of an existing condition in a variety of ways. One way is they contribute to an increase in plaque/biofilm retention. An example of this would be an over hanging margin on a Class II restoration or a Class IV composite restoration at or below the gingival margin. Another way they contribute is to cause direct damage to the periodontium. An example of this would be a partial denture impinging on the periodontium or trauma from misuse of oral health aids (Nield-Gehrig and Willmann 2016).

Biologically sound and functioning dentition as an unmet human need may be caused by restorations that are poorly contoured, have open margins, or overhanging margins. Following are more detailed examples of local contributing factors:

- Figure 2.6.1 shows plaque accumulation around a crown margin. Note the inflammation around the gingival margin. The crown could be bulky or have an open margin. After dental hygiene therapy a re-evaluation appointment to determine the need for further care is recommended.
- Figure 2.6.2 shows calculus accumulation on the root surface of anterior crowns. Note the crowns are fused leading to difficulty in completing oral hygiene self-care. The distal margin of the lateral incisor may have an open and overhanging margin. These restorations contain many of the contributing factors for plaque retention and difficulty in cleaning.

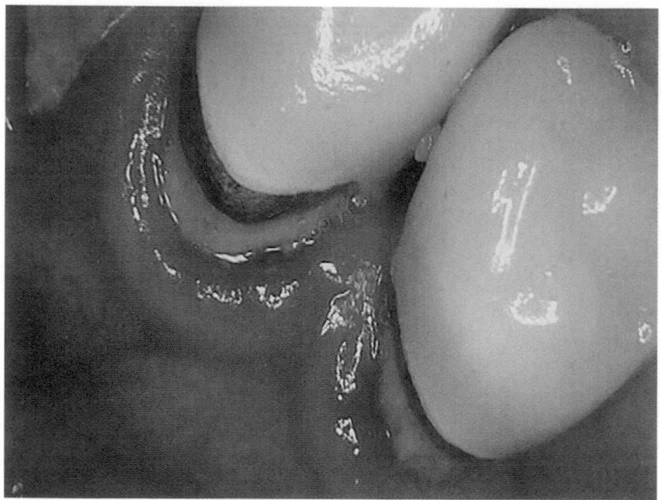

Figure 2.6.1: Note the plaque accumulation around the crown margin and associated gingival inflammation. *Source:* Photo courtesy of Rio Salado College.

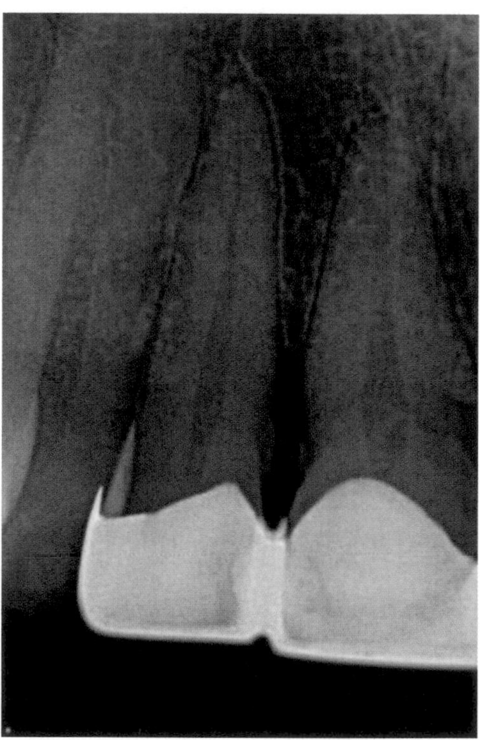

Figure 2.6.2: Calculus formation around anterior crowns. Note the crowns are fused and the margin on the distal of the lateral incisor are local contributing factors. *Source:* Photo courtesy of Rio Salado College.

- Figure 2.6.3 shows gingival inflammation around anterior crown margins. It appears there is minimal plaque accumulation. The margins could be bulky or it could be a tissue reaction to the dental biomaterials used in the fabrication of the crowns.
- Figure 2.6.4 shows a broken tooth/restoration with plaque accumulation. Planned interventions would include dental care to replace the restoration. Pain should also be a consideration when developing a dental hygiene diagnosis and care plan.
- Figure 2.6.5 shows crowding on the mandibular incisors. Crowding is a local contributing factor in different ways. One way is difficulty for the patient to conduct self-care and plaque removal. Another way is root proximity contributing to difficulty in root debridement procedures.

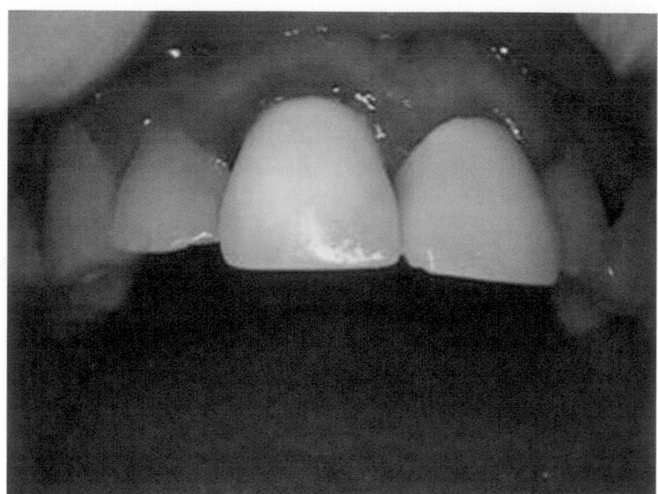

Figure 2.6.3: Gingival inflammation around anterior crowns, may be a result of a tissue reaction to biomaterials used in the fabrication or bulky crown margins. *Source:* Photo courtesy of Rio Salado College.

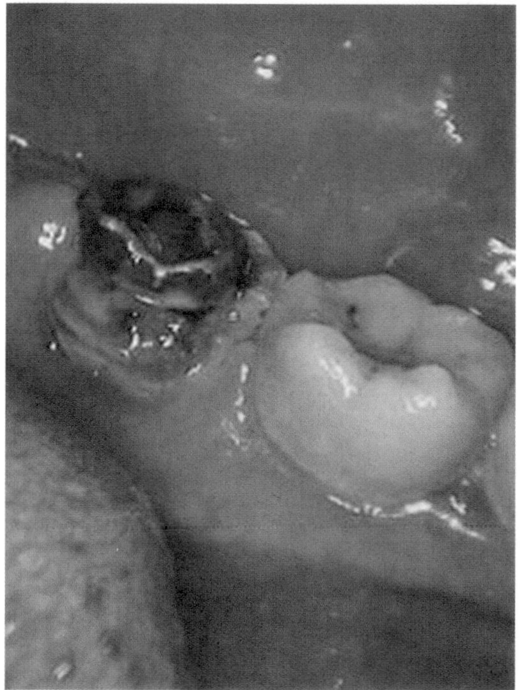

Figure 2.6.4: A broken tooth with plaque accumulation and gingival inflammation. *Source:* Photo courtesy of Rio Salado College.

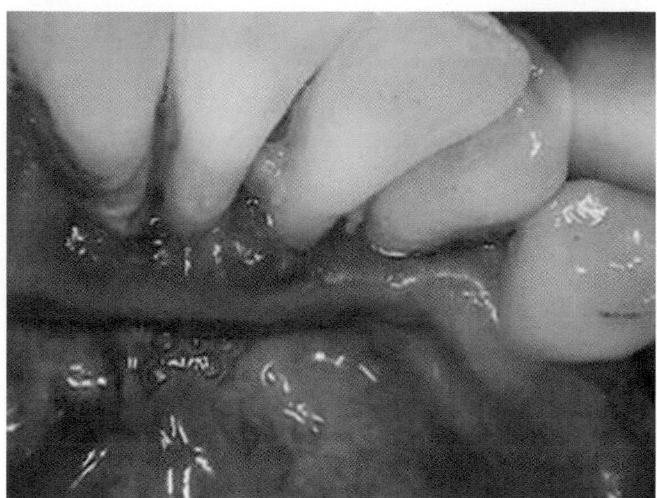

Figure 2.6.5: Crowding on the mandibular incisors resulting in difficulty in plaque removal and root debridement procedures. *Source:* Photo courtesy of Rio Salado College.

Plaque accumulates for many reasons. One reason may be the patient's ability to effectively perform self-care. Another may be the specific dental material used such as a large fill composite that is rough and difficult to polish. Margins that are bulky or have overhangs provide a nexus for plaque accumulation. Broken teeth or restorations have rough margins and lead to plaque accumulation. Realistic goals of educating the patient as to the reason further dental treatment are required as well as oral hygiene care around the restoration. The clinician can use both biologically sound and functioning dentition due to the crown margins being bulky or ill-fitting or skin and mucous membrane integrity due to gingival inflammation. Dental hygienists can perform margination techniques to remove overhangs on Class II restorations and polish restorations that are rough and plaque retentive. Other than these adjunct interventions a referral for dental services to address concerns must be included.

A dental hygiene diagnosis of integrity of skin and mucous membrane is used to plan for dental hygiene care related to inflammation and calculus accumulation. The evidence of plaque or calculus accumulation accompanied by bleeding, reddened, and edematous gingiva allows for a care plan of nonsurgical periodontal therapy. Examples of these are shown in Figures 2.6.4 and 2.6.5.

- Figure 2.6.6 shows calculus accumulation on the lingual of the mandibular incisors with associated edematous papilla and rolled margins. Calculus as a local contributing factor is a plaque retentive factor.
- Figure 2.6.7 shows heavy subgingival calculus leading to plaque retention and difficulty performing oral hygiene self-care.

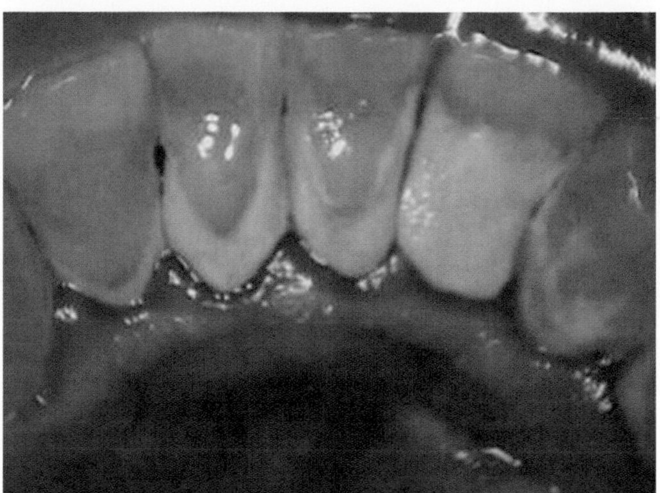

Figure 2.6.6: Calculus formation on the lingual of the mandibular incisors note the edematous papilla and rolled margins. *Source:* Photo courtesy of Rio Salado College.

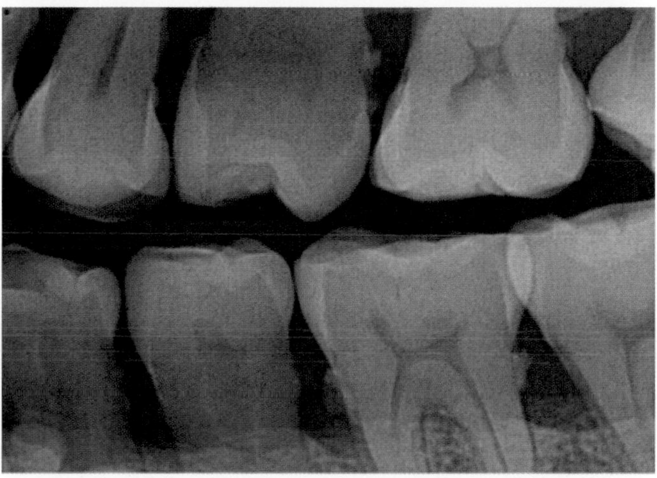

Figure 2.6.7: Heavy subgingival calculus preventing daily plaque removal and contributing to plaque retention. *Source:* Image courtesy of Rio Salado College.

Although calculus is not the cause of periodontal disease, it plays a significant role in increasing the risk for development or exacerbation of an existing condition. Plaque accumulation is associated with calculus. Mature plaque that covers calculus can increase the pathogenicity. Interventions include patient education regarding the removal of the deposits and disease progression. Oral hygiene instructions to reduce plaque accumulation and address the patient's self-care behaviors can also be employed. Nonsurgical periodontal therapy and adjunctive therapies tailored to the individual patient should also be included.

The American Academy of Periodontists added the addition of a category on "Developmental or Acquired Deformities and Conditions" to address localized tooth-related factors. Tooth anatomic factors, dental restorations/appliances, root fractures, and cervical root resorption are specifically listed. They have been included as important modifiers of the susceptibility to periodontal diseases. Addressing these tooth-related factors can affect the outcomes of treatment (Armitage 1999).

Recognizing the risk factors and addressing the patient's unmet human needs are the initial steps in the process of care. Developing a dental hygiene care plan and interventions that include dental referrals is essential to the outcomes of treatment when dealing with local contributing factors.

Take-Home Hints

1. Consideration of the removal of local contributing factors
2. Education of the patient in the disease progression and self-care behaviors
3. Relate the dental hygiene care to the dental hygiene diagnosis
4. Include dental referrals to address biologically sound and functioning dentition.

Self-Study Questions

1. All of the following are local contributing factors except one, which is the exception?

A. Calculus
B. Poor crown margins
C. Diabetes
D. Class II overhang restoration

2. Which dental hygiene diagnosis addresses poor restorations?

A. Biologically sound and functioning dentition
B. Conceptualization and problem solving
C. Integrity of the skin and mucous membrane of the head and neck
D. Responsibility for oral health

3. Local contributing factors influence the development or progression of periodontal disease by:

A. Increasing plaque retention
B. Affecting the host's immune response
C. Causing damage to the periodontium
D. Contributing to systemic conditions
i. A only
ii. A and C
iii. None of the above
iv. All of the above

References

Armitage, G.C. (1999). Development of a classification system for periodontal diseases and conditions. *Annals of Periodontology* 4 (1): 1–6. [Online]. Retrieved from: http://www.joponline.org/doi/pdf/10.1902/annals.1999.4.1.1.

Darby, M. and Walsh, M. (2015). *Dental Hygiene Theory and Practice*. St Louis: Evolve Elsevier.

Nield-Gehrig, J.S. and Willmann, D.E. (2016). *Foundations of Periodontics for the Dental Hygienist*, 4e. Philadelphia: Wolters Kluwar.

Answers to Self-Study Questions

1. C

2. A

3. B

3

Planning and Managing Dental Hygiene Care

Clinical Cases in Dental Hygiene, First Edition. Edited by Cheryl M. Westphal Theile, Mea A. Weinberg and Stuart L. Segelnick.

Case 1

Infection Control

CASE STORY

A 61-year-old female, presented with a chief complaint of: "I am here for my regular check-up. I am very concerned with how you clean your office and instruments. After visiting the oral surgeon, I contracted hepatitis C."

PROBLEM-BASED LEARNING GOALS AND OBJECTIVES

- Describe the risk factors and clinical features of Hepatitis C
- Provide advice and recommendations for patients at risk for Hepatitis C
- List elements of a comprehensive infection control strategy

Medical History

This patient donates blood regularly, and at her most recent visit to the blood center, the screening report was positive for Hepatitis C (HCV). The facility reviewed past donation screening records, going back several years, and the reports were all negative for HCV. As mandated by state legislation, the blood center reported the incidence of HCV to the state health department. The patient was seen by her primary care physician who interviewed her about potential risk factors commonly associated with HCV and confirmed the diagnosis of acute HCV with genotype 1a. The physician reported back to the state health department that the only possible risk factor was her visit to the oral surgeon who extracted two third molars with IV sedation.

The state health department sent investigators to the dental facility that was believed to be the source of infection. After interviewing and testing several thousand patients, the investigators identified 96 people with HCV. Of these people; genetic testing identified the Hepatitis C genotype of the case patient that matched with another individual who had oral surgery on the same day. Further investigation revealed a contaminated sedation medication vial that was used for the infected patient and reused for the case patient. The final report included several infection control violations as probable cause for disease transmission (adapted from OK.gov 2016).

The patient's medical history did not reveal any other significant medical findings or conditions. Vital signs were within normal limits.

Dental History

Patient is aware of her dental health and the importance of regular checkups. She recently visited the oral surgeon for surgical extractions with no oral complications. She is now concerned about transmission of infectious disease.

Social History

Patient is married with two adult children and lives in the suburbs. She is a human resource consultant.

Dental Examination

Extraoral exam revealed no significant findings. Intraorally the patient presents with generalized pink gingiva with light supragingival calculus and biofilm. Class I malocclusion with slight mandibular anterior crowding was noted. Teeth #1 and #16 were removed four months ago. Periodontal examination reveals generalized maxillary and mandibular probing depths of 3–4 mm with bleeding upon probing on posterior quadrants and 1 mm recession on the premolars. Radiographs were current.

Dental Hygiene Diagnosis

Problems	Related to Risks and Etiology
Dental fear of disease transmission	HCV diagnosis
Dental hypersensitivity	Gingival recession
Potential for periodontal disease	Generalized light supragingival calculus and biofilm with bleeding upon probing posteriorly on all quadrants

Planned Interventions

Planned Interventions (to arrest or control disease and regenerate, restore or maintain health)		
Clinical	**Education/Counseling**	**Oral Hygiene Instruction**
Adult Prophylaxis 5% NaF fluoride varnish to prevent root caries	Educate about recession prevention and dentinal sensitivity reduction Educate about periodontal disease and disease prevention Educate on current infection control practices in the dental office	Modified Stillman's brushing technique Interdental cleaning with interproximal brushes Recommend dentinal hypersensitivity toothpaste with fluoride

Progress Notes

The patient arrived for her appointment 30 minutes before her appointment time. Medical, social, and dental history assessed. Review and tour of infection control office practices. Patient felt comfortable, and the hygiene appointment continued. Oral, dental, and periodontal exams were updated. Treatment plan explained and accepted. Biofilm management was reviewed and tailored to her needs. A recall appointment was scheduled.

History and Clinical Pathophysiology

Gastrointestinal symptoms may appear within two weeks to six months after infection with HCV. HCV is acute, asymptomatic, and cleared by the body within six months approximately 15–25% of the time (Takehara and Hayashi 2007; Heymann 2015). Of the remaining acute cases, 75–85% will become chronic, and can go undetected for 20–30 years until symptoms of cirrhosis and hepatocellular carcinoma are diagnosed (Heymann 2015; CDC.gov 2016).

Bloodborne pathogens, Hepatitis A and B were isolated in the 1970s, though an unidentified hepatitis type infection continued to appear in blood transfusions and was labeled Non-A or Non-B Hepatitis (NANBH). The molecular structure of HCV was isolated in 1989 from the plasma of infected chimpanzees (Choo et al. 1989) and subsequent serologic testing provided insight into epidemiologic details and disease transmission. HCV is an acellular, obligate parasite that replicates ribonucleic acid (RNA) genetic material (Figure 3.1.1) within liver hepatocytes and is only transmitted by contact with infected human blood (Chevaliez and Pawlotsky 2006; Takehara and Hayashi 2007; Pfaender et al. 2015). The virus can survive in plasma while drying on fomites for up to 16 hours (Kamili et al. 2007), and cool (40° F) environments for up to five months (Ciesek et al. 2010). HCV is isolated into six genetic groups labeled in chronological order of discovery with Arabic numerals (1–6), and subtypes identified with lower case letters (a, b, c) (Choo et al. 1989).

Diagnosis of HCV is made by the detection of antibodies to the hepatitis virus (anti-HCV) in a blood test called an enzyme immunoassay (EIA). A patient with a positive EIA should confirm the diagnosis with a more sensitive immunoassay that tests specifically for the presence of HCV RNA (CDC.gov 2016).

In 1998 the National Center for Chronic Disease and Health Promotion (CDC) collected epidemiological data on the prevalence of HCV by testing high-risk individuals (Table 3.1.1). The data revealed that the largest cohort, who tested positive, was born between 1945 and 1965; "*five times higher than among adults born in other years*" (CDC.gov 2012). The CDC also reported that 45–85% of these persons were unaware of their HCV status, and in 2012 published recommendations that individuals born between 1945 and 1965 – "baby boomers" – be tested for HCV (CDC.gov 2012).

Undetected chronic HCV is the leading cause of liver transplantation in the United States (CDC.gov 2012). Barriers to risk testing by individuals in this cohort include lack of health insurance, alcoholism, and provider knowledge of recommendations, testing methodology, and current guidelines (CDC.gov 2012).

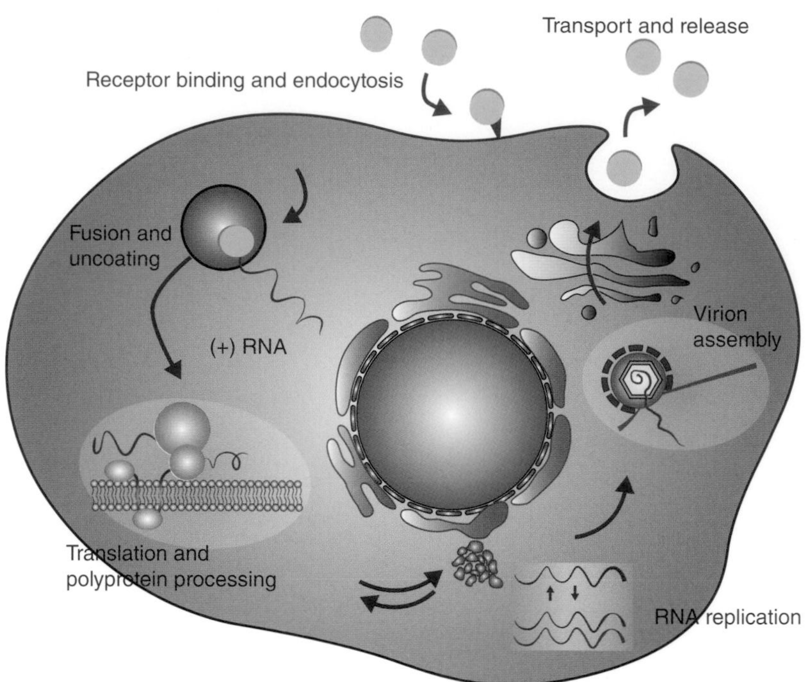

Figure 3.1.1: Schematic representation of the major steps of HCV life cycle. *Source:* Courtesy of Dubuisson (2007).

Table 3.1.1: Individuals with high risk for HCV.

- Persons-Who-Inject-Drugs (PWID)
- Hemodialysis patients
- Patients who had a blood transfusion or organ transplant before July 1992 or received clotting factor concentrates produced before 1987
- Persons with a known exposure to HCV by a needle stick
- Persons born to an HCV-infected mother
- Patients with liver inflammation
- Individuals with HIV

Source: (CDC.gov, 2012).

Employers of health-care providers must abide by the Occupational Safety & Health Administration (OSHA) Bloodborne Pathogens Standard (29 CFR 1910.1030). This federal law mandates that employers of health-care workers provide a plan for exposure control, engineering and safe work practice controls, hepatitis B (HBV) vaccinations, hazard communication and training, and maintain documentation of exposure incidents. This law also requires compliance with universal precaution guidelines to prevent occupational exposure to bloodborne pathogens and cross contamination (OSHA.gov 1991). These guidelines instruct health-care workers to consider all patients as potential carriers of bloodborne disease and thus adhere to precautions in the form of personal protective equipment (PPE) – gloves, masks, and eyewear at all times when caring for them. The reasoning behind this approach was that disclosure by infected patients could not always be corroborated through the process of obtaining medical history information or observing visible symptoms, and health-care providers needed to be protected.

The Standard Precautions Standard, revised Universal Precautions in 2007, by including guidelines for Safe Injection Practices and Respiratory Hygiene/Cough Etiquette (CDC.gov 2007). Safe Injection Practices identified a need to contain outbreaks of HCV and HBV that occur by the "reinsertion of used needles into a multiple-dose vial or solution container (e.g. saline bag) and use of a single needle/syringe to administer intravenous medication to multiple patients" instead (CDC.gov 2007).

The CDC Healthcare Infection Control Practices Advisory Committee (HICPAC) *Guideline for Disinfection and Sterilization in Healthcare Facilities* (CDC.gov 2008) and the *Guidelines for Infection Control in Dental Health-Care Settings* (CDC.gov 2003) include recommended procedures for instrument processing. In general, the guidelines identify and categorize disinfection and sterilization procedures of patient-care items by the risk of disease transmission: critical, semi-critical and non-critical (Table 3.1.2).

Patient-care items that penetrate soft tissue and come in contact with blood are categorized as critical and should be sterilized by heat (Table 3.1.2). Sterilization is defined as the inactivation of cellular

Table 3.1.2: There are three categories of patient-care items depending on their intended use and the potential risk of disease transmission.

Instrument Type	Features	Examples
CRITICAL	Critical items penetrate soft tissue or contact bone, the bloodstream, or other normally sterile tissues of the mouth. They have the highest risk of transmitting infection and should be heat-sterilized between patient uses. Alternatively, use sterile, single-use disposable devices.	Examples include surgical instruments, periodontal scalers, scalpel blades, and surgical dental burs.
SEMI-CRITICAL	Semi-critical items contact only mucous membranes and do not penetrate soft tissues. As such, they have a lower risk of transmission. Because most items in this category are heat tolerant, they should be heat sterilized between patient uses. For heat-sensitive instruments, high-level disinfection is appropriate.	Examples of semi-critical instruments include dental mouth mirrors, amalgam condensers, and impression trays. Dental handpieces are a special case. Even though they do not penetrate soft tissue, it is difficult for chemical germicides to reach the internal parts of handpieces. For this reason, they should be heat sterilized using a steam autoclave or chemical vapor sterilizer.
NON-CRITICAL AND OTHER DEVICES	Non-critical instruments and devices only contact intact (unbroken) skin, which serves as an effective barrier to microorganisms. These items carry such a low risk of transmitting infections that they usually require only cleaning and low-level disinfection. If using a low-level disinfectant, according to OSHA, it must have a label claim for killing HIV and HBV. However, if an item is visibly bloody, it should be cleaned and disinfected using an intermediate-level disinfectant before use on another patient.	Examples of instruments in this category include X-ray head/cones, face bows, pulse oximeter, and blood pressure cuff.

processes and coagulation of proteins resulting in cell death. The most common equipment in dental offices used for sterilization of heat tolerant instruments is either a gravity displacement or high-speed pre-vacuum steam under pressure autoclave. Cleaned and packaged instruments must be definitively placed inside the autoclave to allow for direct contact and steam circulation over a prescribed period of time. Dental health-care providers should follow manufacturer instructions for use, monitoring gauges for the attainment of pressure and temperature, and allow for minimum sterilization time to reach asepsis. Recommended sterilizing times and temperatures are 30 minutes at 250 °F for a gravity displacement autoclave and four minutes at 132 °F for a high-speed pre-vacuum autoclave. Monitoring of sterilization effectiveness is recommended for each procedure. Internal and external indicators, such as heat sensitive tape or internal chemical indicators can verify that a package was exposed to heat for a period, though do not prove that sterilization had been achieved. The placement of heat resistant biological indicators (BIs) containing *Geobacillus stearothermophilus* is used to confirm that sterilization has been achieved. Spores are more resistant and have a higher threshold to heat sterilization than the common microbial population found on patient-care instruments (CDC.gov 2003, 2008). Analysis of the BI with evidence of spore death indicates that any pathogen less resistant had also been inactivated.

As highly infectious diseases emerge and are identified, infection control guidelines are revised to accommodate new information and are upheld by state agencies and federal law. Failure to adhere to these guidelines can often have serious consequences for both the provider and the patient.

Take-Home Hints

- More than 75% of baby boomers in the United States are HCV infected.
- CDC reported that acute (new) cases of HCV have almost doubled since 2012.
- CDC estimated that 2.7–3.9 million people in the United States have chronic HCV.
- Most persons with chronic HCV are asymptomatic.

Self-Study Questions

1. The mode of transmission of HCV is:
- **A. Saliva**
- **B. Infected human blood**
- **C. Airborne particles**
- **D. Inanimate object**

2. Which patients are at risk for HCV that dental hygienists can provide advice and recommendations?
- **A. Those born between 1992 and 2004**
- **B. Those born between 1966 and 1986**
- **C. Those born between 1945 and 1965**
- **D. Those born between 1987 and 1991**

3. Infection control guidelines that assure safe practice in a dental setting are all of the following except one. Which is the exception?
- **A. Monitoring of sterilization**
- **B. Steam heat under pressure autoclave**
- **C. Cold sterilization with Clorox**
- **D. Use of PPE**

4. Persons who are at known risk for HCV are all the following except one. Which one is the exception?
- **A. Hemodialysis patients**
- **B. Persons who injects drugs**
- **C. Known exposure to HVC by a needle stick**
- **D. Chemotherapy patients**

References

CDC.gov. (2003). Guidelines for Infection Control in Dental Health-Care Settings – 2003 [Online] Available at: http://www.cdc.gov/mmwr/preview/mmwrhtml/rr5217a1.htm (August 31, 2016).

CDC.gov. (2007). CDC - 2007 Isolation Precautions: Part 3 – HICPAC [Online] Available at: http://www.cdc.gov/hicpac/2007IP/2007ip_part3.html (September 3, 2016).

CDC.gov. (2008). CDC - 2008 Disinfection & Sterilization Guideline: TOC – HICPAC [Online]. Available at: https://www.cdc.gov/infectioncontrol/guidelines/Disinfection/index.html (Accessed September 1, 2016).

CDC.gov. (2012). Recommendations for the Identification of Chronic Hepatitis C Virus Infection Among Persons Born During 1945–1965 [Online]. Available at: http://www.cdc.gov/mmwr/preview/mmwrhtml/rr6104a1.htm (Accessed August 11, 2016).

CDC.gov. (2016). HCV FAQs for Health Professionals | Division of Viral Hepatitis | CDC [Online]. Available at: http://www.cdc.gov/hepatitis/hcv/hcvfaq.htm (September 3, 2016).

Chevaliez, S. and Pawlotsky, J. (2006). HCV genome and life cycle. In: *Hepatitis C Viruses: Genomes and Molecular Biology*, 1. [online]e (ed. S. Tan). Norfolk (UK): Horizon Bioscience p. Chapter 1 [Online]. Available at: http://www.ncbi.nlm.nih.gov/books/NBK1630 (August 11, 2016).

Choo, Q., Kuo, G., Weiner, A. et al. (1989). Isolation of a cDNA clone derived from a blood-borne non-A, non-B viral hepatitis genome. *Science* 244 (4902): 359–362.

Ciesek, S., Friesland, M., Steinmann, J. et al. (2010). How stable is the hepatitis C virus (HCV)? Environmental stability of HCV and its susceptibility to chemical biocides. *The Journal of Infectious Diseases* 201 (12): 1859–1866.

Dubuisson, J. (2007). Hepatitis C virus proteins. *World Journal of Gastroenterology* 13 (17): 2406.

Heymann, D. (2015). *Control of Communicable Diseases Manual*, 20e, 264–268. Washington, DC: American Public Health Association.

Kamili, S., Krawczynski, K., McCaustland, K. et al. (2007). Infectivity of hepatitis C virus in plasma after drying and storing at room temperature. *Infection Control and Hospital Epidemiology* 28 (5): 519–524.

OK.gov. (2016). Dental Healthcare-Associated Transmission of Hepatitis C: Final Report of Public Health Investigation and Response, 2013 [Online] Available at: https://www.ok.gov/health2/documents/Dental%20Healthcare_Final%20Report_2_17_15.pdf (May 30, 2018).

OSHA.gov. (1991). Bloodborne pathogens. - 1910.1030 [Online]. Available at: https://www.osha.gov/pls/oshaweb/owadisp.show_document?p_table=STANDARDS&p_id=10051 (September 3, 2016).

Pfaender, S., Cavalleri, J., Walter, S. et al. (2015). Clinical course of infection and viral tissue tropism of hepatitis C virus-like nonprimate hepaciviruses in horses. *Hepatology* 61 (2): 447–459.

Takehara, T. and Hayashi, N. (2007). Hepatitis C virus and hepatocellular carcinoma. In: *Hepatitis C Virus Disease Immunobiology and Clinical Applications*, 1e (ed. J. Jirillo), 1–14. New York: Springer.

Tan, S. (2006). *Hepatitis C Viruses*. Wymondham, Norfolk, U.K.: Horizon Bioscience.

Zein, N. (2000). Clinical significance of hepatitis C virus genotypes. *Clinical Microbiology Reviews* 13 (2): 223–235.

Answers to Self-Study Questions

1. B. HCV is a member of the Flaviviridae family, genus Hepacivirus, and is only transmitted by contact with infected human blood (Chevaliez and Pawlotsky 2006).

2. C. In 2012 published recommendations that individuals born between 1945 and 1965 – "baby boomers" – be tested for HCV (CDC.gov 2012).

3. C. Monitoring of sterilization effectiveness is recommended for each procedure.
Since dentistry is also practiced in hospital settings, in 2003 the CDC released a detailed set of guidelines that included expanded standard precautions and the use of PPE in a variety of dental settings (CDC.gov 2003). The most common equipment in dental offices that is used for sterilization of heat tolerant instruments is either a gravity displacement or high-speed pre-vacuum steam under pressure autoclave.

4. D. Individuals with high risk: persons-who-inject-drugs (PWID), hemodialysis patients, patients who had a blood transfusion or organ transplant before July 1992 or received clotting factor concentrates produced before 1987, persons with a known exposure to HCV by a needle stick, persons born to an HCV-infected mother.

Case 2

Emergency Situations and Provision of Appropriate Care

CASE STORY

A 33-year old Caucasian male, smoker, presents for a new patient appointment. He has recently gained employment in a high-stress environment as a stockbroker on Wall Street in New York City. He had been unemployed for the last 10 years, and has not been to the dentist. A benefit of his new job is dental insurance, and he wants to improve his appearance by removing the smoking stain that is present on his teeth. In his dental and social history, he writes about a "bad and painful past experience" at a dental office and is extremely apprehensive about his dental appointment.

PROBLEM-BASED LEARNING GOALS AND OBJECTIVES

- Explain the pathophysiology and differential diagnosis of syncope
- Assess and evaluate the medical, dental, and social history in order to recognize and prepare for a potential syncopal episode
- Recognize symptoms and manage a syncopal patient

Medical History

The patient's medical history did not reveal any significant medical findings or conditions. The patient's vital signs were within normal limits. The patient has smoked since the age of 17. He recently had a physical exam by his primary care physician as a requirement for employment.

Dental History

The patient has not had a dental exam or prophylaxis in 10 years. He brushes daily with a power toothbrush and does not floss. He noticed that his tongue is discolored and coated, along with "bad breath" and eats sugary mints throughout the day. He does not like the heavy, brown stain on his front teeth.

Social History

The patient drinks alcohol on weekends, primarily eats fast food on the run, and smokes a pack of cigarettes daily. He notes that his time is very limited and is very concerned about keeping his new job. He doesn't like doctors, but will see one if he is in pain.

Dental Examination

Extraoral exam revealed no significant findings. Intraorally the patient presents with pale gingiva. The palate appears to have slight nicotine stomatitis. There was: generalized moderate subgingival calculus and moderate stained biofilm with localized bleeding upon probing in the facial and lingual of the lower anterior sextant; generalized maxillary and mandibular probing depths of 3–4 mm; generalized moderate to heavy brown extrinsic stain along the facial and lingual cervical third of the maxillary and mandibular anterior sextants; and Class I malocclusion with slight mandibular anterior crowding.

Dental Hygiene Diagnosis

Problems	Related to Risks and Etiology
Increased caries and periodontal diseases	Dental neglect
Extreme apprehension can lead to syncope	Apprehension
Oral cancer and delayed healing	Smoker
Misuse can lead to cervical abrasion, sensitivity, and ineffective biofilm management	Power toothbrush
Differential diagnosis of causes for halitosis	Halitosis
Increased caries risk	Use of sugary mints
Syncope	Anxiety

Planned Interventions

Planned Interventions
(to arrest or control disease and regenerate, restore or maintain health)

Clinical	Education/Counseling	Oral Hygiene Instruction
Scaling and root planing by quadrant Topical anesthetic as needed Air-Powder Polishing with sodium bicarbonate Full mouth series Initial exam and study models Referral to primary care physician to rule out systemic conditions related to halitosis and syncope	Importance of regular dental visits Increased risk for caries and periodontal diseases Smoking cessation counseling and/or referral Nutritional counseling Importance of healthy living and stress reduction Educate and motivate on the importance of biofilm management	Proper use of power toothbrush Introduce interdental cleaning either with floss or interproximal brushes Use of xylitol gum or candies Use of tongue scraper Nonalcohol antimicrobial mouthrinse

Progress Notes

Patient arrived 20 minutes late for appointment. He was anxious, stressed, and out of breath. Patient was asked to sit in the dental chair and relax before beginning the appointment. Reviewed medical and dental history. Vitals: BP 132/80, 90 BPM, 20 RPM. Extraoral/intraoral examination: An initial comprehensive exam was performed and a full mouth series (FMS) of radiographs was taken. The prophylaxis procedure scheduled for today's appointment was explained to the patient, and as I spoke, I noticed that he was grasping the arm rests and he complained of dizziness and nausea. He shortly thereafter became pale, lost consciousness, and went limp while in an upright position. I placed him in supine position and immediately initiated our office emergency protocol by calling for help. I kept him in supine position with feet slightly elevated and loosened the collar of his shirt. Respiration was monitored and since patient continued breathing, cardiopulmonary resuscitation (CPR) was not indicated. Oxygen tank and mask were brought into the room by designated staff member and I began oxygen administration. Vitals were monitored and were within normal limits. Patient fully recovered after five minutes of oxygen therapy. Patient was asked to sit in reception area for 20 minutes before driving home. The dentist suggested that I speak to him about premedication prior to the next appointment, and that he consider taking an antianxiety medication and/or the addition of nitrous oxide sedation during the appointment. I called the patient that evening to discuss anxiety management. At that time, he was fully recovered with no additional symptoms.

Discussion

Pathophysiology and Differential Diagnosis of Syncope

Syncope is generally categorized as a brief loss of consciousness, related to a drop in arterial blood pressure and subsequent inadequate supply of blood and nutrients to the brain. Loss of consciousness is characterized by a lack of responsiveness, awareness, and postural hypotension. Patients may have prodromal symptoms and complain of dizziness, but most often syncope occurs without any warning, and can last up to 20 seconds. Patients generally recover without knowledge of the episode or the time that has passed (Brignole and Benditt 2011).

Postural hypotension, or collapse, may be confused or reported by the patient as having fainted, when in fact, the cause may be unknown or unrelated to a

Table 3.2.1: Clinical features suggestive of specific causes of syncope.

Type of syncope	Features
Neurally mediated	• Absence of cardiac disease • Long history of syncope • After sudden unexpected unpleasant sight, sound, smell or pain • Prolonged standing or crowded, hot places • Nausea, vomiting associated with syncope • During or in the absorptive state after a meal • With head rotation, pressure on carotid sinus (as in tumors, shaving, tight collars) • After exertion
Orthostatic hypotension	• After standing up • Temporal relationship with start of medication leading to hypotension or changes of dosage • Prolonged standing especially in crowded, hot places • Presence of autonomic neuropathy or parkinsonism • After exertion
Cardiac	• Presence of severe structural heart disease • During exertion, or supine • Preceded by palpitation or accompanied by chest pain • Family history of sudden death
Cerebrovascular	• With arm exercise • Differences in blood pressure or pulse in the two arms

Source: Courtesy of Brignole (2007).

syncopal episode. Olshansky reports (Grubb and Olshansky 2005) on a study with 121 patients who were admitted into an emergency room for having fainted or collapsed. Of the 121 patients, only 15 had a true syncopal episode, 15 patients were diagnosed with cardiac arrest, one patient had fallen asleep, and one patient was dead. The remaining patients' diagnosis was unknown.

The loss or inadequate supply of cerebral nutrients to the brain, is known scientifically as "cerebral hypoperfusion," or the common "faint," and has a quick recovery that distinguishes syncope from loss of consciousness from other causes. A firsthand eyewitness account of a syncopal episode may help with the diagnosis. The American Heart Association recommends referral to a physician who can rule out other conditions that may present similar symptoms and have a more serious pathophysiological origin (American Heart Association.org 2016). A syncopal episode should not be taken lightly, and should be of great concern as it may be a symptom of another more lethal or serious systemic disease, such as cardiac arrest (Grubb and Olshansky 2005). In addition, patients who have a history of some previous trauma such as a concussion, or who are having a seizure or stroke may present similar symptoms and lose consciousness. Patients, who have experienced syncope, may not remember the stimulus or origin of the episode. In addition, episodes of syncope can be related to medications, or withheld from disclosure in the medical history because of embarrassment or drug abuse (Brignole and Benditt 2011).

Differential diagnosis of syncope falls within four general categories (Table 3.2.1): reflex syncope (neurally mediated or neurocardiogenic), syncope from orthostatic hypotension, and cardiac and cerebrovascular related syncope (Grubb and Olshansky 2005; Moya et al. 2009). Unknown or undifferentiated causes may include arrhythmias, seizures, and psychiatric causes (Grubb and Olshansky 2005).

Reflex syncope (neutrally mediated or neurocardiogenic) is further classified as vasovagal (VVS), situational, carotid sinus syncope (CSS), and atypical syncope (Brignole and Benditt 2011). VVS is a response to emotional stress, pain, or fear and is preceded by dizziness, sweating, pallor, and nausea (Sheldon et al. 2015). Situational syncope is more specific with known triggers such as exercise, defecation, or urination. Carotid sinus syncope is rare and involves direct stimulation of the carotid sinuses. Atypical syncope is absent of triggers or known causes (Brignole and Benditt 2011).

VVS is the most common cause of syncope (Grubb and Olshansky 2005; Brignole and Benditt 2011). The vagus nerve is the 10th out of 12 cranial nerves and supplies the involuntary nervous system. In VVS, the vagus nerve is stimulated, causing a vasovagal response that directs blood to the extremities and increases heart rate in order to maintain homeostasis and an adequate supply of blood to the brain. This response is commonly known as the fight or flight response. In the absence of movement, blood pools in the extremities, and venous return decreases. Heart rate slows (bradycardia) to allow for ventricular filling along with a drop in blood pressure. Homeostasis is disrupted, and the brain is deprived of cerebral nutrients, causing cerebral hypoperfusion that results in hypotension and syncope (Malamed 2015). The elderly (≥ 80yo) have the greatest risk for a syncopal episode that would result in an emergency room visit and/or require medical attention (Soteriades et al. 2002; Grubb and Olshansky 2005).

Syncope resulting from orthostatic hypotension may occur when a patient is raised from a supine to an upright position (Figure 3.2.1) and is the second most common cause of syncope (Grubb and Olshansky 2005; Brignole and Benditt 2011). This type of syncope is often related to diabetes, antihypertensive medications, and dehydration. Autonomic nervous system disturbances, such as Parkinson's disease and Addison's disease, may also cause orthostatic syncope (Grubb and Olshansky 2005; Brignole and Benditt 2011).

Cardiovascular syncope is most often related to cardiac arrhythmias and other structural cardiovascular diseases such as myocardial ischemia and infarction (Brignole and Benditt 2011). Findings from the Framingham heart study provide data on the extent and severity of outcomes from syncope. Of the 822 participants included in this subset, VVS was documented as the most common (21.2%) cause of syncope.

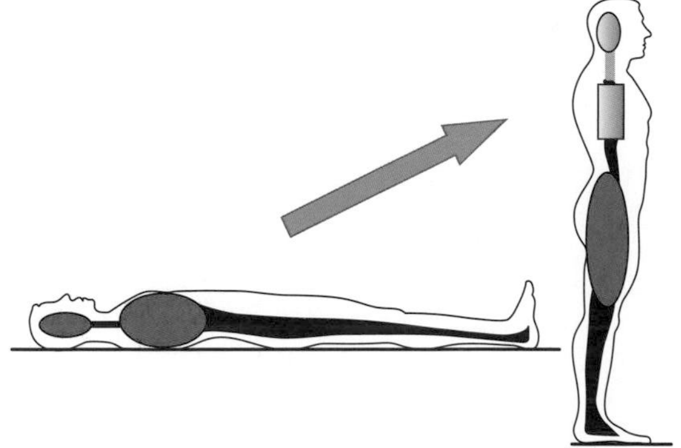

Central Volume is Displaced Caudally with Movement to Upright Posture

Figure 3.2.1: Movement to upright posture reduces intravascular volume in the thorax and diminishes venous return to the heart. Systemic pressure at the level of the brain is placed at risk in the absence of appropriate cardiovascular compensatory responses (*Source:* Brignole and Benditt 2011).

Cardiovascular syncope was determined to be the cause of syncope in only 9.5% of the participants, this type of syncope was associated with an increased risk for cardiovascular events and premature death (Soteriades et al. 2002).

Management of Syncope in the Dental Office

Patients in a dental office environment are exposed to many potential VVS triggers, such as fear of pain, the sight of blood, sharp instruments that include needles, and shrill sounds. In this case study, the patient wrote in his medical history about a painful past experience at a dental office and demonstrated his apprehension while sitting upright, and clutching the arms of the chair tightly. Knowing that the appointment would continue and sensing pain would be imminent – his fear triggered a vasovagal response. Patients may remain frozen with fear, or determined to stay the course, however, without movement or intervention, hypotension and syncope are inevitable. In a fearful situation, children are generally less inhibited and will move or call out decreasing the likelihood of vasovagal syncope (Malamed 2015).

Response and management of a VVS episode is determined by predisposing factors and symptoms – often referred to in stages. The prodromal period of lightheadedness and dizziness is referred to as pre-syncope or near-syncope (Brignole and Benditt 2011; Malamed 2015). The patient is still conscious and is able to breathe on his or her own, therefore, CPR is not indicated. In this situation, the remedy for a patient complaining of dizziness, who is conscious, and who is able to talk, would be to place the patient in supine position until the symptoms are resolved, usually between 15 and 20 seconds. Placing the patient in this position allows gravity to help blood return from the extremities to the heart and brain.

Many dental offices maintain an emergency medical kit that contains ammonia inhalants for use as a secondary measure. Cracking an ammonia inhalant and waving it under the patient's nose releases the strong smell of ammonia to initiate movement in the body and also aid in restoring blood to the heart. The use of ammonia inhalants to revive patients is highly controversial. A case report in the *Journal of Emergency Medical Services* (Jems.com 2016) describes the danger of using an ammonia inhalant on a person suspected of syncope. In this case, the person was lying on the ground. When the ammonia inhalant was used, it caused the person to reflex and recoil snapping his neck on the ground. Ammonia is a respiratory irritant and should not be used on people who have a history of any respiratory distress, such as asthma, bronchitis, or emphysema.

It is worthwhile talking with the patient before treatment to allay any concerns. This discussion might include a description of the procedure and available relief for any discomfort. Patients may benefit from pre-appointment enteral or inhalation sedation (nitrous oxide/oxygen) that would be available during the appointment. In many cases, the trigger for VVS is anxiety, however, ruling out other causes is recommended and referral to a physician is indicated.

Management of a Patient with Reflex Syncope

1. Stop the procedure and initiate office emergency protocol.
2. Place patient in supine position with feet slightly elevated.
3. Patient should recover within 15–20 seconds.
4. If consciousness was not lost, and the patient only felt "faint," treatment may continue if patient and practitioner agree.
5. If consciousness does not return quickly or if the patient loses consciousness, assess for Basic Life Support measures until Emergency Medical Services arrive.

Take-Home Hints

- Elderly patients are more likely to be medically compromised and on various drugs. Some drugs such as hypertensive drugs that increase arterial pressure helps to decrease the risk of vasovagal syncope.
- Children who show signs of restlessness rarely experience syncope.
- Most patients who experience syncope require reassurance and education on the triggers and management of syncope.
- Complete medical history assessment will facilitate the preparedness of a medical emergency.
- Follow-up with referral to physician for evaluation.

Self-Study Questions

1. A common trigger of vasovagal syncope is
  - **A. Tachycardia**
  - **B. Diaphoresis**
  - **C. Anxiety**
  - **D. Mental confusion**

2. Placing a patient in supine position with the legs elevated
  - **A. Increases venous return**
  - **B. Increases oxygen flow**
  - **C. Decreases venous return**
  - **D. Decreases oxygen flow**

3. A differential diagnosis of syncope could be
  - **A. Cerebrovascular**
  - **B. Hypoglycemia**
  - **C. Orthostatic hypotension**
  - **D. Cardiac**

References

American Heart Association.org. (2016). Syncope (Fainting) [Online]. Available at: http://www.heart.org/HEARTORG/Conditions/Arrhythmia/SymptomsDiagnosisMonitoringofArrhythmia/Syncope-Fainting_UCM_430006_Article.jsp# [(December 31, 2016].

Bilich, L., Jackson, S., Bray, B., and Willson, M. (2015). High-fidelity simulation: preparing dental hygiene students for managing medical emergencies. *Journal of Dental Education* 79 (9): 1074–1081.

Brignole, M. (2007). Diagnosis and treatment of syncope. *Heart* 93 (1): 130–136.

Brignole, M. and Benditt, D. (2011). *Syncope*. London: Springer.

Grubb, B. and Olshansky, B. (2005). *Syncope: Mechanisms and Management*, 2e, 1–53. Malden: Wiley.

Jems.com. (2016). Ammonia Inhalants [Online]. Available at: http://www.jems.com/articles/2004/04/ammonia-inhalants.html (July 8, 2016).

Malamed, S. (2015). *Medical Emergencies in the Dental Office*, 7e, 144–152. St. Louis: Elsevier.

Moya, A., Sutton, R., Ammirati, F. et al. (2009). Guidelines for the diagnosis and management of syncope (version 2009): the task force for the diagnosis and management of syncope of the European Society of Cardiology (ESC). *European Heart Journal* 30 (21): 2631–2671.

Sheldon, R., Grubb, B., Olshansky, B. et al. (2015). 2015 Heart Rhythm Society expert consensus statement on the diagnosis and treatment of postural tachycardia syndrome, inappropriate sinus tachycardia, and vasovagal syncope. *Heart Rhythm* 12 (6): e41–e63.

Soteriades, E., Evans, J., Larson, M. et al. (2002). Incidence and prognosis of syncope. *New England Journal of Medicine* 347 (12): 878–885.

Answers to Self-Study Questions

1. C. In many cases, the trigger for syncope is anxiety.

2. A. Placing the patient in supine position with their legs elevated significantly increases venous return while airway maintenance ensures the delivery of oxygen to the blood.

3. B. Differential diagnosis of syncope falls within four categories: reflex (neurally mediated), syncope from orthostatic hypotension, cardiac and cerebrovascular related syncope.

Case 3

Individualized Patient Care

CASE STORY

A 31-year-old Caucasian female presents for a routine checkup and prophylaxis. "I have been referred to your office by my oncologist to have a comprehensive dental exam. I am scheduled to undergo stem cell transplantation and chemotherapy in the next month due to recurrence of lymphoma in the lymph nodes surrounding my spleen."

PROBLEM-BASED LEARNING GOALS AND OBJECTIVES

- Understand how chemotherapy and radiation affect the oral tissues
- Explain the mechanism of hematopoietic stem cell transplant therapy (HSCT) and associated oral manifestations related to immunosuppression
- Understand the role of the dental hygienist in assessing, diagnosis, planning, implementing, and evaluating patients who will undergo an organ or tissue donation

Medical History

In 2001, at age 21, the patient experienced an episode of severe pain and vomiting and was taken to the emergency room for a complete blood work up. Upon subsequent testing a biopsy revealed lymphoma in a neck lymph node. She was diagnosed with Stage 3B Hodgkin's lymphoma affecting lymph nodes from the neck to the pelvis. Prior to the emergency room she was in good health and only experienced nausea and lower back pain which she had ignored. Lymphoma was treated bi-weekly with ABVD combination chemotherapy (A = Doxorubicin Hydrochloride (Adriamycin), B = Bleomycin, V=Vinblastine Sulfate, D = Dacarbazine). After treatment, the patient went into remission, until recently. She had been seen monthly for a routine CAT scan and blood work up. She will undergo stem cell transplantation next month.

Dental History

Patient has not been to the dentist since remission. She experienced nausea and vomiting during treatment phase and was confined for long periods of time to her house or the hospital because of her immunocompromised state. Patient brushes with fluoride toothpaste twice a day and flosses daily.

Social History

Patient is married with one child. She is a stay-at-home mom and primarily cares for her son.

Dental Examination

A thorough extra- and intra-oral exam (EO/IO) was performed with particular attention to lymph nodes. Decreased salivary function was noted. Complete dental charting and radiographic interpretation reveals caries on nine interproximal surfaces. Periodontal examination reveals healthy gingiva and periodontal tissues with probing depths that were within normal limits in all four quadrants. Four bitewing (BTW) x-rays were taken adhering to As Low As Reasonably Achievable (ALARA) principles.

Dental Hygiene Diagnosis

Problems	Related to Risks and Etiology
Potential for xerostomia	Radiation and chemotherapy
Potential for mucositis	Radiation and chemotherapy
Potential for dry cracked lips	Radiation and chemotherapy
Potential for angular cheilitis	Radiation and chemotherapy
Potential for herpetic infection	Radiation and chemotherapy
Potential for periodontal infections	Radiation and chemotherapy
Potential for oral and pharyngeal ulcerations	Radiation and chemotherapy
Increased dental caries	Xerostomia

Planned Interventions

Planned Interventions (to arrest or control disease and regenerate, restore or maintain health)		
Clinical	**Education/Counseling**	**Oral Hygiene Instruction**
Obtain medical clearance from the patient's medical oncologist before commencing with any treatment including periodontal examination and charting Adult prophylaxis	Maintain healthy oral tissues Educate and motivate need to remove potential sites for infection related to biofilm and calculus Educate on oral manifestations due to chemotherapy and radiation Educate about the effects of chemotherapy and oral preventive measures Educate post-transplantation dental care guidelines	Small, soft toothbrushes or sponge tipped brushes (Toothette®) Gentle flossing to avoid floss laceration Saline (nonmedicated) mouthrinses Topical anesthetic mouthrinses Frequent sips of water Use of salivary stimulants (e.g., xylitol gum) Salivary substitutes (e.g., Biotene®)

Progress Notes

Patient arrived for her appointment and a comprehensive medical, dental, and periodontal examination was performed. Patient will undergo autologous HSCT next month. Treatment plan was reviewed and patient consented. Adult prophylaxis was performed and four BTWs were taken. Explained to patient the oral complications of HSCT, chemotherapy, and radiation. Patient was advised to schedule an appointment after treatment.

Discussion

Since the first successful organ transplant in 1954, advancements in medical technology, immunology, and pharmacology have increased the success rate of solid organ transplantation. Data from the United Network of Organ Sharing (UNOS) and the Organ Procurement and Transplantation Network (OPTN) catalog over 175,000 transplants between the years 2000 and 2015 (Optn.transplant.hrsa.gov 2016). Solid organ transplants by frequency and organ type include the kidney, most commonly as a result of end-stage renal failure related to diabetes or high blood pressure, followed by the liver, as a result of hepatitis C or cirrhosis, next the pancreas, heart, lung, and intestine (nidcr.nih.gov 2016; Transplantpro.org 2016). In addition to solid organs, donated blood and bone marrow is used for hematopoietic (blood-forming) stem cell transplantation (LLS.org 2016). A bone marrow transplant (BMT) or HSCT is commonly used in the replacement of bone marrow and blood constituents in the treatment of hematological disease and malignancy, non-Hodgkin and Hodgkin lymphoma, leukemia, autoimmune disease, and solid tumors (Goldman 2006; Henig and Zuckerman 2014). The Center for International Blood and Marrow Transplant Research® reports that 88,064 hematopoietic cell transplants occurred between 2009 and 2013 (Bloodcell.transplant.hrsa.gov 2016) showing an increase each year of 1000 people. All transplant procedures have lifelong consequences that include medication management and infection control. As the numbers of patients who survive either a solid donor transplant or hematopoietic transplant increases, the likelihood that a transplant survivor will visit a dental practice also increases.

In HSCT, high doses of chemotherapy and radiation are initially employed to destroy rapidly proliferating cancerous blood cells, which in turn damage the bone marrow where blood cells originate, replicate, and differentiate. After which, the HSCT aims to replenish blood-forming, immature, stem cells that can differentiate into healthy red blood cells that carry oxygen, white blood cells (lymphocytes) that fight infection, and platelets that stop bleeding (National Cancer Institute 2016).

Stem cells that are used in HSCT are immature blood cells and are not to be confused with embryonic stem cells. Hematologic stem cells are also referred to as grafts and are harvested from either the patient's bone marrow, peripheral blood system, or are donated. A self-donated stem cell harvest is termed autologous or autogenic. Allogenic stem cells are sourced from matched donors or umbilical cord blood. Allogenic stem cells have the advantage of having been screened for contaminants, such as cancer cells, and for having a sufficient supply of healthy lymphocytes that are capable of destroying any remaining disease. The added advantage of these disease-fighting lymphocytes is referred to as a graft versus leukemia (GVL) or a graft versus tumor reaction. However, these same lymphocytes also have the ability to detect the donor tissue as foreign and attempt to destroy it. This severe and often fatal complication is referred to as graft versus host disease (GVHD) (Goldman 2006; Burke et al. 2014).

The process of an autologous or allogenic stem cell transplant begins with chemotherapy treatment to induce remission and the reduction of cancerous blood cells. Stem cells are next collected from the patient and frozen. Once enough stem cells are collected, the patient undergoes a process called "conditioning" whereby high-intensity chemotherapy and radiation are administered that destroys all remaining cells, cancerous and healthy, within the bone marrow. At this stage, patients are extremely immunocompromised and are isolated in a hospital transplant unit. The previously harvested or donated stem cells are then intravenously returned to the patient with the hope that they develop into healthy bone marrow and circulating blood cells (Burke et al. 2014).

The entire process takes several weeks, and complications resulting from a depressed, or absent, immune system occurs. These complications include opportunistic infections, graft rejection, side effects of medication, and most often, complications that take place in the oral cavity.

While there is little evidence to show dental infections complicate recovery after transplantation, pragmatic advice recommends eradication of existing infection prior to a transplant procedure. In many transplant centers across the world, patients are advised to be proactive and seek dental care prior to the transplant procedure, though the provision of cancer treatment is considered to be paramount and take precedence over operative dental procedures (Guggenheimer et al. 2003; Barker et al. 2004). Invasive dental treatment prior to transplant may delay cancer therapy, while at the same time, infections during the pre-transplant and conditioning stages are to be avoided because there is a risk of infection and delayed healing (Guggenheimer et al. 2003; Barker et al. 2004; Goldman 2006).

In all stages of HSCT, the potential exists to develop oral conditions that include mucositis and xerostomia, as well as viral infections such as herpes simplex virus (HSV), fungal infections such as candidiasis, and bacterial infections related to the reduction in white blood cells. The literature describes xerostomia and mucositis as the most frequently encountered and debilitating consequences of chemotherapy and subsequent immunosuppression (Raber-Durlacher et al. 2004; Burke et al. 2014; Nappalli and Lingappa 2015).

Mucositis evolves as epithelial cells lose the ability to divide and regenerate, allowing for tissue atrophy, a breakdown of mucosal integrity, subsequent tissue sloughing, and ulceration (Figure 3.3.1). The nonkeratinized mucosa of the ventral and lateral borders of the tongue, the floor of the mouth, soft palate, and buccal and labial mucosa are most affected (Raber-Durlacher et al. 2004; Nappalli and Lingappa 2015). The ulcerations can be deep enough to permit opportunistic bacteria to penetrate and cause secondary systemic infections and sepsis. As a result of these infections, patients complain of significant pain that effects speech, swallowing, and eating. These conditions may also have an impact on the patient's quality of life, nutritional stability, and recovery.

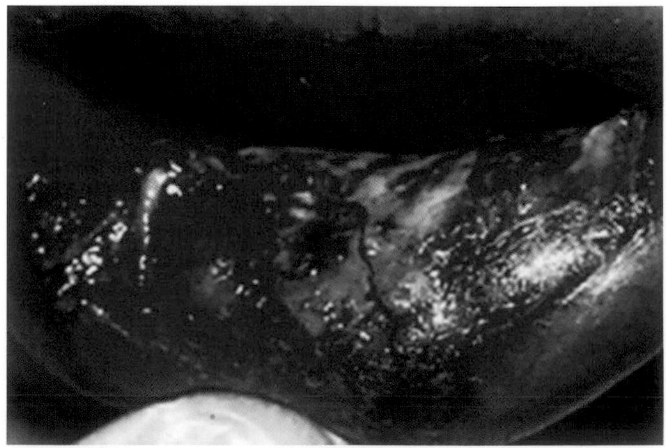

Figure 3.3.1: Severe oral mucositis showing epithelial destruction. *Source:* Raber-Durlacher et al. (2004).

For purposes of documentation and treatment planning, mucositis is classified by the World Health Organization (Nappalli and Lingappa 2015):

Grade 0	No changes
Grade 1	Soreness with or without erythema
Grade 2	Soreness/erythema + ulceration + can eat solid foods
Grade 3	Soreness/erythema + ulceration + can use a liquid diet only
Grade 4	Soreness/erythema + ulceration + oral alimentation is not possible

The Multinational Association of Supportive Care in Cancer and the International Society for Oral Oncology have established oral care guidelines for patients with mucositis (Lalla et al. 2014). Patients will need to change their oral hygiene habits to avoid pain and aggravation of the ulcerated tissues. Small, soft toothbrushes or sponge tipped brushes (Toothette®) are recommended, gentle flossing to avoid floss laceration, and saline (non-medicated) mouthrinses. Pain management includes topical anesthetic mouthrinses.

Decreased salivary gland function or hyposalivation, is related to medication use and chemotherapy/radiation, which results in difficulty swallowing (dysphagia), alteration in taste (dysgeusia), and an increase in dental caries (Raber-Durlacher et al. 2004; Burke et al. 2014; Nappalli and Lingappa 2015).Patient recommendations include frequent sips of water and to stay hydrated, use of salivary stimulants (e.g., xylitol gum), and salivary substitutes (e.g., Biotene®). Prescription use of Pilocarpine as a salivary stimulant may be indicated (sialagogue therapy).

Guidelines (Table 3.3.1 and Table 3.3.2) for oral health management of the organ or stem cell transplant patient are offered by The National Institute of Dental and Craniofacial Research (NIDCR) (Goldman 2006; Nidcr.nih.gov 2014). These guidelines are free and available as brochures from the NIDCR website. Recommendations are separated into management of oral health before transplant and after transplant.

Primarily, the dental hygienist should obtain medical clearance from the patient's medical oncologist before commencing with any treatment. The physician may request a complete blood count (CBC) to determine the patient's ability to develop infection and tendency for excessive bleeding. Patients with a low absolute neutrophil count (ANC) may require prophylactic antibiotic pre-medication (ANC is less than 1,000 μL). Excessive bleeding is determined by the prothrombin time and international normalized ratio (PT/INR) test and should fall within normal limits. Patients who have less than 20,000/μL platelets, may need a platelet transfusion and would need to be referred to a hospital setting for dental treatment (Raber-Durlacher et al. 2004).

A dental hygienist who is fluent in dental oncology and transplant treatment protocols can educate patients and facilitate many of the oral health needs of a prospective and post-treatment transplant patient. As an oral health-care manager, the dental hygienist is part of the cancer care team that includes the patient's primary medical oncologist and primary care physician, nursing staff, dietitian, speech therapist, psychologists, and other supporting members (Figure 3.3.2). The dental hygienist can be the patient's liaison and contact for oral health-care triage and maintenance.

Table 3.3.1: Pre-transplantation dental care guidelines.

Consult with patient's physician.
Perform dental prophylaxis.
Treat all active dental disease.
Postpone elective treatment.
Remove all potential sources of acute or chronic infection, including partially erupted third molars.
Remove all non-restorable teeth.
Perform necessary denture adjustments.
Reinforce oral hygiene and home care instructions.
Initiate daily antibacterial mouthrinses.

Source: Guggenheimer et al. (2003).

Table 3.3.2: Post-transplantation dental care guidelines.

Period	Actions
Immediate post-transplantation	Consultation with the physician/ transplant coordinator Emergency care of dental infections only
Stable post-transplantation	Consultation with the physician/ transplant coordinator Frequent recall and prophylaxis Daily antibacterial mouth rinses All indicated dental care No NSAIDS
Post-transplantation rejection	Consideration of antibiotic prophylaxis for invasive procedures Screening for oral and head and neck cancers Corticosteroid supplementation, if necessary Consultation with the physician/ transplant coordinator

Source: Guggenheimer et al. (2003).

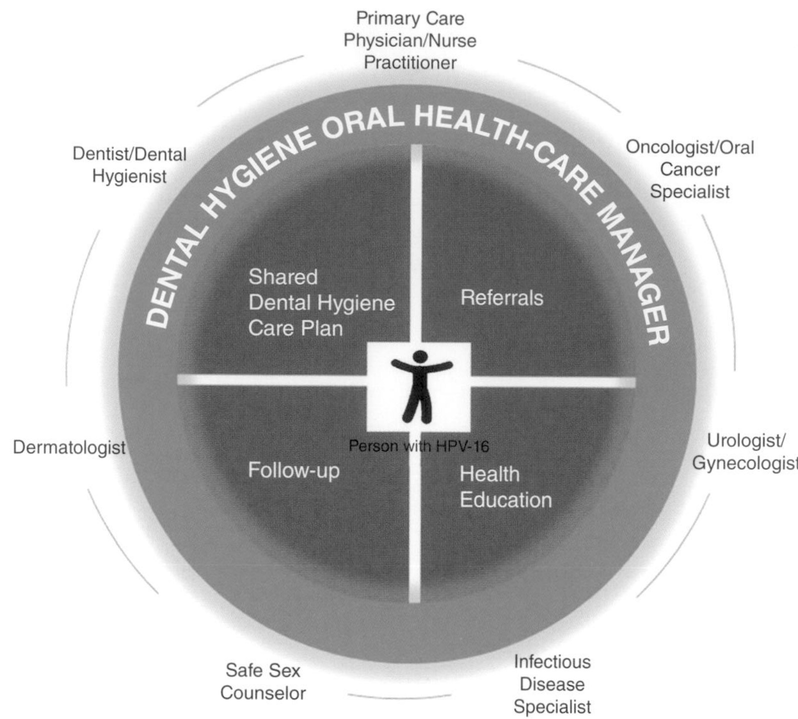

Figure 3.3.2: The dental hygienist as an oral health-care manager. *Source:* Theile et al. (2016).

Take-Home Hints

- Current medication, herbal supplements, and any over the counter medications must be updated at every dental hygiene visit.
- The dental hygienist plays an important role in educating patients' effective oral hygiene care pre- and post-transplantation to reduce oral infections.
- It is important to realize that patients are concerned about their condition, have higher stress levels, and have difficulty in dealing with interpersonal communication.

Self-Study Questions

1. Hematologic stems cells that are harvested from matched donors are:
A. Autogenic
B. Allogenic
C. Autologous
D. Xenogenic

2. The most frequently encountered and debilitating consequence of chemotherapy in the oral cavity is:
A. Candida
B. HSV
C. Mucositis
D. Aspergillus

3. A potential oral secondary infection as a result of ulcerations that permit opportunistic bacteria to cause secondary systemic infection and sepsis:
A. Endodontic infections
B. HSV
C. HPV
D. Mucositis

4. The effects of hyposalivation include all of the following except:
A. Dysphagia
B. Dysgeusia
C. Polydipsia
D. Dental caries

References

Barker, G., Epstein, J., Williams, K. et al. (2004). Current practice and knowledge of oral care for cancer patients: a survey of supportive health care providers. *Support Care Cancer* 13 (1): 32–41.

Bloodcell.transplant.hrsa.gov. (2016). Transplant Activity Report [Online]. Available at: http://bloodcell.transplant.hrsa.gov/research/transplant_data/transplant_activity_report/index.html#summary (August 3, 2016].

Burke, S., Kwasnicki, A., and Macpherson, J. (2014). Dental management during stem cell transplantation. *Dental Nursing* 10 (1): 25–29.

Goldman, K. (2006). Dental management of patients with bone marrow and solid organ transplantation. *Dental Clinics of North America* 50 (4): 659–676.

Guggenheimer, J., Eghtesad, B., and Stock, D. (2003). Dental management of the (solid) organ transplant patient. *Oral Surgery, Oral Medicine, Oral Pathology, Oral Radiology, and Endodontology* 95 (4): 383–389.

Henig, I. and Zuckerman, T. (2014). Hematopoietic stem cell transplantation—50 years of evolution and future perspectives. *Rambam Maimonides Medical Journal* 5 (4): e0028.

Lalla, R., Bowen, J., Barasch, A. et al. (2014). MASCC/ISOO clinical practice guidelines for the management of mucositis secondary to cancer therapy. *Cancer* 120 (10): 1453–1461.

Nappalli, D. and Lingappa, A. (2015). Oral manifestations in transplant patients. *Dental Research Journal* 12 (3): 199–208.

National Cancer Institute. (2016). Blood-Forming Stem Cell Transplants [Online]. Available at: http://www.cancer.gov/about-cancer/treatment/types/stem-cell-transplant/stem-cell-fact-sheet#q1 (August 3, 2016).

National Institute of Dental and Craniofacial Research National Institutes of Health. (NIDCR.NIH.gov.) (2016). Dental Management of the Organ or Stem Cell Transplant Patient [Online]. Available at: www.nidcr.nih.gov/sites/default/files/2017-09/dental-management-organ-stem-cell-transplant.pdf (May 29, 2018).

Organ Procurement and Transplantation Network. Optn.transplant.hrsa.gov. (2016). National Data – OPTN [Online]. Available at: https://optn.transplant.hrsa.gov/data/view-data-reports/national-data (August 2, 2016).

Raber-Durlacher, J., Barasch, A., Peterson, D. et al. (2004). Oral complications and management considerations in patients treated with high-dose chemotherapy. *Supportive Cancer Therapy* 1 (4): 219–229.

The Leukemia & Lymphoma Society. LLs.org. (2016). Normal Blood and Marrow | Leukemia and Lymphoma Society [Online]. Available at: https://www.lls.org/managing-your-cancer/understanding-blood-marrow-and-the-lymphatic-system/normal-blood-and-marrow (August 3, 2016).

Theile, C., Strauss, S., Northridge, M., and Birenz, S. (2016). The oral health care manager in a patient-centered health facility. *The Journal of Evidence-Based Dental Practice* 16: 34–42.

Transplantpro.org. (2016). Transplant trends | Transplant Pro [Online] Available at: https://www.transplantpro.org/technology/transplant-trends/#transplants_by_organ_type+year+2015 (August 3, 2016).

Answers to Self-Study Questions

1. B. Allogenic stem cells are sourced from matched donors or umbilical cord blood.

2. C. The literature describes xerostomia and mucositis as the most frequently encountered and debilitating consequences of chemotherapy and subsequent immunosuppression.

3. B. Reactivation of HSV and acute necrotizing ulcerative gingivitis are examples of potential secondary infections.

4. C. The effects of decreased salivary gland function or hyposalivation include difficulty swallowing (dysphagia), alteration in taste (dysgeusia), and an increase in dental caries as a result of the reduced buffering of acids produced by dental biofilm.

Case 4

Nutritional Counseling

CASE STORY

An 82-year-old Caucasian female, recently widowed, presented with a chief complaint of: "My tongue doesn't feel right. It sometimes burns when I eat certain foods and looks fiery red." She has not been to the dentist in five years due to finances and lives alone. Her children live out of state and only visit her on holidays.

PROBLEM-BASED LEARNING GOALS AND OBJECTIVES

- Explain the pathophysiology and differential diagnosis of Vitamin B12 deficiency
- Identify the oral manifestations of Vitamin B12 deficiency
- Recommend interventions and supportive treatment

Medical History

The patient's medical history revealed high blood pressure diagnosed five years ago and takes clonidine 0.2 mg twice daily (b.i.d). She has hypothyroidism diagnosed 10 years ago and takes levothyroxine 0.88 mcg once a day. Also she has been taking omeprazole, a proton pump inhibitor, 20 mg orally once a day for seven years. She is postmenopausal. The patient is compliant with her medication and her vital signs were within normal limits.

Height: 5′2″
Weight: 100 lbs
BMI: 18.3

Dental History

Patient has not had a dental exam or prophylaxis in five years. She brushes daily with a soft toothbrush and uses an interdental brush. She had full mouth periodontal surgery over 10 years ago. She noticed that her tongue is red, feels funny, and burns after eating certain foods. She is concerned about her periodontal health.

Social History

Patient has been a vegetarian for seven years. She drinks one glass of red wine daily. She purchases her produce at the local farm market and cooks for herself. She does not eat any processed food or animal products. Her diet consists mainly of plant based foods and some grains. She does not take any vitamin supplements. Due to limited finances, she has a very restricted budget.

Her oral symptoms have impacted her social life because she finds it difficult to eat and talk. She finds that her attention span has diminished and has been feeling fatigued. She was a member of a bridge group but has not attended in the last month.

Dental Examination

Extraoral exam revealed no significant findings. Intraorally the patient presents with the appearance of a red enlarged tongue, denuded papilla on dorsum of tongue, and pale oral mucosa. Generalized moderate biofilm, slight supra, and subgingival calculus with bleeding upon probing posteriorly on all quadrants. Generalized maxillary and mandibular probing depths of 3–4 mm with generalized 1–2 mm recession. Class I malocclusion with slight mandibular anterior crowding.

Dental Hygiene Diagnosis

Problems	Related to Risks and Etiology
Increased caries and periodontal diseases	Dental neglect
Significant xerostomia, orthostatic hypotension	Clonidine
Glossitis with papillary atrophy	Proton pump inhibitor >seven years
Vitamin deficiency, low BMI, fatigue	Plant-based diet
Cervical abrasion, root caries, and root sensitivity	Loss of clinical attachment from periodontal surgery
Increased caries and periodontal diseases	Generalized moderate biofilm, slight supra and subgingival calculus with bleeding upon probing posteriorly on all quadrants
Differential diagnosis of Vitamin B12 deficiency	Medication and diet
Noncompliance with medication	Hypertension

Planned Interventions

Planned Interventions (to arrest or control disease and regenerate, restore or maintain health)		
Clinical	**Education/Counseling**	**Oral Hygiene Instruction**
Take blood pressure at every visit; monitor chair position for orthostatic hypotension Periodontal maintenance Topical anesthetic as needed for sensitivity 5% NaF fluoride varnish to prevent root caries Air polish with glycine powder Initial exam, radiographs, and study models Referral to primary care physician for complete physical exam and blood tests (to rule out systemic disease)	Importance of regular dental visits Increased risk for caries and reoccurrence of periodontal disease Nutritional counseling, journaling for dietary analysis Educate and motivate about the importance of healthy lifestyle Educate and motivate on the importance of biofilm management	Modified Stillman's brushing technique Interdental cleaning with interproximal brushes Recommend use of fluoride toothpaste Recommend frequent sips of water during the day or salivary substitute to minimize xerostomia

Progress Notes

Patient arrived early for her appointment but was seen at the appointed time. A complete medical, social, and dental history was taken. Initial exam, FMS, dental, and periodontal exams were performed. Patient agreed to a periodontal maintenance procedure and air polishing with glycine powder. Biofilm management was explained and tailored to her needs. A seven-day nutrient dietary assessment journal was explained and given to the patient. Patient was instructed to return in one week for dietary analysis and counseling. Patient was advised to see primary care physician for a differential diagnosis of Vitamin B12 deficiency.

Discussion

Pathophysiology and Differential Diagnosis of Vitamin B Deficiency

The appearance of a red, denuded tongue and diminished attention span may be symptoms of a Vitamin B deficiency (Field et al. 1995). The B complex vitamins are water-soluble and include: Thiamin (B_1), Riboflavin (B_2), Niacin (B_3), Pantothenic acid (B_5), Pyridoxine (B_6), Biotin (B_8), Folate (B_9), Cobalamin (B_{12}), and Choline (B_{13}). Since the body cannot synthesize water-soluble vitamins, dietary consumption of meat, fish, eggs, and dairy products is necessary. Specifically, glossitis, cognitive impairment and other neurological manifestations are cited in the literature as symptoms of a B12 or cobalamin deficiency (Field et al. 1995; Andres 2004; Pontes et al. 2009; Hoffbrand et al. 2010; Goosen 2016).

Vitamin B12 or cobalamin, is necessary for sound deoxyribonucleic acid (DNA) metabolism in cells of tissues that are constantly reproducing, such as skin, blood, and the lining of the gastrointestinal tract (Peckenpaugh 2010). For example, B12 acts as a coenzyme in DNA biosynthesis for developing blood cells in the bone marrow (hematopoiesis) (Goosen 2016). Impaired DNA cripples cell division, which allows immature cells to become enlarged and often multinucleated resulting in megaloblastic anemia (ineffective hematopoiesis) (Stabler 2013). These enlarged cells are ineffective in carrying oxygen to the peripheral tissues resulting in anemia, from the Greek *anaimia* or "without blood" and a disruption in homeostasis (Goosen 2016).

Additional clinical manifestations of Vitamin B12 deficiency and oxygen deficit includes "demyelination of the cervical and thoracic dorsal and lateral columns of the spinal cord," (Stabler 2013) fatigue, jaundice, paresthesia, memory loss, and peripheral nervous system interferences (walking) (Pontes et al. 2009; Stabler 2013; Goosen 2016). Abnormal epithelial cell proliferation interferes with keratinization and causes smoothing of the tongue, which would appear red and inflamed, along with reduced taste and a burning sensation (Pontes et al. 2009).

In this case, a referral to a primary care physician is indicated for a differential diagnosis. The physician will conduct blood tests to determine whether the deficiency is due to inadequate diet, food-cobalamin malabsorption in the stomach, or lack of intrinsic factor (IF), otherwise known as pernicious anemia (Andres 2004).

Once consumed, cobalamin passes through a series of "hand-offs" (Figure 3.4.1) as it makes its way through the digestive system to the liver where cobalamin is stored (Andres 2004). Aśok Antony describes the process as an "odyssey … [whereby] cobalamin is accompanied by several chaperones that sequentially bind, sequester, and thereby ensure that cobalamin does not participate in side reactions. This ensures its fitness for service [sic] for critical enzymes" (Antony 2016). Though, failure or damage to any function or process along the way can cause a deficiency.

Dietary Deficiency

Dietary deficiency in healthy adults is less than 5%, while studies conducted with the elderly reveal up to a 50% incidence of cobalamin deficiency (Andres 2004). Plants do not synthesize B12, and strict vegetarians, who do not supplement with B12, are susceptible for a dietary B12 deficiency (Goosen 2016).

Food-Cobalamin Malabsorption

Cobalamin is initially bound to the animal protein as it enters the mouth and forms a bolus when chewed and swallowed. Absorption of cobalamin begins in the stomach where pepsin and hydrochloric acid (HCl) are released to break apart the cobalamin from the animal protein (Andres 2004; Antony 2016; Goosen 2016). Malabsorption of cobalamin can occur if the release of pepsin and HCL are impaired resulting in gastric atrophy, thus failing to break apart cobalamin from the protein (hypoclorhydria or achlorhydria) (Andres 2004; Goosen 2016). Reasons for impairment and subsequent food-cobalamin malabsorption include, an overgrowth of Helicobacter pylori (*H. pylori*) and ulcerations of the stomach lining; as well as long-term use of antacids, and medications used to treat gastric reflux (GERD), such as H_2 receptor agonists (Zantac, Pepcid) and proton pump inhibitors (Prilosec, Nexium) that interfere with production of HCL and pepsin (Andres 2004; Goosen 2016). Andres writes that "food-cobalamin malabsorption is caused primarily by gastric atrophy … in 40% of patients older than 80" (Andres 2004).

Lack of Intrinsic Factor

Free cobalamin is next picked up by a protein released by the salivary glands –"haptocorrin, also known as R protein or transcobalamin" (Antony 2016; Goosen 2016) and is carried through the stomach to the lower part of the stomach or duodenum. In the duodenum, pancreatic enzymes weaken this transport mechanism in order to allow for the freed cobalamin to bind with IF that is produced by the parietal cells in the stomach. Intrinsic factor is a glycoprotein with only one important function, and that is to carry cobalamin through the lower regions of the stomach – the jejunum to the ileum (Figure 3.4.2) where it is absorbed into the circulatory system (Andres 2004; Antony 2016). Lack of IF is considered an autoimmune disease that is associated with the presence of anti-intrinsic factor antibodies and chronic atrophic gastritis that results in the (Andres 2004; Antony 2016) "destruction of gastric parietal cells" (Stabler 2013) that produce IF. These combined symptoms present a cobalamin deficiency disease known as pernicious anemia (PA). Other autoimmune diseases such as hyperthyroidism (Graves disease), hypothyroidism (Hashimoto thyroiditis), Type 1 diabetes mellitus, and vitiligo are also associated with pernicious anemia (Andres 2004; Stabler 2013). Serious illnesses that require gastrectomy or cancer, may also affect production of IF (Andres 2004; Goosen 2016). Stabler writes about the prevalence of pernicious anemia as, "The most frequent cause of severe vitamin B_{12} deficiency … that ranges from 50 to 4000 cases per 100 000 persons. All age groups are affected … with a median age of 70–80 years" (Stabler 2013).

Management of Vitamin B12 Deficiency in the Dental Office

The liver stores an abundant amount of cobalamin, and a deficiency may take two to five years to develop (Field et al. 1995, Pontes et al. 2009). Symptoms are most frequently observed in the elderly population and strict vegetarians. Oral and peri-oral manifestations, such as

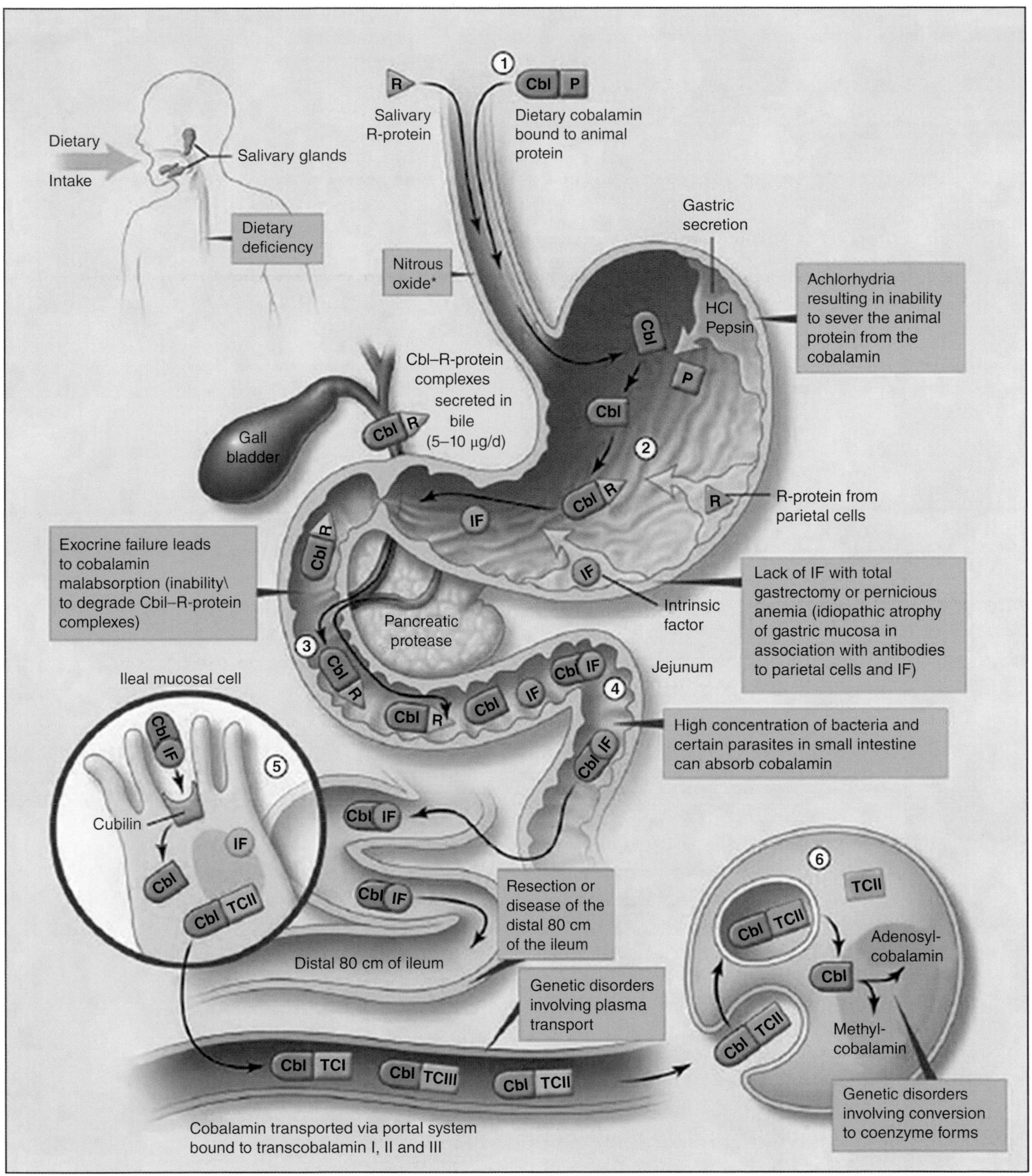

Figure 3.4.1: Cobalamin metabolism and corresponding causes of deficiency. Causes of cobalamin deficiency are shown in blue. The metabolic pathway starts when (1) dietary cobalamin (Cbl), obtained through animal foods, enters the stomach bound to animal proteins (P). (2) Pepsin and HCL in the stomach sever the animal protein, releasing free cobalamin. Most of the free cobalamin is then bound to R-protein (R), which is released from the parietal and salivary cells. IF is also secreted in the stomach, but its binding to cobalamin is weak in the presence of gastric and salivary R-protein. (3) In the duodenum, dietary cobalamin bound to R-protein is joined by cobalamin–R-protein complexes that have been secreted in the bile. Pancreatic enzymes degrade both biliary and dietary cobalamin–R-protein complexes, releasing free cobalamin. (4) The cobalamin then binds with IF. The cobalamin–IF complex remains undisturbed until the distal 80 cm of the ileum, where (5) it attaches to mucosal cell receptors (cubilin) and the cobalamin is bound to transport proteins known as transcobalamin I, II and III (TCI, TCII, and TCIII). TCII, although it represents only a small fraction (about 10%) of the transcobalamins, is the most important because it is able to deliver cobalamin to all cells in the body. The cobalamin is subsequently transported systemically via the portal system. (6) Within each cell, the TCII–cobalamin complex is taken up by means of endocytosis and the cobalamin is liberated and then converted enzymatically into its two coenzyme forms, methylcobalamin and adenosylcobalamin.

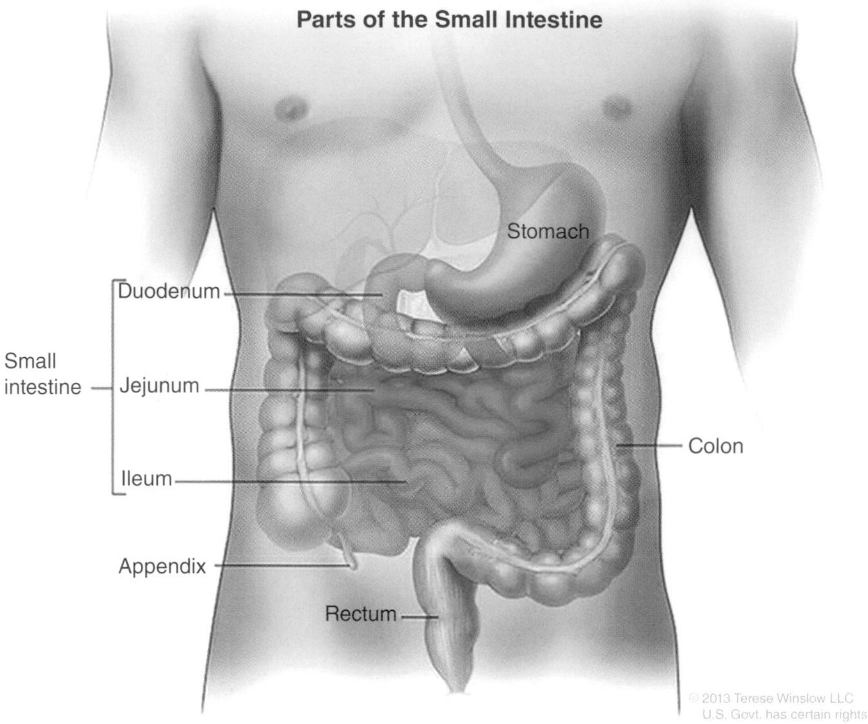

Figure 3.4.2: The small intestine connects the stomach and the colon. It includes the duodenum, jejunum, and ileum.

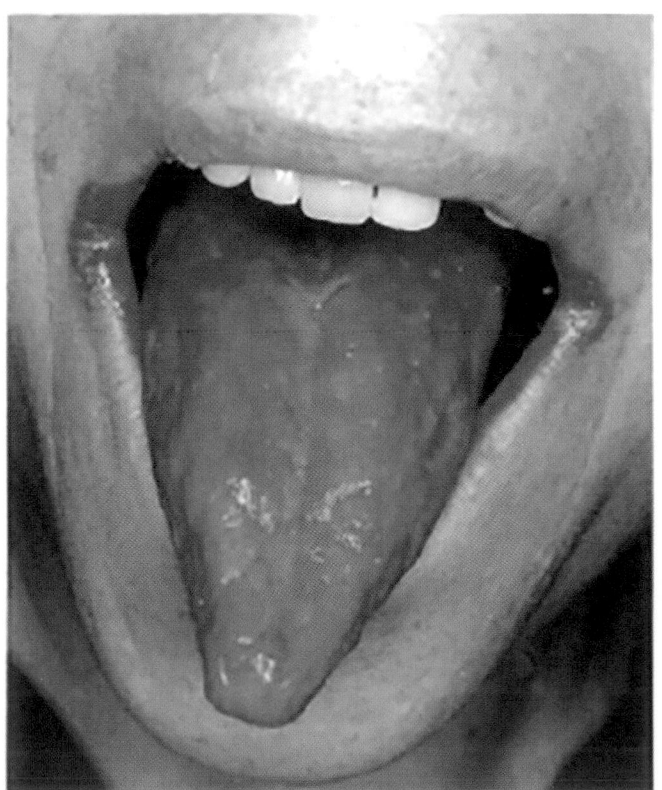

Figure 3.4.3: Angular cheilitis and depapillation of the tongue in a patient with pernicious anemia. *Source*: Ibsen, 1992. Reproduced with permission of Elsevier.

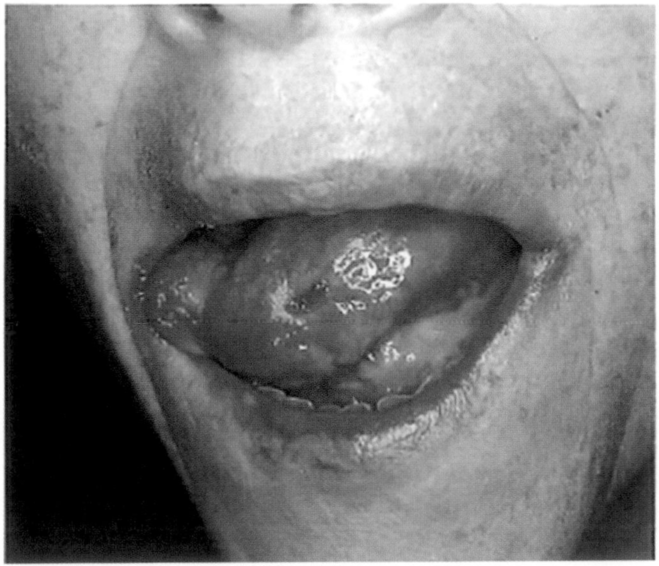

Figure 3.4.4: The mucosa becomes atrophic in pernicious anemia and easily ulcerated. Note ulcer on left lateral aspect of the tongue. *Source*: Ibsen, 1992. Reproduced with permission of Elsevier.

glossitis, angular cheilitis (Figure 3.4.3 and 3.4.4), and candidiasis, are frequently observed prior to other more significant symptoms of a vitamin B12 deficiency (Pontes et al. 2009).

This patient's oral symptoms, along with a history of hypothyroidism, strict vegetarianism, and fatigue may all be related to a vitamin B12 deficiency. Patient discussion would include a referral to her primary care physician for blood tests to determine the cause of her symptoms. A physician would need to determine first, that the anemia is present. This is usually done by evaluating the complete blood count (CBC). Once anemia is confirmed, the physician would need to identify the anatomic location and cause for the deficiency and rule out any underlying disease (Antony 2016).

Dietary counseling would include the role of vitamin B12 in cell maintenance and homeostasis. In most instances, dietary deficiency can be alleviated with vitamin supplements or parenteral injections.

Take-Home Hints

- An average nonvegetarian Western diet contains 5–7 mcg per day of cobalamin, which adequately sustains normal cobalamin equilibrium.
- A vegetarian diet supplies between 0.25 and 0.5 mcg per day of cobalamin, so most vegetarians do not receive adequate dietary cobalamin and are at risk for cobalamin deficiency.
- The recommended daily allowance is 2.4 mcg for men and nonpregnant women, 2.6 mcg for pregnant women, 2.8 mcg for lactating women, and 1.5–2 mcg for children aged 9–18.
- When placing radiographic holders or sensors be careful of patient's sensitivity due to the condition of the oral mucosa.
- Vitamin B12 is found naturally only in foods of animal origin, such as liver, meats, and milk. Some cereals are fortified with Vitamin B12.

Self-Study Questions

1. Foods that are high in B complex are
- **A. Fruits**
- **B. Green leafy vegetables**
- **C. Meats**
- **D. Legumes**

2. A symptom of cobalamin deficiency is
- **A. Chancre**
- **B. Xerostomia**
- **C. Glossitis**
- **D. Herpes labialis**

3. A differential diagnosis of Vitamin B12 deficiency would include
- **A. Food-cobalamin malabsorption**
- **B. Inadequate diet**
- **C. Lack of intrinsic factor**
- **D. All of the above**

4. Malabsorption of cobalamin can occur with use of
- **A. Serotonin uptake inhibitor**
- **B. Proton pump inhibitors**
- **C. Aminoquinoline**
- **D. ACE inhibitor**

References

Andres, E. (2004). Vitamin B12 (cobalamin) deficiency in elderly patients. *Canadian Medical Association Journal* 171 (3): 251–259.

Antony, A. (2016). Megaloblastic anemias. In: *Hematology Basic Principles & Practice*, 6e (ed. R. Hoffman, E. Benz, L. Silberstein, et al.), 473–504. Philadelphis: Elsevier/Saunders.

Field, E., Speechley, J., Rugman, F. et al. (1995). Oral signs and symptoms in patients with undiagnosed vitamin B12 deficiency. *Journal of Oral Pathology & Medicine* 24 (10): 468–470.

Goosen, L. (2016). Anemias caused by defects of DNA metabolism. In: *Rodak's Hematology: Clinical Principles and Applications*, 5e (ed. E. Keohane, L. Smith and J. Walenga), 314–329. St. Louis: Elsevier.

Hoffbrand, A., Pettit, J., and Vyas, P. (2010). *Color Atlas of Clinical Hematology*, 99–114. Philadelphia, PA: Mosby/Elsevier.

Peckenpaugh, N. (2010). *Nutrition Essentials and Diet Therapy*. St. Louis, Mo: Saunders/Elsevier.

Pontes, H., Neto, N., Ferreira, K. et al. (2009). Oral manifestations of vitamin B12 deficiency: a case report. *Journal of the Canadian Dental Association* 75 (7): 533–537.

Stabler, S. (2013). Vitamin B 12 deficiency. *New England Journal of Medicine* 368 (2): 149–160.

Answers to Self-Study Questions

1. C. Dietary consumption of meat, fish, eggs, and dairy products are high in Vitamin B12.

2. C. Glossitis, cognitive impairment and other neurological manifestations are cited in the literature as symptoms of a Vitamin B12 or cobalamin deficiency.

3. D. Differential diagnosis could be due to an inadequate diet, food-cobalamin malabsorption in the stomach, or lack of intrinsic factor, otherwise known as pernicious anemia.

4. B. Reasons for impairment and subsequent food-cobalamin malabsorption include, an overgrowth of Helicobacter pylori (*H. pylori*) and ulcerations of the stomach lining; long term use of antacids, and medications used to treat gastric reflux (GERD), such as H2 receptor agonists (Zantac, Pepcid) and proton pump inhibitors (Prilosec, Nexium) that interfere with production of HCL and pepsin.

Case 5

Dental Hygiene Treatment Strategies

CASE STORY

An 18-year-old male presented for a dental check up with a chief complaint of: "I feel some pain in between my teeth every time I eat candy or drink soda. I think I have a cavity." He has not been to the dentist in three years.

PROBLEM-BASED LEARNING GOALS AND OBJECTIVES

- Explain how to manage and prevent the disease of dental caries using caries management by risk assessment (CAMBRA)
- Evaluate and apply patients' status for caries risk using CAMBRA
- Recommend dental hygiene treatment strategies using CAMBRA

Medical History

The patient's medical history revealed no significant findings and vital signs were within normal limits.

Dental History

Patient has not had a dental exam or prophylaxis in three years. He just moved to the area and previously did not visit the dentist on a regular basis. He brushes once a day with a soft toothbrush and nonfluoridated toothpaste and does not use interdental cleaners or mouthrinses. He frequently snacks during school and drinks sugary beverages throughout the day.

Social History

Patient lives with his mother and three younger siblings. He has started a new job after school at a convenience store to help with family finances.

Dental Examination

Extraoral exam revealed no significant findings. Intraorally the patient presents with cheek biting and Class II malocclusion. Gingiva appears red, enlarged with generalized moderate biofilm with bleeding upon probing. Patient has posterior occlusal deep pits and fissures and Class V white spot lesions on teeth #5, #6, #11 and #12.

Dental Hygiene Diagnosis

Problems	Related to Risks and Etiology
Gingival bleeding/inflammation	Biofilm accumulation
Increased caries risk (CAMBRA) level high	Consumption of sugar-sweetened foods and beverages frequently throughout the day
	Irregular dental visits
	Irregular personal oral-care habits
	Frequent sugar intake
	Current cavitated lesions

Planned Interventions

Planned Interventions (to arrest or control disease and regenerate, restore or maintain health)		
Clinical	**Education/Counseling**	**Oral Hygiene Instruction**
CAMBRA assessment Adult Prophylaxis every 3–4 months NaF varnish every 3–4 months BTW x-rays every 6–18 months until no cavitated lesions are evident Baseline salivary flow and bacterial culture and again at every recare appt. Sealants posterior teeth (ICDAS [International Caries Detection and Assessment System] protocol)	Importance of regular dental visits Educate about the relationship between fermentable carbohydrates and caries; recommend dietary analysis Educate and motivate on the importance of biofilm management Educate and motivate on the importance of a healthy lifestyle	Proper use of toothbrush and interdental cleaning 1.1% NaF toothpaste b.i.d. Xylitol (6–10 g day) 2 tabs of gum or candies four times a day Chlorhexidine gluconate 0.12% mouthrinse, 10 ml for 1 minute daily, 1 week each month Optional: 0.2% NaF rinse daily OTC 0.05% NaF rinse daily CPP paste daily

Progress Notes

The patient was seated for his appointment, and a complete medical, social, and dental history was taken. An initial exam, FMS, dental exam, and periodontal exam was performed and revealed white spot lesions, deep pits, and fissures. Radiographs revealed interproximal decay on teeth #30 and #19. The periodontal exam revealed generalized gingival inflammation with probing depths of 1–4 mm. A caries management by risk assessment (CAMBRA) was performed, and the patient was determined to be at high risk. The treatment plan was explained, and consent obtained. Bacterial culture and salivary flow rate were obtained. Caries risk and biofilm management were explained, and oral hygiene methods were demonstrated and reviewed with patient. An adult prophylaxis was performed, and topical fluoride varnish was applied. It was recommended that the patient brush twice a day with a high fluoride toothpaste, rinse with an antibacterial mouth rinse for one week each month and suck or chew xylitol candies or gum four times a day. Dietary recommendations were explained and patient was put on a three-month recall. The patient was scheduled for his next appointment.

Discussion

A cornerstone model of disease progression is the epidemiological triad. This model proposes that disease does not occur randomly – disease is only spread among populations at risk for the disease. Risk factors include the immune status of the host, the presence of the infectious agent, and the environment in which the disease is most likely to occur (CDC.gov 2012). The likelihood for and the extent that dental caries causes destruction in healthy teeth is also dependent on risk factors and can be viewed in a similar manner. Dental caries is an infectious, and communicable, disease that is dependent on several variables, each of which can be modulated to arrest further progression or occurrence. These risk factors include the ability of the tooth to resist demineralization (immunity), the presence of infectious organisms (agent), the consumption of cariogenic foods, and the quality and quantity of salivary components (environment) (Diagnosis and Management of Dental Caries Throughout Life 2001; Wilkins et al. 2016).

Historically, the incidence of dental caries in children 13–15 years of age declined 68% by 1970 after fluoridated water was adopted as a public health measure in 1962. The rate of decline in caries slowed in the 1980s and left a significant number of children aged 5–17 years with caries in their permanent teeth. Dental caries continues to be a significant global problem, and the risk for dental caries is exacerbated in populations who are limited or without access to care. Research then revealed that fluoride alone was not sufficient in controlling the disease and other risk factors needed to be addressed (CDC.gov 1999; Featherstone 2000; Diagnosis and Management of Dental Caries Throughout Life 2001).

A seminal article written by Featherstone (2000) presented a compelling argument to support the stance that the risk for progression of dental caries may be assessed as a balance between "pathological factors" and "protective factors" (Featherstone 2000).

Table 3.5.1: Indicators for increased risk of dental caries.

Indicator	Example
Past caries experience	Most consistent predictor
Presence of caries in the mother and siblings	Matrilineal transmission
Inadequate exposure to fluoride	Use of fluoride dentifrice
Conditions that compromise maintenance of good oral hygiene practices	Illness, physical, and mental challenges, existing restorations, oral appliances
Fermentable carbohydrates consumption associated with acid formation and demineralization	Amount, consistency, frequency
Xerostomia	Saliva provides calcium, phosphate, and neutralizes acids formed by bacterial metabolism

Source: Adapted from Diagnosis and Management of Dental Caries Throughout Life (2001).

Pathological factors include elements that increase the propensity for the disease, for example, cariogenic bacteria and the presence of fermentable carbohydrates. Protective factors are elements that may provide protection or arrest the caries process, for example, fluoride and adequate saliva. It is this balance between pathological factors and protective factors, which mitigate the tooth's ability to resist the development of dental caries. Featherstone appreciated the need for prevention of the disease through caries risk management and refuted the premise that caries can be stopped by surgical removal or restoration. He instead provided evidence that fluoride by way of the saliva can interrupt the demineralization of tooth enamel and become a vehicle for calcium and phosphorus to remineralize the affected area (Featherstone 2000).

Subsequently, the National Institutes of Health (NIH) convened a panel of experts to review research on the best practices for diagnosis and the management of dental caries. The panel identified many disease indicators (Table 3.5.1) and provided a list of recommended treatment modalities to prevent, arrest, or reverse the disease process, for example, fluoride, chlorhexidine, sealants, salivary enhancers, and oral-health education (Diagnosis and Management of Dental Caries Throughout Life 2001). In addition, research suggested increased remineralization of the tooth surface by application of amorphous calcium phosphate (ACP) and complex casein phosphopeptides (CPP) on the tooth surface (Zero et al. 2009).

These findings were later used in the development of a clinical protocol so named for its purpose: caries management by risk assessment (CAMBRA). The protocol included a form and diagram that would enable the clinician to identify risk factors, disease indicators, and protective factors, which would ultimately determine the level of caries risk for the patient and recommended treatment strategies (Featherstone et al. 2007). An illustration (Figure 3.5.1) assigning acronyms for the three elements included in caries risk assessment (WREC, BAD, SAFE), captures the essence of the disease process and the balance of attenuating factors (Featherstone et al. 2007). The risk factors are tallied and categorized at extreme, high, moderate, or low risk. For example, patients with severe salivary hypofunction are automatically deemed at extreme risk for developing caries and patients with current dental caries are deemed at high risk. Moderate risk includes patients who have some disease indicators and risk factors that without intervention could move into the high-risk category. Low-risk patients have no history of dental caries and whose protective factors outweigh any disease indicators (Table 3.5.2). The patient referenced in this case was found to have interproximal cavitated lesions on radiographs, which would place him in the high-risk category. Existing caries or restorations, along with the observation of white spot lesions, are strong indicators that the likelihood or risk for developing caries will continue to progress (Featherstone et al. 2007).

Once a risk level is identified, the CAMBRA protocol recommends specific therapeutic interventions and strategies (Jenson et al. 2007). Clinical guidelines for patients in the high-risk category are reflected in the Dental Hygiene Care Plan Recommended Interventions for this patient. Guidelines for patients in other risk levels are presented in Table 3.5.3 (Jenson et al. 2007).

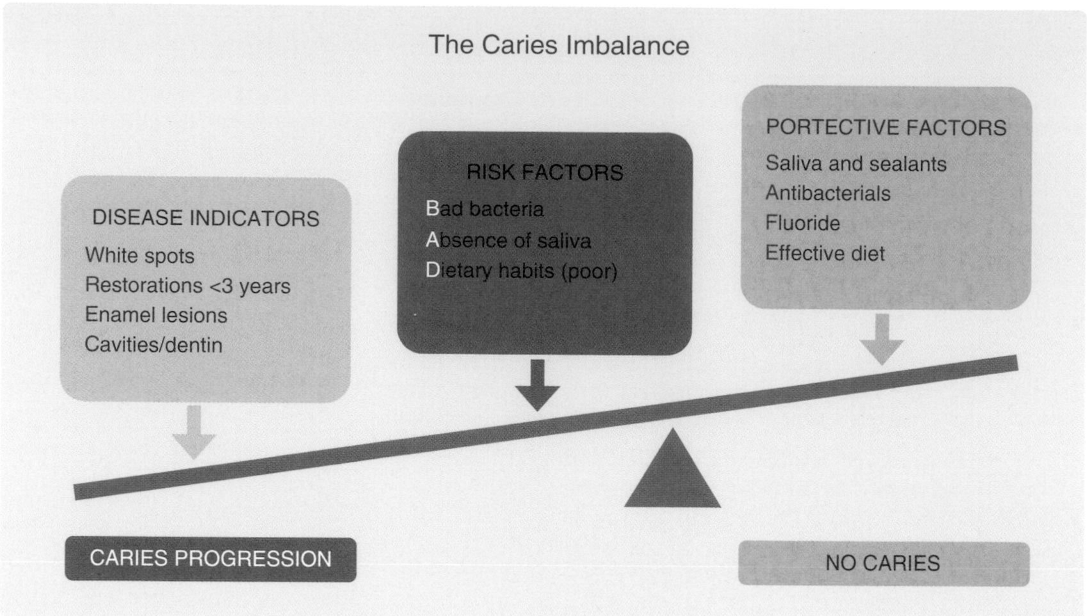

Figure 3.5.1: The caries "imbalance." The balance among disease indicators, risk factors, and protective factors determines whether dental caries progresses, halts, or reverses. Cavities/dentin refers to frank cavities or lesions to the dentin by radiograph. Restorations < three years means restorations placed in the previous three years. This figure has been updated from previous versions of the "caries balance" with the very important addition of the disease indicators. If these indicators are present they weigh heavily on the side of predicting caries progression unless therapeutic intervention is carried out. The abbreviations that help recall of the imbalance (WREC; BAD; SAFE) are shown as well as sealants as a protective factor. Dietary habits (poor) indicate frequent ingestion of fermentable carbohydrates (greater than three times daily between meals). *Source:* Reprinted with permission from the California Dental Association, copyright October 2007.

Research to support or refute the therapeutic interventions recommended in the CAMBRA protocol is ongoing. The clinical efficacy of fluoride and sealants in the prevention of dental caries is well-documented. Definitive clinical evidence to support additional therapeutic strategies, for example, CPP-ACP, xylitol, chlorhexidine, are not confirmed. The clinician must use reasonable care when proposing a treatment plan that is not completely grounded in evidence-based research and weigh the risks, and costs against the benefits for the patient (Jenson et al. 2007; Fontana et al. 2009; Zero et al. 2009). With this in mind, Hurlbutt and Young (2014) provide a literature review of CAMBRA best practices and current research on the efficacy of each of the recommended treatment strategies for the dental hygienist. The traditional caries imbalance graphic is wisely updated to include "Risk Based Reassessment" as a protective factor and offers guidance when research to support clinical efficacy for a marketing claim is not available. A revised CAMBRA clinical protocol (Table 3.5.4) includes these considerations in treatment planning (Hurlbutt and Young 2014).

Take-Home Hints

- The role of the dental hygienist in CAMBRA includes medical history review, risk assessment, radiographs, intraoral photos, saliva assessment and bacterial testing, patient education in biofilm management, and fluoride varnish and sealant application.
- Dental caries is an infectious and communicable disease that is dependent on several variables, each of which can be modulated to arrest further progression or occurrence.
- The most consistent predictor of caries risk in children is past caries experience.
- Salivary gland hypofunction poses an extreme risk for dental caries. Subjective complaints of xerostomia must be corroborated with a differential diagnosis and salivary flow rate test.

Table 3.5.2: Caries Risk Assessment Form — Children Age 6 and Over/Adults. Featherstone et al. (2007).

Patient Name:_____________ Chart #:________________ Date:_____________________
Assessment Date: Is this (please circle) base line or recall

Disease Indicators (Any one "YES" signifies likely "High Risk" and to do a bacteria test)**	**YES = CIRCLE**	**YES = CRCLE**	**YES = CRCLE**
Visible cavities or radiographic penetration of the dentin	YES		
Radiographic approximal enamel lesions (not in dentin)	YES		
White spots on smooth surfaces	YES		
Restorations last three years	YES		
Risk Factors (Biological predisposing factors)			
MS and LB both medium or high (by culture**)		YES	
Visible heavy plaque on teeth		YES	
Frequent snack (> 3x daily between meals)		YES	
Deep pits and fissures		YES	
Recreational drug use		YES	
Inadequate saliva flow by observation or measurement (**If measured note the flow rate below)		YES	
Saliva reducing factors (medications/radiation/systemic)		YES	
Exposed roots		YES	
Orthodontic appliances		YES	
Protective Factors			
Lives/work/school fluoridated community			YES
Fluoride toothpaste at least once daily			YES
Fluoride toothpaste at least 2x daily			YES
Fluoride mouthrinse (0.05% NaF] daily			YES
5000 ppm F fluoride toothpaste daily			YES
Fluoride varnish in last six months			YES
Office F topical in last six months			YES
Chlorhexidine prescribed/used one week each of last six months			YES
Xylitol gum/lozenges four times daily last six months			YES
Calcium and phosphate paste during last six months			YES
Adequate saliva flow (> 1 ml/min stimulated)			YES

****Bacteria/Saliva Test Results: MS: LB; Flow Rate: ml/min. Date:**

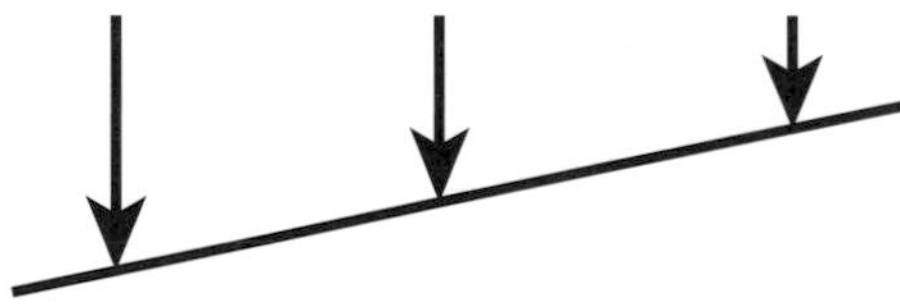

VISUALIZE CARES BALANCE
(Use circled indicators/factors above)
(EXTREME RSK – HIGH RISK + SEVERE SALIVARY GLAND HYPOFUNCTION)
CARIES RISK ASSESSMENT (CIRCLE): EXTREME HIGH MOOERATE LOW
Doctor signature/#:______________________________ Date:________________

Table 3.5.3: Clinical guidelines for patients age six and older. Jenson et al. (2007).

Risk Level[###,***]	Frequency of Radiographs	Frequency of Caries Recall Exams	Saliva Test (Saliva Flow and Bacterial Culture)	Antibacterials Chlorhexidine Xylitol[****]	Fluoride	pH Control	Calcium Phosphate Topical Supplements	Sealants (Resin-based or Glass Ionomer)
Low risk	Bitewing radiographs every 24–36 months	Every 6–12 months to re-evaluate caries risk	May be done as a base line reference for new patients	Per saliva test if done	OTC fluoride-containing toothpaste twice daily, after breakfast and at bedtime. Optional: NaF varnish if excessive root exposure or sensitivity	Not required	Not required Optional: for excessive root exposure or sensitivity	Optional or as per ICDAS sealant protocol (TABLE 2 [in original])
Moderate risk	Bitewing radiographs every 18–24 months	Every 4–6 months to re-evaluate caries risk	May be done as a base line reference for new patients or if there is suspicion of high bacterial challenge and to assess efficacy and patient cooperation	Per saliva test if done Xylitol (6–10 grams/day) gum or candies. Two tabs of gum or two candies four times daily	OTC fluoride-containing toothpaste twice daily plus: 0.05% NaF rinse daily. Initially, 1–2 app of NaF varnish; 1 app at 4–6 month recall	Not required	Not required Optional: for excessive root exposure or sensitivity	As per ICDAS sealant protocol (TABLE 2 [in original])
High risk[*]	Bitewing radiographs every 6–18 months or until no cavitated lesions are evident	Every 3–4 months to re-evaluate caries risk and apply fluoride varnish	Saliva flow test and bacterial culture initially and at every caries recall appt. to assess efficacy and patient cooperation	Chlorhexidine gluconate 0.12% 10 ml rinse for one minute daily for one week each month. Xylitol (6–10 grams/day) gum or candies. Two tabs of gum or two candies four times daily	1.1% NaF toothpaste twice daily instead of regular fluoride toothpaste. Optional: 0.2% NaF rinse daily (1 bottle) then OTC 0.05% NaF rinse 2X daily. Initially, 1–3 app of NaF varnish; 1 app at 3–4 month recall	Not required	Optional: Apply calcium/ phosphate paste several times daily	As per ICDAS sealant protocol (TABLE 2 [in original])
Extreme risk[**] (High risk plus dry mouth or special needs)	Bitewing radiographs every 6 months or until no cavitated lesions are evident	Every 3 months to re-evaluate caries risk and apply fluoride varnish.	Saliva flow test and bacterial culture initially and at every caries recall appt. to assess efficacy and patient cooperation	Chlorhexidine 0.12% (preferably CHX in water base rinse) 10 ml rinse for one minute daily for one week each month. Xylitol (6–10 grams/day) gum or candies. Two tabs of gum or two candies four times daily	1.1% NaF toothpaste twice daily instead of regular fluoride toothpaste. OTC 0.05% NaF rinse when mouth feels dry, after snacking, breakfast and lunch. Initially, 1–3 app. NaF varnish; 1 app at 3 month recall.	Acid-neutralizing rinses as needed if mouth feels dry, after snacking bedtime and after breakfast. Baking soda gum as needed	Required Apply calcium/ phosphate paste twice daily	As per ICDAS sealant protocol (TABLE 2 [in original])

Source: Reprinted with permission of the California Dental Association, copyright October 2007.

[*] Patients with one (or more) cavitated lesion(s) are high-risk patients.

[**] Patients with one (or more) cavitated lesion(s) and severe hyposalivation are extreme-risk patients.

[***] All restorative work to be done with the minimally invasive philosophy in mind. Existing smooth surface lesions that do not penetrate the DEJ and are not cavitated should be treated chemically, not surgically. For extreme-risk patients, use holding care with glass ionomer materials until caries progression is controlled. Patients with appliances (RPDs, prosthodontics) require excellent oral hygiene together with intensive fluoride therapy e.g., high fluoride toothpaste and fluoride varnish every three months. Where indicated, antibacterial therapy to be done in conjunction with restorative work.

[****] Xylitol is not good for pets (especially dogs).

[###] For all risk levels: Patients must maintain good oral hygiene and a diet low in frequency of fermentable carbohydrates.

Table 3.5.4: SAFER Protocol: An example of clinical guidelines based on caries risk for patients 6 years through adult.

	S		A	F		E	R	
Caries Risk Level	**Sealants**	**Saliva**	**Antibacterials**	**Fluoride (Topical)**	**Factors favorable for remineralization (pH, Ca^{2+} & PO_4^{3-})**	**Effective Lifestyle Habits**	**Radiographs**	**Recare Interval**
Low Risk	Not indicated. (Optional for primary prevention of at risk deep pits and fissures).	Saliva testing is optional or may be done for purposes of baseline records.	Not indicated.	OTC fluoride toothpaste used b.i.d.	Recession or sensitive roots may indicate need for supplementation.	Encourage healthy dietary habits, low frequency of fermentable carbohydrates, adequate protein intake & effective oral hygiene practices using motivational interviewing techniques. Substitute xylitol for sucrose.	Every 24–36 months.	Every 6 months.
Moderate Risk		Measure resting and stimulated flow and pH, especially if hypo salivation is suspected.	Xylitol therapy at least 2–3 times/day for a total daily dose of 6–10 grams	OTC fluoride toothpaste used b.i.d. NaF rinse b.i.d. Varnish applied every 4–6 months.	Low resting pH, low stimulated flow or pH may indicate need for supplementation.		Every 18–24 months.	Every 4–6 months.
High Risk	Sealants have been proven to be effective.	Objective measurement of acidogenic bacterial load via culturing or direct measurement of plaque ATP.	It must be understood the evidence is limited for antibacterials and pH neutralization with agents such as chlorhexidine, sodium hypochlorite, povidone iodine, and essential oils. If high levels of acidogenic bacteria are present, using such agents, per manufacturer's instructions, should be monitored closely. Retest bacterial load after initial treatment, discuss and motivate patient, and repeat as needed.	5000 ppm toothpaste used qd or b.i.d. NaF rinse b.i.d. Varnish applied every 3 to 4 months	Consider supplementing if topical fluoride alone is not effective.		Every 6–18 months.	Every 3–4 months.
Extreme Risk					Required if hyposalivation is present.		Every 6 months until no new caries lesions.	Every 3 months.

Source: © Michelle Hurlbutt

Note: Patients with one (or more) cavitated lesion(s) are High Risk patients. Patients with one (or more) cavitated lesion(s) and hyposalivation are Extreme Risk patients. All restorative work to be done with the minimally invasive philosophy in mind. Existing smooth surface lesions that do not significantly penetrate the DEJ and are not cavitated should be treated chemically not surgically. For Extreme Risk patients with multiple cavitations, caries control procedures with glass ionomer materials until caries progression is halted and/or reversed may be used and followed with more permanent restorative care. Patients at risk with appliances (RPDs, Orthodontics) require excellent oral hygiene together with intensive fluoride therapy (e.g. high fluoride toothpaste and fluoride varnish every 3 months). If antibacterial therapy is tried, it should be done in conjunction with fluoride therapy (and every attempt be made not to interfere with the fluoride intervention). A 1-month initial treatment evaluation may be helpful for positive reinforcement. Patients must maintain good oral hygiene (a powered toothbrush may be helpful for High and Extreme Risk patients). A diet low in frequency of fermentable carbohydrates is recommended. It is important to know the amount of xylitol in the product being recommended. Xylitol products should contain 100% xylitol (daily dosages of a total of 6–10 grams across the day for antimicrobial effects).

Self-Study Questions

1. A patient with extensive restorative history, missing teeth, generalized attachment loss, new carious lesions, and salivary hypofunction would be placed into what risk category?
- **A. Low risk**
- **B. Moderate risk**
- **C. High risk**
- **D. Extreme risk**

2. What does the acronym for CAMBRA represent?
- **A. Caries methods by risk assessment**
- **B. Caries mapping by risk assessment**
- **C. Caries maintenance by risk assessment**
- **D. Caries management by risk assessment**

3. When assessing a patients' risk for dental caries using CAMBRA and the risk assessment form (CRA) a single YES under Disease Indicators signifies:
- **A. Likely a moderate risk**
- **B. Likely a low risk**
- **C. Likely a high risk**
- **D. Likely extreme risk**

4. A dental hygienist would recommend to a patient with a moderate risk for dental caries:
- **A. 1.1% NaF toothpaste twice daily**
- **B. 0.05% NaF rinse daily**
- **C. 0.2% NaF rinse daily**
- **D. 0.05% NaF twice daily**

References

CDC.gov. (1999). Achievements in Public Health, 1900–1999: Fluoridation of Drinking Water to Prevent Dental Caries [Online]. Available at: https://www.cdc.gov/mmwr/preview/mmwrhtml/mm4841a1.htm (September 23, 2016).

CDC.gov. (2012). Principles of Epidemiology | Lesson 1 - Section 8 [Online]. Available at: http://www.cdc.gov/OPHSS/CSELS/DSEPD/SS1978/Lesson1/Section8.html#TXT116 (September 25, 2016).

Diagnosis and Management of Dental Caries Throughout Life (2001). *National Institutes of Health consensus development conference statement. Journal of Dental Education* 65 (10): 1162–1168.

Featherstone, J. (2000). The science and practice of caries prevention. *The Journal of the American Dental Association* 131 (7): 887–899.

Featherstone, J., Domejean-Orliaguet, S., Jenson, L. et al. (2007). Caries risk assessment in practice for age 6 through adult. *Journal of the California Dental Association* 35 (10): 703–713.

Fontana, M., Young, D., and Wolff, M. (2009). Evidence-based caries, risk assessment, and treatment. *Dental Clinics of North America* 53 (1): 149–161.

Hurlbutt, M. and Young, D. (2014). A best practices approach to caries management. *The Journal of Evidence-Based Dental Practice* 14: 77–86.

Jenson, L., Burdenz, A., Featherstone, J. et al. (2007). Clinical protocols for caries management by risk assessment. *California Dental Journal* 35 (10): 714–713.

Wilkins, E., Wyche, C., and Boyd, L. (2016). *Clinical Practice of the Dental Hygienist*, 12e, 581. Philadelphia: Wolters Kluwer.

Zero, D., Fontana, M., Martínez-Mier, E. et al. (2009). The biology, prevention, diagnosis and treatment of dental caries. *The Journal of the American Dental Association* 140: 25S–34S.

Answers to Self-Study Questions

1. D. Salivary gland hypofunction poses an extreme risk for dental caries. Subjective complaints of xerostomia must be corroborated with a differential diagnosis and salivary flow rate test.

2. D. Caries Management by Risk Assessment (CAMBRA).

3. C. Refer to Table 3.5.2.

4. B. Refer to Table 3.5.3.

4

Nonsurgical Periodontal Procedures

Clinical Cases in Dental Hygiene, First Edition. Edited by Cheryl M. Westphal Theile, Mea A. Weinberg and Stuart L. Segelnick.

Case 1

Periodontal Debridement (Hand, Ultrasonic, Sonic Instrumentation)

CASE STORY
A 38-year-old female presents with the chief complaint "I need a cleaning." She complains of pain and bleeding while brushing.

PROBLEM-BASED LEARNING GOALS AND OBJECTIVES

- Identify the need for nonsurgical periodontal therapy based on the periodontal assessment
- Recommend appropriate dental hygiene interventions based on key factors including probing depths, extent of calculus present, root anatomy, and patient factors such as need for topical anesthesia, local anesthesia, and/or use of nitrous oxide
- Recognize possible effects of improper instrumentation
- Select correct instruments for nonsurgical periodontal instrumentation

Dental History

The patient's last dental examination, prophylaxis, and radiographic assessment occurred five years ago. The patient states she is dental phobic. Currently the patient brushes once daily with a manual, soft-bristled toothbrush and does not use any interdental aides.

Medical History

The patient and is currently breastfeeding after giving birth six months ago. She is in good health, taking no medications at this time. She reports no known allergies.

- Vital Signs:
- Blood pressure: 130/70 mmHg
- Pulse: 74 beats/min
- Respiratory Rate: 15 breaths/min

Social History

The patient is a nonsmoker and reports never using tobacco products. She drinks socially, having two to four glasses of wine per week. Her current diet includes starchy vegetables, carbohydrate rich foods, and caffeinated soda to help her stay awake and have energy for her newborn baby.

Dental Examination

The extra- and intraoral examinations are within normal limits. The gingival examination reveals bright red, shiny gingiva with generalized moderate inflammation, and bleeding on probing for all sites. The gingival margins on the maxillary anterior sextant are rolled with blunted papilla between teeth #8 and #9. There is heavy generalized supragingival biofilm and calculus accumulation with heavy interproximal subgingival calculus in all posterior quadrants. Probing depths range from 3–5 mm. Localized gingival recession is present on the facial of #22 and #27. No tooth mobility or furcation involvement is detected.

Radiographic Examination

Radiographs reveal slight generalized horizontal bone loss with a slight vertical bony defect on the mesial of tooth #31. Interproximal calculus appears radiographically in all four quadrants (see Figures 4.1.1, 4.1.2, 4.1.3, and 4.1.4).

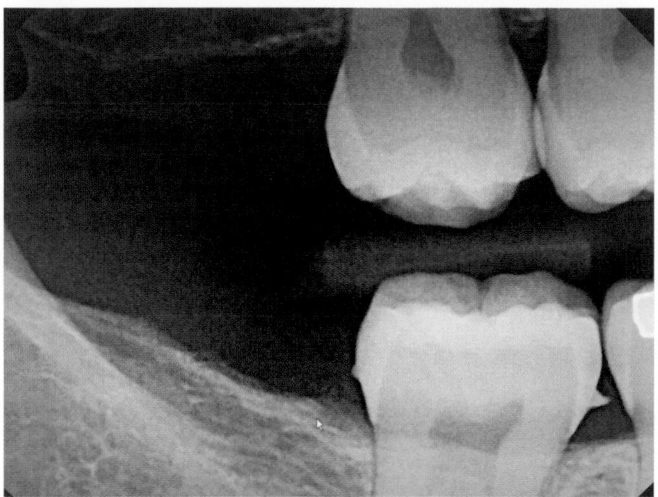

Figure 4.1.1: Radiograph showing heavy subgingival calculus deposits #31 – Mesial.

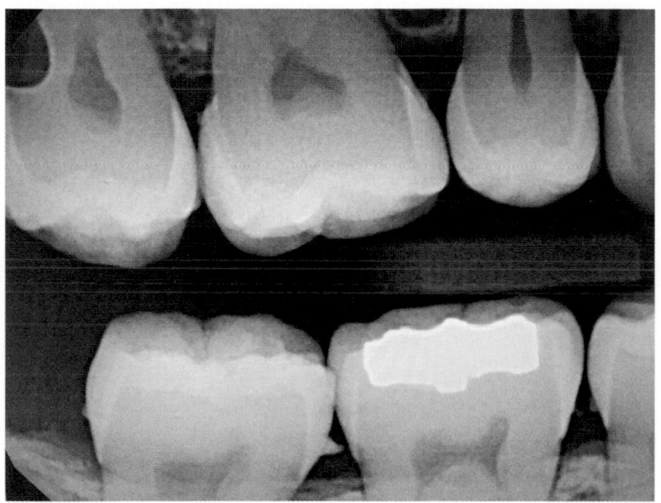

Figure 4.1.2: Bitewing radiograph of right side showing heavy interproximal subgingival calculus deposits.

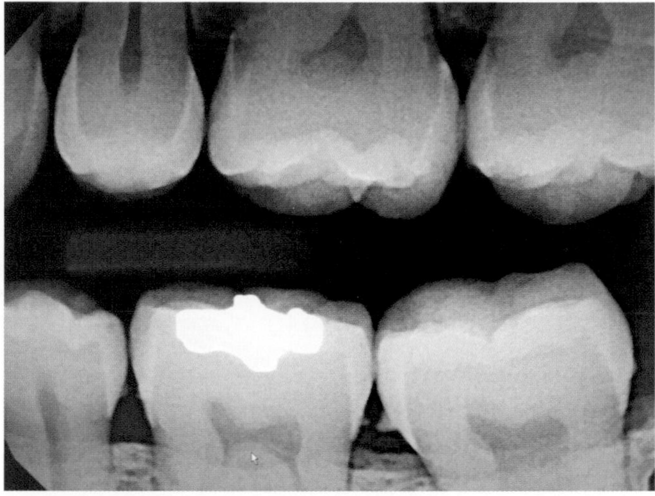

Figure 4.1.3: Bitewing radiograph of left side showing heavy interproximal subgingival calculus deposits. Note the slight periodontal ligament widening on the distal of the maxillary premolar.

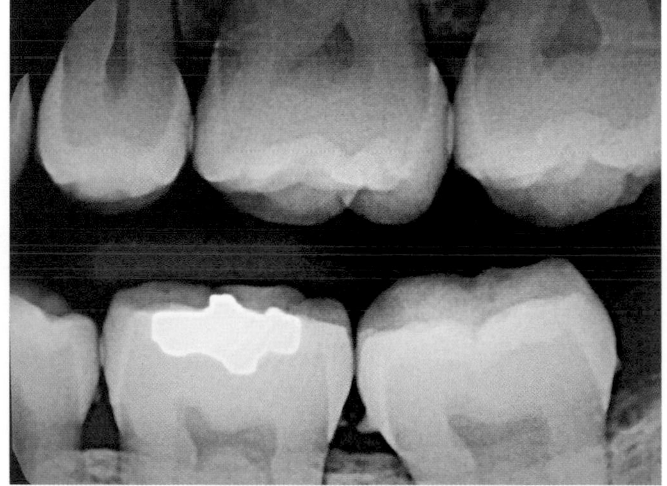

Figure 4.1.4: Bitewing radiograph of left side showing heavy interproximal calculus.

Dental Hygiene Diagnosis

Problems	Related Etiology
Increased risk for periodontal disease	Dental neglect; moderate biofilm; once daily brushing without interproximal aids. heavy interproximal calculus, bleeding upon probing, and probing depths >4 mm existing in all quadrants
Increased risk for caries	Irregular dental care, starchy and carbohydrate diet, and soda
Generalized gingival sensitivity and possible gingival recession post-dental hygiene treatment	Gingival inflammation related to biofilm accumulation, lack of proper oral hygiene instruction (OHI) and homecare

Planned Dental Hygiene Interventions

Clinical	Education	Oral Hygiene Instruction
Four quadrants scaling and root planing with ultrasonic and hand instrumentation Use of local anesthesia and nitrous oxide for pain management and ease dental anxiety Four to eight week (Segelnick and Weinberg 2006) re-evaluation of periodontal tissue and probing depths Three to four month periodontal maintenance appointments	Progression and etiology of periodontal disease Increased risk for dental caries Nutritional Counseling Reinforce importance of regular dental visits Educate on techniques available to ease patient anxiety for future treatments Follow-up/review of OHI	Electric, battery powered, or manual toothbrush with emphasis on two-minute brushing at least twice daily C-shaped flossing or use of a floss handle for interdental cleaning or other interdental aides per patient preference Use of antimicrobial rinse twice daily Healthy snacks and beverages

Progress Notes

During her initial visit the patient was instructed on plaque control and oral hygiene home care. The patient brushed only once daily and did not use interproximal cleaning aids at the initial visit. An electric toothbrush with a two minute timer or a manual toothbrush for twice daily use was recommended for plaque control. Thin, waxed floss and a floss handle for improved access to posterior interproximal areas was provided and the patient was instructed with c-shaped flossing technique. Use of a 0.12% chlorhexidine rinse was recommended twice daily after completion of scaling and root planing for two weeks. The patient consented to four quadrants of scaling and root planing with local anesthesia and nitrous oxide for pain and anxiety control. A three-to-four month maintenance recall was recommended upon completion of nonsurgical periodontal treatment. The patient appeared motivated to continue with efforts for further improvement of her oral health.

Discussion

The patient presents with generalized moderate biofilm, supra, and heavy interproximal subgingival calculus located in all four posterior quadrants. Upon effective removal of calculus and biofilm, and considering no tooth mobility, lack of furcation involvement, nonsmoking history, and a positively motivated patient, the periodontal prognosis for this patient is favorable.

The goal of periodontal instrumentation includes the removal of plaque and calculus, the elimination of bleeding upon probing, reduction in probing depths, reduction of inflammation, improvement in gingival health and appearance, and resolution of patient discomfort (Carnio et al. 2015; Kumar 2015). Any biofilm or calculus remaining on a tooth's surface may increase the risk for future plaque retention and increased risk for attachment loss (Aspriello et al. 2011; Krishna and De Stefano 2016). Effective nonsurgical periodontal therapy involves the combination of both manual and ultrasonic instrumentation, including the selection of appropriate instruments. These depend upon periodontal probing depths, amount of calculus, and biofilm present, detection of root surface irregularities prior to scaling, and radiographic interpretation of tooth and root anatomy (Carnio et al. 2015; Krishna and De Stefano 2016; Kumar 2015; Wilkins 2009). Consideration of all of these factors prior to instrumentation allows the clinician to minimize risk for potential periodontal abscess formation and any alteration to the root surface structure. Years of inappropriate instrumentation and minor tooth structure removal may create cumulative damage to the root increasing the rate of plaque retention and toxin formation (Kumar 2015, p. 56). A number of factors contribute to root surface roughness including the type of ultrasonic tip, curette tip design, force applied, angulation, and duration of instrumentation (Henchman et al. 2016; Kumar 2015).

Manual instrumentation for scaling and root planing is the established protocol for successful treatment of periodontal disease and dental caries. This protocol provides the advantage of better instrument control and tactile perception for the clinician (Henchman et al. 2016; Kumar 2015). Universal curets, depending on their design, may be used in all areas of the mouth for scaling and root planing (Darby and Walsh 2003, p. 387). Area specific curets may be used in all areas of the mouth, but the clinician must assess the specific design for use on anterior versus posterior surfaces (Darby and

Walsh 2003, p. 387). In general the more acute the angle and the greater the number of bends, the more access the instrument provides for posterior teeth (Darby and Walsh 2003, p. 387). A key to effective instrumentation includes the sharpness of an instrument's cutting edge, with sharp instruments providing the clinician with more tactile sensitivity, more control for working efficiency and lateral pressure, and increased patient comfort (Darby and Walsh 2003, p. 397). Sharpening instruments at the first sign of dullness helps to ensure blade effectiveness while preserving the original contours and design (Darby and Walsh 2003, p. 396). Once appropriate instruments are selected, the clinician chooses the correct working end for nonsurgical manual instrumentation. For ideal calculus and biofilm removal, the angulation of the blade adapts from 45° to 90° with the tooth's surface (Darby and Walsh 2003, p. 394). A more open angulation is recommended for a smoothing, root planing stroke, while a closer angulation grabs the root surface for heavy deposit removal (Darby and Walsh 2003, p. 394). However, manual instrumentation is timely, skill dependent, and with limitations when utilized in deep periodontal pockets or hard to navigate furcation areas (Henchman et al. 2016; Kumar 2015; Wilkins 2009).

Ultrasonic and power instrumentation provides less fatigue to the operator while effectively removing dental debris from difficult to reach areas (Kumar 2015; Wilkins 2009). The three modes of action for power instrumentation include mechanical action, cavitation, and acoustic mainstreaming (Darby and Walsh 2003, p. 473). The types of ultrasonic instrumentation, magnetostrictive and piezoelectric, refer to the range of acoustical vibrations that are a unit of frequency referred to as cycles per second (Darby and Walsh 2003, p. 474). Magnetostricitve tips act with alternating electromagnetic fields causing the tip of the insert to vibrate in an elliptical or orbital motion (Darby and Walsh 2003, p. 476). The piezoelectric units differ in that vibration occurs when alternating currents are applied to the transducer, creating a dimensional change transmitted to the tip where the tip moves in a linear pattern with only two sides of the tip activated to the adapted tooth surface (Darby and Walsh 2003, p. 481). Effective power and ultrasonic instrumentation requires deliberate, multidirectional strokes, keeping the tip constantly moving (Henchman et al. 2016, p. 137). Overlapping vertical, horizontal, and oblique strokes, in a cross-hatching pattern and working circumferentially allow for effective removal of pathogens (Henchman et al. 2016, p. 137). A power or ultrasonic insert designed for subgingival periodontal debridement has a tip that is 40–47% thinner than the standard diameter tip with a longer shank that can reach 1 mm deeper than hand instruments, into subgingival areas, furcations, root concavities, and interproximal areas (Henchman et al. 2016, p. 136).

After complete patient assessment, the suggested treatment for nonsurgical periodontal instrumentation begins with use of the ultrasonic or other power driven scaler on high to medium power to remove heavy calculus deposits, moving to thinner insert tips on lower power settings for residual deposits and biofilm removal (Henchman et al. 2016; Wilkins 2009). The use of multidirectional, short overlapping strokes using vertical, horizontal, and oblique motions in a cross-hatching pattern on the entire surface of tooth and root structure is necessary for removal of biofilm pathogens (Henchman et al. 2016, p. 137). The lavage and mechanical vibrations in addition to the use of ultrasonic scalers, act to disrupt biofilm and flush endotoxins from the sulcus (Henchman et al. 2016, p. 136). When debriding moderate to heavy supragingival calculus, a heavy insert tip set on moderate to high power allows for proper fragmenting of heavy calculus deposits (Henchman et al. 2016; Wilkins 2009). If used on a low setting, the heavy insert becomes more likely to burnish calculus or damage the existing tooth structure. Slim insert tips used on low to medium power are able to reach 1 mm deeper into subgingival pockets, furcations, and root concavities than hand instruments (Henchman et al. 2016, p. 136). When choosing an ultrasonic tip insert for instrumentation the clinician must adjust the power setting accordingly.

Take-Home Hints

1. Effective removal of biofilm and calculus accumulation is necessary for successful nonsurgical periodontal therapy.
2. Ultrasonic or power driven scaler tips used on the incorrect power setting may damage existing tooth structure.
3. Goals for selecting appropriate instrumentation techniques include minimizing risks for root structure damage and improving tissue health.
4. Manual instrumentation provides greater instrument control and tactile sensitivity but is clinician skill dependent.

Self-Study Questions

1. True or False: Manual instrumentation provides less clinician fatigue and better access to difficult to reach areas such as furcations.

A. True

B. False

2. Prior to manual or power-driven instrumentation, periodontal probing depths and radiographs must be used as a guide by the clinician. Identifying the level of calculus, root irregularities, and furcation involvement prior to scaling allows the clinician to select the proper curets and tips for instrumentation.

A. Both statements are true.

B. Both statements are false.

C. The first statement is false. The second statement is true.

D. The first statement is true. The second statement is false.

3. Cumulative damage may occur to the tooth structure from years of improper instrumentation. Damage to the root surface increases plaque retention and toxin formation to the root surface.

A. Both statements are true.

B. Both statements are false.

C. The first statement is false. The second statement is true.

D. The first statement is true. The second statement is false.

4. All of the following strokes are part of proper instrumentation for subgingival scaling except one. Which one is the exception?

A. Oblique

B. Vertical

C. Parallel

D. Horizontal

5. Slim ultrasonic tips are used on a medium to high setting only for moderate to heavy supragingival calculus. Thinner, longer ultrasonic, or power-scaler tips provide better access to subgingival surfaces in periodontal pockets.

A. Both statements are false.

B. The first statement is false. The second statement is true.

C. The first statement is true. The second statement is false.

D. Both statements are true.

References

Aspriello, S., Piemontese, M., Levrini, L., and Sauro, S. (2011). Ultra morphology of the root surface subsequent to hand-ultrasonic simultaneous instrumentation during non-surgical periodontal treatments: an *in vitro* study. *Journal of Applied Oral Science* 19 (1): 74–81.

Bower, R. (1979). Furcation morphology relative to periodontal treatment: furcation entrance architecture. *Journal of Periodontology* 50 (1): 23–27.

Carnio, J., Moreira, A., Jenny, T. et al. (2015). Nonsurgical periodontal therapy to treat a case of severe periodontitis. *The Journal of the American Dental Association* 146 (8): 631–637.

Darby, M. and Walsh, M. (2003). *Dental Hygiene Theory and Practice*, 2e. Philadelphia: W.B. Saunders.

Henchman, S., Funk, A., Debiase, C., and Frere, C. (2016). Ultrasonic instrumentation instruction in dental hygiene programs in the United States. *The Journal of Dental Hygiene* 90 (2): 135–141.

Krishna, R. and De Stefano, J. (2016). Ultrasonic vs. hand instrumentation in periodontal therapy: clinical outcomes. *Periodontology 2000* 71 (1): 113–127.

Kumar, P. (2015). Comparison of root surface roughness produced by hand instruments and ultrasonic scalers: an invitro study. *Journal of Clinical and Diagnostic Research* 9 (11): ZC56–ZC60.

Segelnick, S. and Weinberg, M. (2006). Reevaluation of initial therapy: when is the appropriate time? *Journal of Periodontology* 77 (9): 1598–1601.

Wilkins, E. (2009). *Clinical Practice of the Dental Hygienist*. Philadelphia: Wolters Kluwer Health/Lippincott Williams & Wilkins.

Answers to Self-Study Questions

1. False/B. Manual instrumentation provides greater instrument control and tactile sensitivity, but ultrasonic instrumentation provides less user fatigue and better access to difficult areas such as furcations and root concavities. Slim insert ultrasonic tips are able to reach 1 mm further subgingivally.

2. A. Periodontal probing depth charting and radiographs provide a guide for instrumentation for biofilm and calculus removal. Prior to scaling, use of a subgingival explorer allows the clinician to identify the location and level of calculus, root surface irregularities and furcations. After this assessment the clinician will be able to select the proper instruments and ultrasonic tip inserts for successful instrumentation.

3. A. Years of improper instrumentation and minor tooth structure removal may cause root surface irregularities. These irregularities may increase plaque retention and toxin formation.

4. C. Directional strokes for scaling include vertical, oblique, and horizontal strokes done in an overlapping, crosshatching motion. Universal curets, depending on their design, may be used in all areas of the mouth for scaling and root planing. Area specific curets may be used in all areas of the mouth but, the clinician must assess the specific design for use on anterior versus posterior surfaces. For calculus and biofilm removal, the angulation of the blade adapts from 45° to 90° with the tooth's surface. Effective instrumentation by the clinician includes the sharpness of an instrument's cutting edge, with sharp instruments providing the clinician with more tactile sensitivity, more control for working efficiency and lateral pressure, and increased patient comfort.

5. B. Thin ultrasonic tip inserts are used on low to medium settings for residual calculus and biofilm. Insert tips used on the incorrect power setting may lead to burnished calculus or damage to tooth structure. Thinner, narrower ultrasonic or power tips allow for better access to deeper subgingival periodontal pockets. Since the average furcation entrance is 0.7 mm or less 58% of the time, and the average curette width is 0.75 mm, the curette will not enter most furcations (Bower 1979). A power or ultrasonic insert designed for subgingival periodontal debridement has a tip that is 40–47% thinner than the standard diameter tip with a longer shank that can reach 1 mm deeper than hand instruments, into subgingival areas, furcations, root concavities, and interproximal areas. The modes of action for power instrumentation include mechanical action, cavitation, and acoustic mainstreaming. Magnetostricitve tips act with alternating electromagnetic fields causing the tip of the insert to vibrate in an elliptical or orbital motion. The piezoelectric units differ in that vibration occurs when alternating currents are applied to the transducer, creating a dimensional change transmitted to the tip where the tip moves in a linear pattern with only two sides of the tip activated to the adapted tooth surface.

Case 2

Reassessment and Maintenance

CASE STORY

A 61-year-old female with a history of surgical and nonsurgical treatment of periodontal disease presents for evaluation.

PROBLEM-BASED LEARNING GOALS AND OBJECTIVES

- Describe evaluation and assessment after initial dental hygiene treatment such as scaling and root planing
- Determine key indicators for evaluating oral health goals set forth for each patient within the dental hygiene care plan
- Create individualized maintenance plan for patient dependent upon patient's individual needs
- Understand contributing factors to recurring periodontal disease

Dental History

After years of undergoing periodontal treatment, the patient states that she does not want to return to a specialist, does not want periodontal surgery and is "just looking to maintain" her periodontal condition. The patient has a history of both surgical and nonsurgical periodontal treatments, with the most recent scaling and root planing completed in 2012 on the upper right (UR) and upper left (UL) quadrants. She complains of bleeding and food trapping between implant tooth #12 and a mesial-occlusal (MO) restoration on #13.

Medical History

The patient is being treated for type I diabetes and hypothyroidism. Both conditions are controlled. She sees her physician regularly and takes her medications as prescribed. No known allergies reported.

- Medications
  - Novolog 100 units/mL,
  - Januvia 100 mg, and
  - levothyroxine (Synthroid)100mcg
- Vital Signs:
  - Blood pressure: 135/80 mmHg
  - Pulse: 70 beats/min
  - Respiration: 14 breaths/min
  - A1C (glycosylated hemoglobin test): 7

Social History

The patient reports a history of smoking as a teenager. She states currently no tobacco or alcohol use. The patient works full time and prefers her appointments to be scheduled early in the morning after finishing work.

Dental Examination

Extraoral examination and intraoral soft tissue examination are within normal limits. The gingival examination reveals moderate facial inflammation, an implant crown replacing tooth #7 and crown on #8. The remaining gingiva on the maxillary arch is light pink, stippled with 4–5 mm gingival recession on both facial and lingual aspects. Bleeding on probing occurs on all surfaces of tooth #8 and tooth #13. The patient presents with light generalized interproximal plaque accumulation. Moderate localized subgingival calculus is present on #8 distal lingual and distal facial surfaces. The deepest probing depth on this tooth is an 8 mm pocket on the distal surface measured from both the facial and lingual. Threads of the adjacent implant replacing tooth #7 are detectable from the mesial surface with a plastic probe. A large open contact exists between implant replacing tooth #12 and #13 MO restoration. Tooth #15 presents

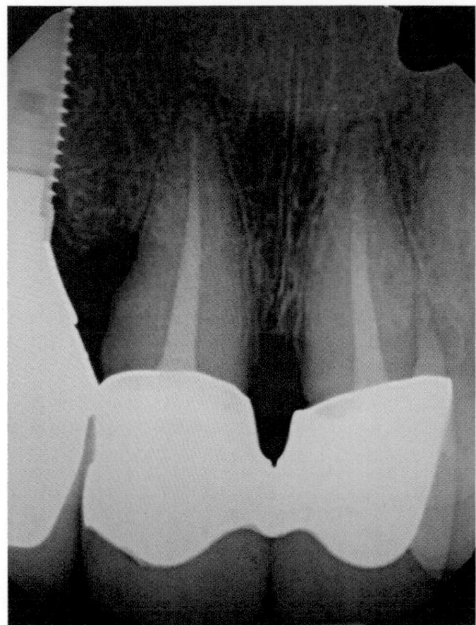

Figure 4.2.1: Radiograph showing severe bone loss between #7 and 8.

with Class III mobility. The patient currently uses a power toothbrush twice daily and interdental brushes three to four times per week.

Radiographic Examination

Generalized moderate to severe horizontal bone loss is present on the maxillary arch (see Figure 4.2.1). A severe vertical bony defect is present on #8 distal and #7 mesial. Implants replace teeth #5 and #7 (see Figure 4.2.2) and #12.

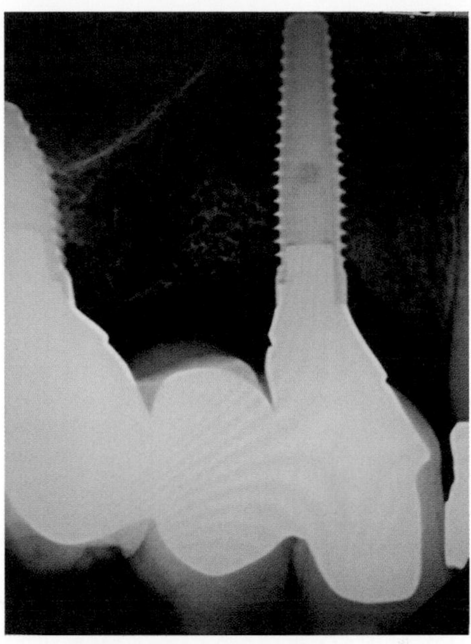

Figure 4.2.2: Implant supported bridge for teeth #5 to #7. Note the vertical bone loss occurring on the mesial of implant #7.

Dental Hygiene Diagnosis

Problems	Related Etiology
Increased periodontal disease	Systemic relationship with type I diabetes; irregular recare and dental maintenance
Root caries and sensitivity	Loss of clinical attachment due to surgical and nonsurgical periodontal procedures
Xerostomia	Medication use and type I Diabetes
Bleeding upon probing	Generalized biofilm accumulation, localized subgingival calculus, open contact between restorations

Planned Dental Hygiene Interventions:

Clinical	Education	Oral Hygiene Instruction
Review most recent HBAC1 (glycated hemoglobin) level at each visit; review medical history; ensure patient ate prior to the appointment Selective scaling and root planing implant #7 and tooth #8 with ultrasonic, hand instrumentation, and plastic implant scalers and plastic tipped ultrasonic insert Subgingival placement of minocycline HCl, 1 mg (Arestin) tooth #8 Periodontal maintenance of remaining dentition Four to eight week re-evaluation #7 and #8 5% fluoride varnish on exposed root surfaces Three-month periodontal maintenance	Systemic relationship between diabetes and periodontal disease (wound healing) Stress the importance of regular medical evaluations for control of systemic diseases Educate on healthy lifestyle, diet, and exercise Increased susceptibility for caries and root sensitivity due to exposed root surfaces Educate on proper biofilm control for natural and implant supported teeth Educate on the benefits of periodontal nonsurgical therapy Educate on importance and necessity of frequent dental recall visits for periodontal maintenance Explain benefits of varnish	Modified Stillman's technique at least twice daily with manual or powered tooth brush Interdental brushes and waxed or unwaxed floss with floss threaders for removal of debris under the bridge. Use of saliva substitute oral rinse twice daily and additional saliva substitute products as needed for xerostomia Use of fluoridated toothpaste or a desensitizing toothpaste Provide instruction post fluoride varnish application Use of oral irrigator for removal of food particles from interproximal areas.

Progress Notes

The patient presents with advanced periodontal disease and a history of surgical and nonsurgical periodontal therapies. There is severe vertical bone loss and active localized periodontal disease on tooth #8. The patient prefers to forego further surgical procedures and commits to periodontal maintenance. She currently brushes two to three times per day, alternating between electric and manual toothbrushes. She uses interproximal brushes for interdental cleaning and rinses occasionally with an antimicrobial rinse. Upon initial oral hygiene instructions, the use of oral irrigation in addition to use of interproximal brushes and floss threaders is recommended for daily use for cleaning under her bridge and implant bridge areas. The patient is informed on the systemic relationship between periodontal disease and diabetes, as it relates to creating a viable dental hygiene maintenance program.

Discussion

Initial assessment includes medical history, dental history, social history radiographic interpretation and clinical findings (See Figure 4.2.3). Considering all of these factors allows the clinician to create a viable care plan and maintenance plan for continuing care and optimal oral health (Costa et al. 2015, p. 2). Factors contributing to maintenance planning include risk for periodontal disease activity, risk for caries, risk for oral

Review Medical History

- Evaluate current state of health
- Assess any changes
- Vital Signs
- Systemic diseases controlled

Poor health or uncontrolled systemic disease = defer tx and refer

Intra/Extraoral Examination

- Assess increased risks for oral cancer
- Tobacco/Alcohol/Drug use (current use or hx of)
- Evaluation of other oral conditions (xerostomia, candidiasis, atrophy of papilla)

Dental Assessment

- Caries Risk
- Plaque Retentive Factors (defective restorations, overhangs, open contacts, etc)
- Radiographic Assessment

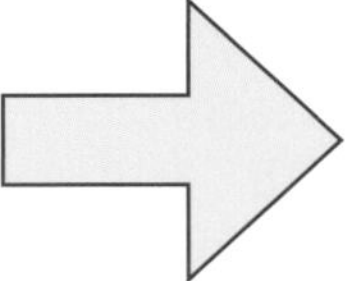

Number and frequency of radiographs taken are based on the patient's risk factors/ needs at the dentist's discretion

Periodontal Assessment

- Periodontal Charting (probing depths, bleeding sites, presence of exudate)
- Gingival Assessment (size, shape, consistency)
- Plaque Index
- Furcation Involvement
- Tooth mobility

Oral Hygiene Assessment

- Current state of oral hygiene health
- Relationship of biofilm present to patient's ability to remove
- Adherence and compliance to recommended dental hygiene care plan

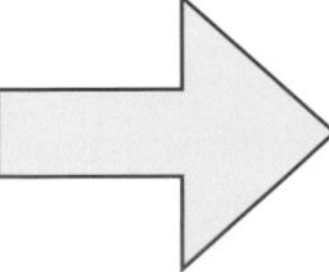

Patient must act as co-therapist for successful maintenance and dental hygiene care

Figure 4.2.3: Reassessment and maintenance for dental hygiene process of care.

cancers, predisposing conditions such as HIV/AIDS, history of dental treatments, ability for biofilm control, and compliance (Wilkins 2009, pp. 755–757). Current guidelines for maintenance of implants and implant restorations are not clearly defined or based on recommendations for patients with natural dentitions rather than what is best for implant maintenance and supporting tissues (Bidra et al. 2015, p. 61). Often patient compliance becomes a key obstacle in both appointment scheduling and biofilm control (Costa et al. 2015; Wilkins 2009). Neglect of regular recare appointments is associated with a higher risk of recurrence and progression of periodontitis (Costa et al. 2015, p. 2). Studies observing the progression of periodontal disease note the cumulative nature of the disease over time (Bidra et al. 2015, p. 61).

"Numerous numbers of pathogens may be left in the oral environment after instrumentation. Repopulation of these may occur within 60 days after periodontal debridement. Periodontal pathogens also populate the oral environment in areas such as the tongue, tonsils, saliva and buccal mucosa, and other non-periodontal sites. The overall treatment must consider the possibility that these sites may be responsible for reinfection. There have been some chemical agents shown to be effective in suppressing dental plaque when used with periodontal debridement and surgery. It is known today that periodontal diseases are infectious diseases and treatment is focused on the reduction and the removal of specific bacteria. Antimicrobial products may be utilized as additional agents but not replacement of non-surgical or surgical procedures. It is not the therapist's goal to eliminate all oral bacteria, as many bacteria living in the oral environment are beneficial." (Weinberg et al. 2015, p. 334)

The primary risk factor for failure of an implant is attributed to certain bacteria. The loss of an implant may occur from a bacterial infection caused by the repopulation of bacteria around the implant after being successfully placed (Weinberg et al. 2015, p. 131). The term used to describe soft-tissue inflammation around an implant is known as peri-implant mucositis. The term used to describe the inflammation of soft and hard tissue around an implant leading to bone loss is called peri-implantitis. The treatment for this disease may include periodontal instrumentation, individualized instruction for oral hygiene, rinses, systemic antibiotics, peri-implant surgery, or implant removal as a last resort (Weinberg et al. 2015, p. 131). Patients with complex tooth- and implant-borne restorations, as the patient above in this case study (2), require long term professional individualized care and recall regimens for long-term success (Bidra et al. 2015, p. 61).

For scaling and plaque removal around dental implant surfaces the clinician chooses from plastic or Teflon-coated manual instruments and/or plastic tipped power instruments approved for implant use (Darby and Walsh 2003, p. 1038). Metal instruments, metal power instruments, or abrasive air polishers may scratch or form irregularities on the implant surface and should not be used on dental implants (Darby and Walsh 2003, p. 1038). Titanium scalers can be used. Periodontal probes may be used for assessment around the dental implant but should be used with caution so as to not disrupt the biologic seal (Darby and Walsh 2003, p. 1038).

Take-Home Hints

1. A patient's ongoing compliance is required for successful maintenance.
2. Metal instruments are not recommended for dental implants because they may damage the surface of the implant.
3. Control of systemic diseases is necessary for optimal oral health.
4. Gingival assessment, periodontal probing, and plaque indices allow the clinician to evaluate patient progress at maintenance appointments.

Self-Study Questions

1. True or False: After scaling and root planing for a patient with controlled diabetes the appropriate recall interval is always scheduled for six months.
- **A. True**
- **B. False**

2. Which of the following are contributing factors for recurring periodontal disease?
- **A. Systemic diseases**
- **B. Lack of patient compliance**
- **C. Insufficient plaque control**
- **D. Faulty restorations**
- **E. All of the above**

3. After scaling and root planing is completed, the progression of disease stops and does not recur. Dental hygiene maintenance intervals may fluctuate based on a variety of factors including any disease progression.
- **A. Both statements are true.**
- **B. The first statement is true and the second statement is false.**
- **C. The first statement is false and the second statement is true.**
- **D. Both statements are false.**

4. True or False. Plastic and titanium instruments and plastic-tip power instrumentation inserts maybe used on dental implants.
- **A. True**
- **B. False**

5. True or False: Inflammation and bacterial repopulation around an implant after successful placement may ultimately cause the implant to fail.
- **A. True**
- **B. False**

References

Bidra, A., Daubert, D., Garcia, L. et al. (2015). Clinical practice guidelines for recall and maintenance of patients with tooth-borne and implant-borne dental restorations. *Journal of Prosthodontics* 25 (S1): S32–S40.

Costa, F., Cota, L., Cortelli, J. et al. (2015). Surgical and non-surgical procedures associated with recurrence of periodontitis in periodontal maintenance therapy: 5-year prospective study. *PLoS One* 10 (10): e0140847.

Darby, M. and Walsh, M. (2003). *Dental Hygiene Theory and Practice*, 2e. Philadelphia: W.B. Saunders.

Weinberg, M., Westphal Thiele, C., From, S., and Segelnick, S. (2015). *Comprehensive Periodontics for the Dental Hygienist*, 4e. Upper Saddle River, N.J: Pearson Education.

Wilkins, E. (2009). *Clinical Practice of the Dental Hygienist.* Philadelphia: Wolters Kluwer Health/Lippincott Williams & Wilkins.

Answers to Self-Study Questions

1. False/B. There is no set recall interval for patients. An optimal maintenance program evaluates the individual needs of each patient. The patient's medical history, social history, periodontal examination, radiographic examination, and goals set forth in the dental hygiene care plan determine the recall interval.

2. E. The recurrence of periodontal disease includes systemic diseases such as diabetes or HIV, lack of patient compliance either in keeping appointments or biofilm control, insufficient plaque control from lack of patient motivation or lack of patient's manual ability, or faulty restorations.

3. C. Nonsurgical dental hygiene treatment may arrest the progression of disease, but the patient must be educated to understand the possibility of recurrence of periodontal disease and the importance for compliance and maintenance. The maintenance schedule interval is based on numerous factors including any signs of disease progression.

4. True/A. Metal instruments are not recommended for dental implants because they may damage the surface of the implant.

5. True/A. Inflammation around an implant due to bacterial repopulation may lead to failure of the implant.

Case 3

Oral Hygiene Instruction with Limited Dexterity

CASE STORY

A 59-year-old female presents at the dental office for complete dental evaluation and states, "I feel like some of my teeth are loose." One year ago the patient suffered a spinal cord injury, seriously damaging her C5 and C6 vertebrae. She uses a walker for balance, has moderate functioning level, with limited mobility on the right side of the body. A home health aid is present with the patient and helps her with household duties three to four days a week. The patient states that prior to her accident she was physically fit and active. She was an avid runner, swimmer, and tennis player and states she had no health or dental problems, and only visited health-care providers when she experienced pain.

PROBLEM-BASED LEARNING GOALS AND OBJECTIVES

- Identify potential barriers to patient care when creating plan for oral hygiene instruction after nonsurgical periodontal therapy
- Create a dental hygiene instruction plan to include the patient and caregivers as cotherapists
- Identify when changes in oral hygiene educational instruction are necessary
- Provide positive feedback and instruction for the patient

Dental History

The patient reports no dental treatment for at least five years. Unless she experienced pain or discomfort, the patient did not routinely seek dental care. She brushes one to two times per day with a powered toothbrush and occasionally uses waxed floss for interproximal cleaning. Since noticing tooth mobility, the patient avoids chewing on her right side.

Medical History

One year ago the patient suffered a spinal cord injury after a car accident. The accident left the patient paralyzed from the chest down due to injury to the C5 and C6 vertebrae. After intense physical and occupational therapy, the patient has regained some of her mobility with the use of a walker. She currently takes no medication, but following her accident she was prescribed and took corticosteroids for inflammation of the spinal cord caused by the accident. She continues to receive physical and occupational therapy. She reports no known allergies.

- Vital Signs:
  - Blood pressure: 124/ 76 mmHg
  - Pulse: 68 beats/min
  - Respiration: 14 beats/min

Social History

The patient is a nonsmoker and reports no prior tobacco use. She consumes alcohol occasionally, having one to two drinks a week. Prior to her accident she was physically active. She ran three to four times a week, swam, and played tennis. Currently, she swims for exercise during her physical therapy sessions and continues to work with occupational therapists focusing on improvement with her manual dexterity. The patient runs a small business from her home and has not returned to previous full-time employment due to her limited mobility. The patient who claims to be a lover of sweets, often snacks on a variety of candy and chocolate treats throughout the day.

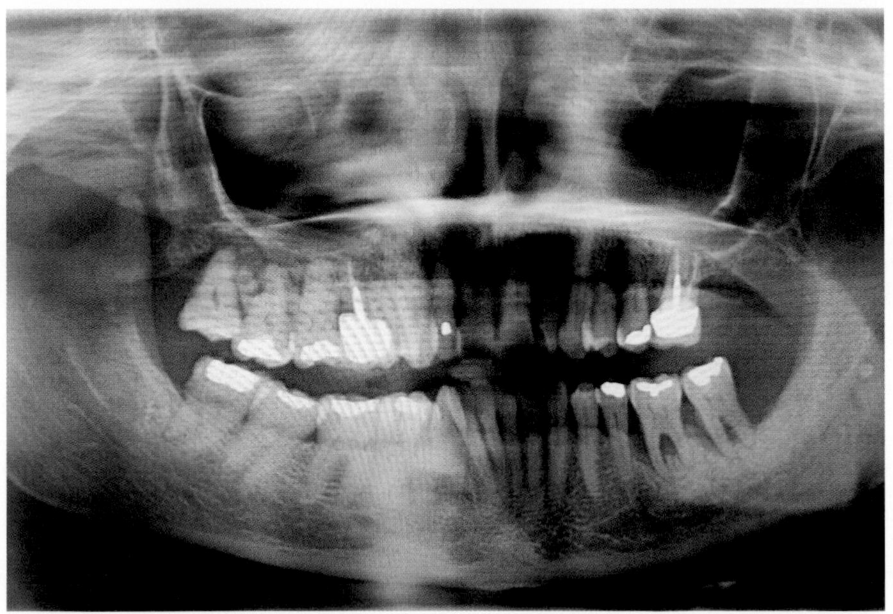

Figure 4.3.1: Panoramic radiograph.

Dental Examination

The intra- and extraoral examinations of the patient is within normal limits. The generalized appearance of the gingiva is deep red with blunted gingival margins in the upper right (UR) and lower left (LL) quadrants. Generalized recession ranging from 2 to 4 mm is noted on the mandibular arch. The patient complains of moderate root sensitivity to temperature and to the touch. Localized severe inflammation appears on teeth #1, #2, #3, #18, and #19. Generalized bleeding on probing occurs throughout the dentition with localized supragingival calculus located on the lower anterior teeth. Generalized moderate interproximal calculus is present. Slight crowding of the mandibular anterior teeth is noted. Exudate is present upon probing teeth #1, #2, #3, and #19. Class III mobility on #1, #2, #3, #18, and #19. Recurrent decay is present on tooth #20 and under the distal margin of the crown on tooth #4.

Radiographic Examination

Radiographic examination reveals severe bone loss surrounding teeth #1, #2, #3, #18, and #19. (See Figure 4.3.1).

Dental Hygiene Diagnosis

Problems	Related Etiology
Periodontal disease and tooth mobility	Dental and oral health neglect; possible side effects of long-term steroid prescription use
Recurrent dental caries	Past dental neglect; sugar rich diet; possible side effects of long-term steroid use and patient disability
Root exposure and sensitivity	A loss of attachment, and biofilm accumulation

Planned Interventions

Clinical	Education	Oral Hygiene Instruction
Periodontal debridement and localized scaling and root planing Topical and local anesthetic for patient sensitivity Antimicrobial therapy 5% fluoride varnish for root sensitivity and caries prevention Four to eight-week re-evaluation of gingiva and reinforcement of homecare routine Three-month periodontal maintenance recall	Progression of periodontal disease Educate on importance of periodontal maintenance visits as required or 2 to 3 months Educate on adjunct therapies. and incorporate into daily oral home care Nutritional counseling Educate on relationship between past medication use, diet, and dental caries	Modified Stillman's technique with modification of toothbrush handle for patient grasp to accommodate patient's disability Floss holder with modification of handle for interproximal cleaning including additional periodontal aides to accommodate patient's ability Use of fluoridated toothpaste and fluoride rinse

Progress Notes

The patient in case study three presented with severe periodontal involvement in the UR and LL posterior quadrants. Due to severe tooth mobility, presence of exudate, and the extent of bone and gingival attachment loss, extractions were the dentist's recommendation for teeth #1, #2, #3, #18 and #19 (see Figure 4.3.2). The patient consented to extractions of teeth #1, #2, #3, #18 and #19 and full mouth periodontal debridement with localized scaling and root planing of teeth #12–#14, #20 and #30–#32 (See Figures 4.3.3 and 4.3.4).

Discussion

Creating an oral hygiene care plan for a special needs patient after completing nonsurgical periodontal therapy involves complete assessment of the patient's abilities and motivation. The healthy maintenance of the periodontium and supporting tissues continues to be imperative. Attitude and physical barriers may hinder compliance and personal oral hygiene care (Wilkins 2009, pp. 382–383). Upon initial examination the severity of the periodontal disease and expected outcomes must be considered as it relates to patient compliance, successful completion of treatment, and creation of an acceptable oral hygiene homecare regimen (Wilkins 2009, pp. 374–375). For optimal success, positive reinforcement and motivation are necessary and must be consistently provided throughout maintenance (Wilkins 2009, p. 383). This increases the opportunity for successful periodontal disease management and oral hygiene care.

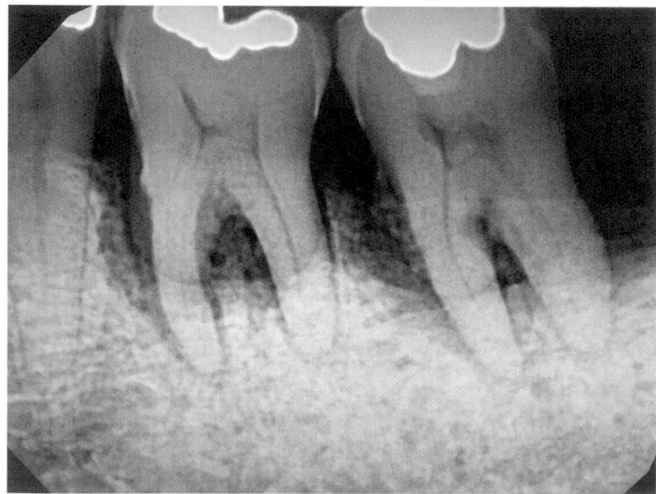

Figure 4.3.2: Lower left radiograph of teeth #18 and #19 revealing furcation involvement.

The Modified Stillman's toothbrushing technique is recommended over the Bass Method due to the patient's gingival recession and root sensitivity. The Stillman's method is considered less traumatic because the bristles are not directed towards the sulcus (Darby and Walsh 2003, p. 355). The modification adds a roll stroke, where the bristles are rolled occlusally to clean the entire facial and lingual surfaces after the cervical areas are cleaned (Darby and Walsh 2003, p. 355). For this patient, customizing oral self-care devices is necessary. There are a variety of objects such as bicycle handle grips, soda cans, and tennis or soft rubber balls that may be used to enlarge the diameter of a handle and create an adaptive oral hygiene device to fit the

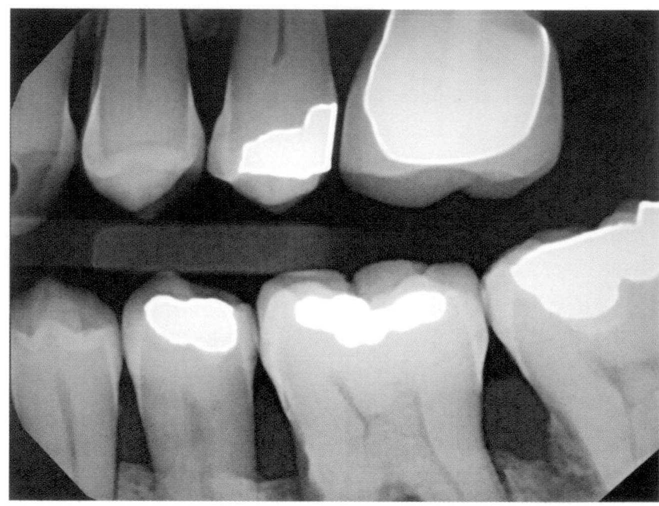

Figure 4.3.3: Bitewing radiograph of left side showing advanced horizontal bone loss.

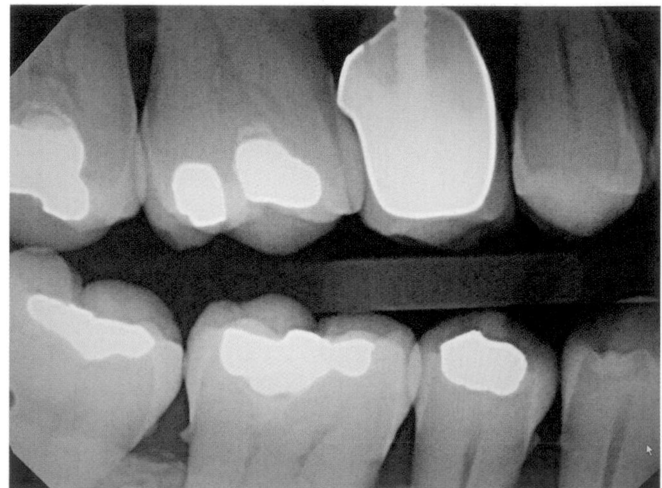

Figure 4.3.4: Bitewing radiograph of right side showing interproximal calculus with horizontal bone loss.

patient's grasp and closure abilities (Darby and Walsh 2003, p. 774). A wide variety of interdental aids are available for debris removal. When the interdental gingiva fills the embrasure space, biofilm removal is best accomplished with dental floss or dental tape. Manipulating the regular dental floss to form the c-shaped flossing for wrapping around interproximal surfaces is impossible for this patient. For interproximal cleaning flossholders with enlarged diameter handles allow this patient to remove debris from areas that are not periodontally involved. If interdental gingiva is reduced or missing, the embrasure space is larger, as seen in between #18 and #19 (see Figure 4.3.2), and other methods of debris removal are needed (Darby and Walsh 2003, p. 361). Interdental brushes provide access to larger interdental spaces and come in a variety of shapes and sizes (Blue 2017, p. 497). The conical or tapered design is inserted into a handle and may be angled to fit interproximal spaces (Darby and Walsh 2003, p. 371). A single session of oral hygiene instruction is not sufficient for long-term periodontal management or behavior change (Yuen 2013, p. 2). Frequent visits to monitor patient progress including written oral hygiene instruction on homecare are necessary aspects of patient care for a successful end result.

Take-Home Hints

1. Barriers to consider for patient care include mental and physical barriers.
2. Patient compliance in daily oral hygiene self-care is key to the success of oral hygiene health following nonsurgical periodontal therapy.
3. For effective debris removal for a patient with special needs, modifications may need to be made to toothbrushes and oral hygiene aides for grasping and use.

Self-Study Questions

1. True or False. When creating a plan for oral hygiene instruction it is important for the clinician to consider any barriers to care such as cost of an electric toothbrush or the patient's physical ability to grasp the handle.

A. True.
B. False.

2. True or False. Interproximal brushes are best used for interproximal areas where gingiva completely fills the embrasure space.

A. True
B. False

3. True or False. During recare appointments, the clinician assesses the effectiveness of patient's oral hygiene compliance and determines when any modifications are necessary.

A. True
B. False

4. True or False. The Modified Stillman's method is recommended for patients with recession.

A. True.
B. False.

References

Blue, C. (2017). *Darby's Comprehensive Review of Dental Hygiene*, 8e. St. Louis: Elsevier.

Darby, M. and Walsh, M. (2003). *Dental Hygiene Theory and Practice*, 2e. Philadelphia: W.B. Saunders.

Wilkins, E. (2009). *Clinical Practice of the Dental Hygienist*. Philadelphia: Wolters Kluwer Health/Lippincott Williams & Wilkins.

Yuen, H. (2013). Effect of a home telecare program on oral health among adults with tetraplegia: a pilot study. *Spinal Cord* 51 (6): 477–481.

Answers to Self-Study Questions

1. True/A. Barriers to care can include physical, mental, and financial barriers. When recommending oral aides or tools for patient homecare routines it is important for the clinician to consider any barriers to care that may impact on the patient.

2. False/B. When the interdental gingiva fills the embrasure space, biofilm removal is best accomplished with dental floss or dental tape.

3. True/A. Effectiveness of plaque control depends on patient ability. It is the job of the clinician to note when any educational or instructional techniques are in need of review or modification.

4. True/A. The Modified Stillman's method is considered less traumatic because the bristles are not directed towards the sulcus.

5

Pharmacology

Clinical Cases in Dental Hygiene, First Edition. Edited by Cheryl M. Westphal Theile, Mea A. Weinberg and Stuart L. Segelnick.

Case 1

Pain and Anxiety Control: Analgesics

CASE STORY

A 59-year-old Asian male presented with a complaint of occasional pain and food impaction around his maxillary right fixed bridge.

PROBLEM-BASED LEARNING GOALS AND OBJECTIVES

- Understand the appropriate use of systemic analgesics in the relief of oral pain
- Understand the concerns associated with the use of systemic analgesics

Medical History

The patient's medical history was significant for hypertension. Current medications included hydrochlorothiazide 25 mg and atenolol 25 mg.

Review of Systems

- Vital signs
  - Blood pressure: 134/72 mmHg
  - Pulse: 69 beats/min
  - Respiration: 12 breaths/min

Dental History

The patient reports that he has not seen a dentist in over 25 years. Previous active dental treatment had involved extractions and fabrication of maxillary right and mandibular left fixed bridges. The patient reports that he brushes once a day and has never flossed.

Social History

The patient has smoked a pack of cigarettes a day since he was 11 years old (48 pack years). He does not drink alcohol.

Extraoral and Intraoral Examination

There were no significant extraoral findings, no swellings, or masses detected. Intraoral examination revealed generalized poor oral hygiene and a very strong scent of tobacco on breath. The gingiva was generally fibrotic with minimal bleeding upon probing. Periodontal probing depths ranged from 5 to 12 mm, with generalized advanced furcation defects on all molar teeth. Unopposed tooth #16 was extruded and grossly carious (see Figure 5.1.1).

Diagnosis

Generalized severe chronic periodontitis (Armitage 1999).

Treatment Plan

The initial treatment plan for the patient included smoking cessation counseling, home care education, and extraction of teeth #1, #3, #14, #16, #18, #29, and #30. Postoperative pain was effectively managed with a combination of 400 mg ibuprofen and 500 mg acetaminophen every six hours. Following scaling and root planing therapy, transitional removable partial dentures were fabricated.

Discussion

The relief of oral pain is one of the primary obligations of a dental professional. Dental diseases and the treatment of dental diseases both have the potential to cause pain. Most dental pain has an inflammatory component. The most effective analgesics used for dental pain have anti-inflammatory properties (see Table 5.1.1).

Nonsteroidal anti-inflammatory drugs (NSAIDs) are the most common agents used to relieve oral pain, with both prescription (Rx) and over the counter (OTC) products available. NSAIDs have analgesic,

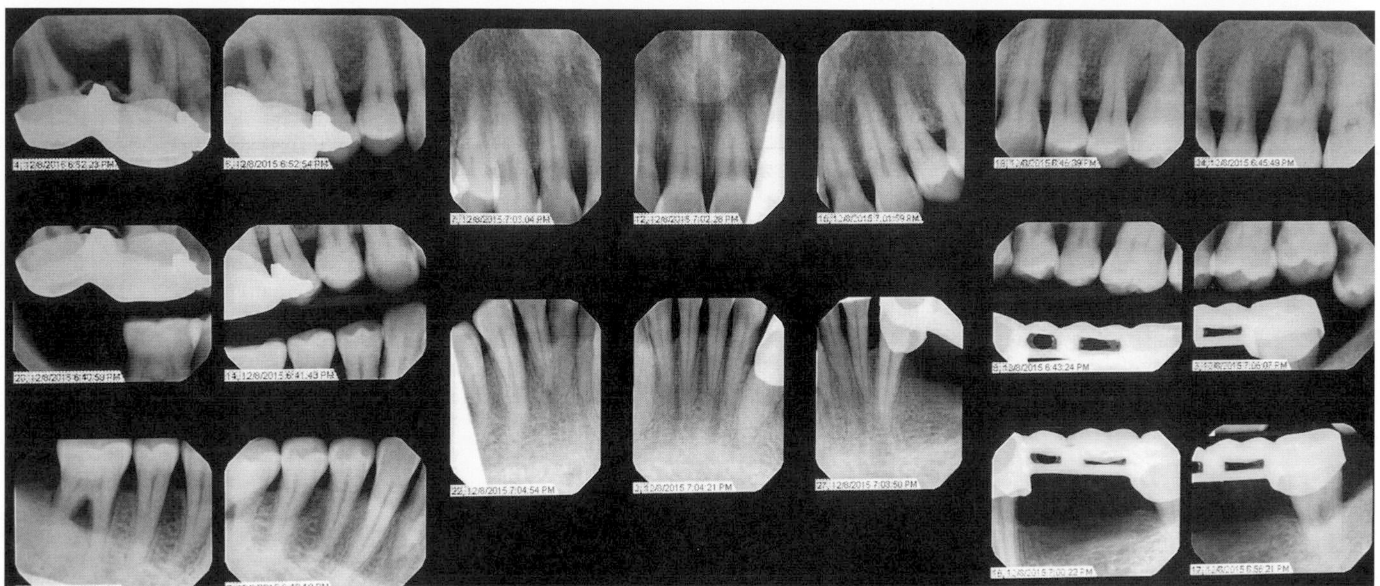

Figure 5.1.1: Full mouth series.

Table 5.1.1: Commonly used systemic analgesics.

Drug	Brand Name	Does	Concerns	OTC/RX
Aspirin	Bayer	325–650 mg Q6H	Antiplatelet effect GI bleeding Aggravation of asthma Interaction with warfarin Tinnitus/ototoxicity	OTC
Ibuprofen	Motrin	200–600 mg Q6H	Antiplatelet effect GI bleeding Aggravation of asthma Altered kidney function	OTC/RX
Naproxen sodium	Aleve	220–550 mg Q8H	Antiplatelet effect GI bleeding Aggravation of asthma Altered kidney function	OTC/RX
Diflunisal	Dolobid	500 mg Q12H	Antiplatelet effect GI bleeding Interaction with warfarin Aggravation of asthma Tinnitus/ototoxicity	RX
Acetaminophen	Tylenol	325–650 mg Q6H	Liver toxicity	OTC

anti-inflammatory, antipyretic, and antiplatelet properties (see Table 5.1.2). The principle mechanism of action of NSAIDs is the competitive, reversible inhibition of the conversion of arachidonic acid to prostaglandins by cyclooxygenase (COX) enzymes. There are two isoforms of COX enzymes, COX-1, and COX-2. Arachidonic acid is converted to thromboxane A2 by the COX-1 enzyme, leading to platelet aggregation. Arachidonic acid is converted to prostaglandins by the enzyme COX-2, leading to inflammation and pain. There are several NSAID products, each with subtle differences in their abilities to block COX-1 and COX-2. These differences account for the products variability in potency, dosing, adverse

Table 5.1.2: Effects of cyclooxygenase inhibition by aspirin and NSAIDs ("4 A's of NSAIDs").

Analgesia
Anti-inflammatory
Antipyretic (anti-itch)
Antiplatelet effects

Table 5.1.3: Potential drug interactions due to cyclooxygenase inhibition and prostaglandin reduction.

- Decreased effectiveness of both thiazide and loop diuretics (used for hypertension)
- Decreased effectiveness of beta-blockers (used for hypertension)
- Decreased effectiveness of angiotension converting enzymes inhibitors (used for hypertension)
- Increased effectiveness of sulfonylureas (used for diabetes)
- Increased blood levels and toxicity of lithium (used for bipolar disorder)

drug reactions, and clinical therapeutic indications. NSAIDs, as a class, are known as having the side effects of gastrointestinal (GI) bleeding, altered renal (kidney) effects, an aggravation of asthma in susceptible individuals, and antiplatelet effects that may cause postoperative bleeding. Newer NSAIDs have been developed that are selective COX-2 inhibitors; however they have been implicated as having increased risk of cardiovascular events (Laskarides 2016).

NSAIDs have the potential of drug interactions due to their effects on the COX enzymes (see Table 5.1.3). NSAIDs may decrease the hypotensive effects of certain antihypertensive medications (beta-blockers, angiotension converting enzyme inhibitors, and diuretics). NSAIDs may increase the hypoglycemic effects of the sulfonylurea class of oral antidiabetic agents. NSAIDs may also increase the blood levels of the psychiatric medication lithium, leading to potential lithium toxicity.

The most commonly used NSAIDs are ibuprofen and naproxen sodium. Ibuprofen is available in both OTC and RX formulations, with common dosing of 200–600 mg every six hours. Naproxen sodium is available in both OTC and RX formulations with common dosing of 220–550 mg every eight hours.

Aspirin is a salicylate nonnarcotic analgesic with analgesic, anti-inflammatory, antipyretic, and antiplatelet properties. Aspirin irreversibly blocks both COX-1 and COX-2 and is known as having greater antiplatelet activity than NSAIDs. Low-dose aspirin (81 mg per day) is frequently recommended by physicians for prevention of stroke or heart attack due to its antiplatelet properties. The usual analgesic dose of aspirin is 325–650 mg every six hours. The prescription drug diflunisal is a salicylate used at a dose of 500 mg every 12 hours. In addition to the common side effects of GI

Table 5.1.4: Special patient populations that may complicate the choice of an analgesic.

Condition	Concern
Peptic ulcer disease	Aspirin and NSAIDs may cause GI bleeding
Alcoholism	Aspirin and NSAIDs may cause GI bleeding. Acetaminophen is hepatoxic
Kidney disease	NSAIDs may alter kidney function
Patient on warfarin	Aspirin may reduce protein binding of warfarin. Aspirin and NSAIDs have antiplatelet effects
Hypertension	NSAIDs may reduce efficacy of antihypertensives
Diabetes	NSAIDs may increase efficacy of sulfonylureas
Arthritis	Patient may be taking other OTC or RX NSAIDs

bleeding, aggravation of asthma, altered renal function, and antiplatelet effects, salicylates have the unique side effects of vertigo, tinnitus, and ototoxicity. The risk of ototoxicity is increased when salicylates are used along with other ototoxic medications such as loop diuretics (Weinberg et al. 2013).

Salicylates share the same potential for drug side effects as other cyclooxygenase blocking agents. Salicylates have the side effect of displacing the anti-Vitamin K blood thinner warfarin from its plasma protein binding sites, increasing therapeutic blood levels of active warfarin. Aspirin should be used with great caution in patients taking therapeutic levels of warfarin due to a significant risk of postoperative bleeding related to both the increased blood levels warfarin and the antiplatelet actions of aspirin (see Table 5.1.4).

Acetaminophen is a drug that does not fall into a specific category. It is not a salicylate; it is not an NSAID; it does not block COX. The exact mechanism of action of acetaminophen is not known. Theories of its action include a possible inactivation of COX enzymes, inhibition of nitric acid production, or blockade of prostaglandin (Guggenheimer and Moore 2011; Moore and Hersh 2013; Laskarides 2016). Acetaminophen has analgesic and antipyretic properties, but does not have anti-inflammatory or antiplatelet properties. Its acute pain relief properties are less than that achieved by NSAIDs. Acetaminophen is commonly dosed at 325–650 mg every six hours, with occasional dosing of 1000 mg every six hours. It is generally considered safe for most patients, including children and pregnant women, when used as directed. Unlike salicylates or NSAIDs, it is not associated with GI bleeding and does not inhibit platelet aggregation. Acetaminophen is hepatotoxic, causing severe liver damage (possibly fatal) when used at excessive dosage, when used along with other hepatotoxic drugs, or when used by individuals who consume three or more alcoholic beverages daily (Guggenheimer and Moore 2011). The maximum daily dose of acetaminophen as recommended by the US Food and Drug Administration (FDA) is 4000 mg per day. Recently, a leading drug manufacturer of acetaminophen changed its packaging instructions to reflect a maximum daily dose of 3000 mg per day due to concerns over liver toxicity (Moore and Hersh 2013).

The risk of a patient taking an inappropriate dose of acetaminophen and suffering a hepatic event is complicated by the fact that multiple OTC products containing acetaminophen are marketed for a variety of symptoms (cough and cold products, migraine pain products, arthritis pain products, etc.). The inclusion of acetaminophen as an ingredient is frequently listed in small print on the back the product packaging. Many patients do not read ingredient labeling and assume that the product is safe because it is available OTC. Patients may be unaware of the potential of duplicating medication if they take acetaminophen for relief of dental pain (see Table 5.1.5). The prudent clinician regularly asks his patients about all medications (RX and OTC) they are taking in an attempt to avoid inappropriate use.

Combination analgesic therapy is frequently used in the management of postoperative oral pain. The use of ibuprofen at a dose of 200–600 mg combined with acetaminophen at a dose of 500–1000 mg every six hours has been evaluated in multiple pain studies. The combination has been shown to provide pain relief that is superior to that provided by either product alone and at lower doses (Ong et al. 2010; Moore and Hersh 2013). Ibuprofen-acetaminophen combination therapy has also been demonstrated to provide pain relief comparable to that provided by common acetaminophen-opioid combinations (acetaminophen and codeine, acetaminophen and hydrocodone, acetaminophen and oxycodone) for moderate to severe pain without the inherent risks of opioid therapy (Ong et al. 2010; Moore and Hersh 2013).

Table 5.1.5: OTC products that may contain acetaminophen.

Cough and cold products
Cold and flu products
Migraine relief products
Arthritis pain relief products
Menstrual cramp relief products
Back pain relief product

Take-Home Hints

1. Acetaminophen is not known to be a teratogen and is generally considered safe for use during pregnancy when used as directed. Acetaminophen is not a narcotic and does not contribute to narcotic (opioid) addiction. Acetaminophen is a known hepatotoxin and may cause severe liver damage. This risk is greatly increased in individuals who consume three or more alcoholic beverages a day or use other medications that are hepatoxic. The salicylate class of medications (such as aspirin) is known to cause tinnitus.
2. The combination of an NSAID with acetaminophen provides superior relief of pain at lower dosages than that provided by either product alone. The reason for this is not known, as the mechanism of action of acetaminophen is unknown. While NSAIDs act by competing with arachidonic acid and blocking the actions of the cyclooxygenase enzymes, acetaminophen may function by inactivating the cyclooxygenase enzymes themselves. The combination of an NSAID and acetaminophen provides comparable pain relief to that achieved by a combination of acetaminophen with an opioid narcotic, while avoiding the adverse effects of sedation and impaired functioning.
3. Atrial fibrillation is a type of cardiac arrhythmia. Cardiac stents are utilized in the management of coronary artery disease. Both atrial fibrillation and coronary artery disease are treated with blood thinners. Warfarin is an anti-Vitamin K anticoagulant that alters the clotting cascade. Warfarin is a highly protein-bound medication. Nonprotein bound warfarin inhibits the synthesis of Vitamin K dependent clotting factors II, VII, IX, and X. Aspirin displaces warfarin from protein binding sites, increasing the levels of active free warfarin. Active free warfarin increases potential for bleeding. Clopidogrel is an antiplatelet agent. It inhibits platelet aggregation, as does aspirin and naproxen sodium. The combination increases the potential for bleeding. Acetaminophen does not have antiplatelet activity and it is not highly bound to plasma protein.

Self-Study Questions

1. A major drug manufacturer has recently reduced the recommended maximum daily dose of acetaminophen from 4000 to 3000 mg per day. This change was due to which of the following concerns?

- **A. Acetaminophen is a known teratogen.**
- **B. Acetaminophen contributes to narcotic addiction.**
- **C. Acetaminophen may cause severe liver damage.**
- **D. Acetaminophen may cause tinnitus.**

2. Which of the following statements justifies the use of a combination of an NSAID and acetaminophen for the management of postoperative dental pain?

- **A. The combination provides pain relief superior to that obtained by either drug alone.**
- **B. The combination provides pain relief comparable to that obtained by a combination of acetaminophen and an opioid narcotic.**
- **C. The combination provides superior pain relief while utilizing lower doses of either drug.**
- **D. All of the above.**

3. Your patient presents with a diagnosis of generalized moderate chronic periodontitis. Clinical examination reveals periodontal probing depths of 6–7 mm, with generalized pain and bleeding upon probing. Review of medical history reveals atrial fibrillation and a cardiac stent placement. Current medications include warfarin 5 mg and clopidogrel 75 mg once a day. Your patient is concerned about postoperative discomfort. Which of the following analgesic regimens would be most appropriate?

- **A. Aspirin 650 mg every six hours**
- **B. Naproxen sodium 220 mg every eight hours**
- **C. Acetaminophen 500 mg every six hours**
- **D. None of the above**

References

Armitage, G. (1999). Development of a classification system for periodontal diseases and conditions. *Ann. Periodontol.* 4: 1–6.

Guggenheimer, J. and Moore, P.A. (2011). The therapeutic applications of and risks associated with acetaminophen use. A review and update. *J. Am. Dent. Assoc.* 142 (1): 38–44.

Laskarides, C. (2016). Update on analgesia medication for adult and pediatric dental patients. *Dent. Clin. N. Am.* 60: 347–366.

Moore, P.A. and Hersh, E.V. (2013). Combining ibuprofen and acetaminophen for acute pain management after third-molar extractions. Translating clinical research to dental practice. *J. Am. Dent. Assoc.* 144 (8): 898–890.

Ong, C.K., Seymour, R.A., Lirk, P., and Merry, A.F. (2010). Combining paracetamol (acetaminophen) with nonsteroidal anti-inflammatory drugs: a qualitative systemic review of analgesic efficacy for acute postoperative pain. *Anesth. Analg.* 110 (4): 1170–1179.

Weinberg, M.A., Theile, C.M., and Fine, J.B. (2013). Drugs for pain control. In: *Oral Pharmacology for the Dental Hygienist, 2e*, 87–109. Upper Saddle River, NJ: Pearson.

Additional Resources

Moore, R.A., Wiffen, P.J., Derry, S. et al. (2015). Non-prescription (OTC) oral analgesics for acute pain-an overview of Cochrane reviews. *Cochrane Database Syst. Rev.* (11): CD010794. doi: 10.1002/14651858.CD010794.pub2.

Answers to Self-Study Questions

1. C

2. D

3. C

Case 2

Pain and Anxiety Control: Topical and Local Anesthetics

CASE STORY

A 67-year-old Hispanic female patient presented with a tender, bleeding gingival swelling on the maxillary right side.

PROBLEM-BASED LEARNING GOALS AND OBJECTIVES

- Understand the mechanism of action of local anesthetics
- Recognize the signs and symptoms of anesthetic toxicity
- Be able to choose the appropriate anesthetic agent to accomplish the proposed procedure

Medical History

The patient's medical history was unremarkable. The patient takes conjugated estrogens 0.625 mg for postmenopausal symptoms.

Review of Systems

- Vital signs
  - Blood pressure: 128/70 mmHg
  - Pulse: 68 beats/min
  - Respiration: 12 breaths/min

Dental History

The patient reports that she sees her general dentist one to two times per year for examination and prophylaxis. She brushes twice a day and does not floss. She reports that her gingival swelling had developed about five weeks ago. She had visited her dentist after development of the swelling and a prophylaxis was performed. The lesion has since decreased in size, but tenderness and bleeding persist.

Social History

The patient has never smoked. She occasionally drinks wine with dinner.

Extraoral and Intraoral Examination

There were no significant extraoral findings, no extraoral swellings or masses detected. Intraoral examination revealed suboptimal interproximal oral hygiene. An edematous, erythematous, pedunculated swelling of the buccal interproximal gingiva between teeth #6 and #7 was noted (see Figure 5.2.1). Periodontal probing of the area ranged from 5 to 6 mm, with bleeding and discomfort upon probing pressure.

Clinical Diagnosis

A reactive gingival lesion, pyogenic granuloma vs. peripheral giant cell granuloma was suspected (Armitage 1999).

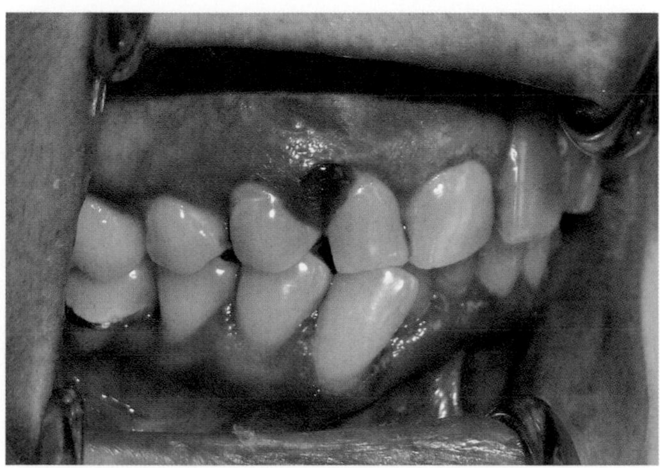

Figure 5.2.1: Pyogenic granuloma.

Treatment Plan

The patient was instructed on appropriate dental home care. Consent was obtained for an excisional biopsy of the gingival lesion. Benzocaine 20% topical anesthesia was placed. The area was anesthetized with one carpule 2% lidocaine with 1:100000 epinephrine. An excisional biopsy of the lesion was performed and the specimen was submitted for histopathological examination. The area healed without incident. Histopathologic diagnosis of the lesion came back as a pyogenic granuloma.

Discussion

The care and treatment of dental patients often involve procedures that are uncomfortable. Fortunately, topical and local anesthetic products are available to decrease the discomfort of the needle experience and to allow for relative pain free treatment (see Table 5.2.1). Benzocaine 20% gel is the most commonly used dental topical anesthetic. It is classified chemically as an ester and is also available OTC in lower concentrations to treat teething pain and soft tissue ulceration. Benzocaine may cause methemoglobinemia. Lidocaine is chemically an amide and is used at a 5% concentration as a preinjection anesthetic gel. It is also available as a prescription 0.5% viscous solution in the treatment of chemotherapy induced mucositis. Dyclonine 0.5% topical solution is available for use in patients allergic to esters and amides. A combination gel containing 2.5% lidocaine and 2.5% prilocaine intended to be placed in periodontal pockets has been developed. Marketed as the product Oraqix, it allows for scaling and root planing therapy under topical anesthesia (Boyce et al. 2016). Kovanaze a new FDA approved intranasal spray of 3% tetracaine and 0.05% oxymetazoline was found to be effective for restorative procedures in adults and provided satisfactory maxillary local anesthesia on premolars, canines, and incisors (Hersh et al. 2016).

Local anesthetics allow for relative pain free dental treatment. Local anesthetics act by decreasing the permeability of the sodium ion channels, which decreases the rate of nerve depolarization preventing the generation of the action potential. Several local anesthetic preparations are available for dental use. Selection of a local anesthetic may be based on the patient's medical history, the anticipated duration of the procedure, the need for hemostasis, and the need for postoperative pain control. A clinician should strive to use the lowest dose of anesthetic necessary to accomplish the proposed procedure, while being aware of the patient's medical status and individual pain tolerance.

Historically, dental local anesthetics have been available from both the ester and amide chemical classes. Ester local anesthetics are metabolized to para-aminobenzoic acid (PABA), which causes allergic reactions, dermatitis, and sloughing of oral mucosal tissue. Ester local anesthetics are potent vasodilators, which decrease duration of action and increase the risk of overdose. Due to these risks, injectable ester local anesthetics are no longer available for dental use. All commercially available dental local anesthetics are from the amide class (Moore and Hersh 2010; Boyce et al. 2016).

Commonly used amide local anesthetics include lidocaine 2% with 1:100,000 epinephrine, mepivacaine 3%, mepivacaine 2% with 1:20,000 levonordefrin, articaine 4% with 1:100,000 epinephrine, prilocaine 4% with 1:200,000 epinephrine, and bupivacaine 0.5% with 1:200,000 epinephrine (see Table 5.2.2). They are metabolized in the liver, and are primarily excreted by the kidneys. Concerns and dosage adjustments would be appropriate in patients with altered liver function. All commercially available dental local anesthetics are packaged as 1.7 ml carpules.

The most commonly used local anesthetic and the one most widely studied for safety is lidocaine 2% with 1 : 100,000 epinephrine. The low dose of anesthetic, combined with vasoconstrictor allow for reasonable working time and small risk of systemic absorption and toxicity when used with proper aspiration technique. Mepivacaine 3% is a popular choice when shorter procedures are planned or for when hypertensive patients are being treated, as it does not contain a vasoconstrictor. This lack of vasoconstrictor does allow for systemic absorption, with greater potential for toxicity. Mepivacaine 2% with 1 : 20,000 levonordefrin allows for longer working time than mepivacaine 3%, however its vasoconstrictor levonordefrin is known to stimulate alpha adrenergic receptors. This may be of concern in patients taking alpha receptor blocking agents for hypertension or prostate problems. Articaine 4% with 1 : 100,000 epinephrine is a popular choice for mandibular infiltration anesthesia when mandibular block anesthesia is unwanted or insufficient. Prilocaine 4% with 1 : 200,000 has effects similar to lidocaine 2% with 1 : 100,000

Table 5.2.1: Common topical anesthetic products.

Product	Use
Benzocaine 20%	Reduce injection discomfort
Lidocaine 5%	Reduce injection discomfort
Dyclonine 0.5%	Reduce injection discomfort
Lidocaine 2.5%/Prilocaine 2.5%	Place in periodontal pocket prior to SRP

Table 5.2.2: Commonly used local anesthetics in dentistry.

Drug	Vasoconstrictor	Duration of Action	
		Pulpal	Soft Tissue
Lidocaine 2%	1 : 100,000 epinephrine	1–1.5 hours	3–5 hours
Mepivacaine 3%	none	20–40 minutes	2–3 hours
Mepivacaine 2%	1 : 20,000 levonordefrin	1–1.5 hours	3–5 hours
Articaine 4%	1 : 100,000 epinephrine	1–1.5 hours	3–6 hours
Prilocaine 4%	1 : 200,000 epinephrine	1–1.5 hours	3–8 hours
Bupivacaine 0.5%	1 : 200,000 epinephrine	1.5–3 hours	4–9 hours

Table 5.2.3: Concerns associated with dental anesthetic products.

Drug	Concern
Topical Benzocaine	Methemoglobinemia
All local anesthetics	Toxicity (CNS stimulation, then CNS and respiratory depression)
Prilocaine	Methemoglobinemia
Levonordefrin	alpha adrenergic stimulation in patients on alpha-blockers
Epinephrine	beta stimulation in patients on nonselective beta-blockers

epinephrine. It has been associated with methemoglobinemia. Bupivacaine 0.5% with 1 : 200,000 epinephrine is infrequently used in general dental practice due to its long duration of action. It is occasionally used in oral surgery practice (Boyce et al. 2016).

As with the use of any medications, there are concerns about potential toxicity or overdose of local anesthetics (see Table 5.2.3). These can be easily avoided by using common-sense guidelines. Most restorative and soft-tissue dental procedures are nonemergency procedures. These procedures can be terminated and the patient reappointed if adequate local anesthesia cannot be achieved with a maximum of three to possibly four carpules. Using this guideline, the maximum doses of anesthetic should never be approached. The use of higher doses should be reserved for patients undergoing complex surgical procedures. Use of proper anesthetic technique, with aspiration and the use of block anesthesia when possible, can reduce the risk of anesthetic toxicity.

All clinicians should be aware of the signs of local anesthetic toxicity. Initially, excitatory central nervous system (CNS) stimulation effects are seen, such as tremors, twitching, shivering, and tonic–clonic convulsive seizures. This is followed by signs of CNS depression including sedation, lethargy, and respiratory depression. At extremely elevated doses, altered cardiac rhythm, bradycardia, and hypotension may occur. There is risk of death due to respiratory failure (Moore and Hersh 2010).

The vasoconstrictor components of local anesthetic preparations may be of concern in certain patient populations. Review of the patient's medical history is imperative to reduce the risk of an untoward event. Most patients who take beta-blockers for hypertension use cardioselective beta-blockers, such as atenolol or metoprolol. However, nonselective beta-blockers (propranolol, nadolol, timolol, sotalol, and pindolol) are still used by some physicians to treat hypertension or migraine headaches. Significant increases in both systolic and diastolic blood pressures have been reported in patients taking nonselective beta-blockers after injections of lidocaine with epinephrine. It is recommended that epinephrine or levonordefrin be completely avoided in patients taking nonselective beta-blockers (Hersh and Giannakopoulos 2010).

Medication use in the pregnant patient is always a concern. Local anesthetic use is no exception. The use of local anesthetics in pregnant patients in generally considered safe if common sense guidelines are followed. Elective care is usually avoided during the first trimester when teratogenic risks are the greatest, although emergency care (treatment of pain or infection) should never be deferred. Routine care can be provided during the second trimester, while most treatment is deferred during the late third trimester. Lidocaine 2% with 1 : 100,000 epinephrine is the most studied local anesthetic and the one least reported to have untoward events. The low concentration of lidocaine and use of the vasoconstrictor minimizes the risk of anesthetic toxicity. Use of the lowest dose, with careful aspiration technique, utilizing block anesthesia whenever possible is recommended (Fayans et al. 2010).

Recently a product has become available to reverse the soft-tissue anesthesia effects of local anesthetic agents. Phentolamine mesylate is marketed as the product Ora-Verse and is intended to decrease prolonged anesthesia in patients at risk for soft-tissue injury or in individuals who may have a speaking engagement or those who may need to return to work (Boyce et al. 2016).

Take-Home Hints

1. Articaine and lidocaine are amides. Dyclonine is neither an amide nor an ester. Benzocaine is an ester.
2. Levonordefrin should be avoided in patients taking alpha blockers.
3. Articaine and lidocaine are local anesthetics agents. Benzocaine is a topical anesthetic agent. Phentolamine mesylate can reverse soft tissue anesthesia.
4. Lidocaine 2% with 1 : 100,000 epinephrine would be poor choice of anesthetic as it is advisable to avoid the use of a vasoconstrictor in a patient using a nonselective beta-blocker such as propranolol, especially if the patient is known to have hypertension. Bupivacaine 0.5% with 1 : 200,000 epinephrine would have similar concerns of using a vasoconstrictor in a patient taking a nonselective beta-blocker. Bupivacaine would also be inappropriate due to the long duration of soft-tissue anesthesia in a patient having a simple procedure. Mepivacaine 3% would provide appropriate duration of anesthesia without the concerns of vasoconstrictor use (Hersh and Giannakopoulos 2010; Moore and Hersh 2010).
5. Early identification of the signs of local anesthetic toxicity is important to allow for appropriate emergency response. An initial CNS stimulation may or may not be clearly evident as signs can range from minor twitching, shivering, to full blown tonic–clonic seizures. This may be followed by sedation, CNS depression, bradycardia, and respiratory depression. Death may occur due to respiratory failure (Moore and Hersh 2010).

Self-Study Questions

1. Which of the following anesthetic agents is chemically classified as an ester?
- **A. Lidocaine**
- **B. Articaine**
- **C. Dyclonine**
- **D. Benzocaine**

2. Your patient is 73-year-old man who is taking the alpha adrenergic blocker doxazosin to manage symptoms of benign prostatic hyperplasia (BPH). Which of the following agents has the potential to stimulate the alpha receptors resulting in an increased blood pressure?
- **A. Epinephrine**
- **B. Lidocaine**
- **C. Levonordefrin**
- **D. Articaine**

3. Which of the following products may be utilized to decrease prolonged anesthesia in patients at risk for soft-tissue injury or in patients that may need to return to work?
- **A. Articaine**
- **B. Lidocaine**
- **C. Phentolamine mesylate**
- **D. Benzocaine**

4. A 46-year-old female patient presents for scaling and root planing therapy of the maxillary and mandibular left quadrants. Review of medical history reveals that the patient is taking 50 mg of hydrochlorothiazide once a day for hypertension and 40 mg propranolol twice a day for migraines. Which of the following local anesthetics would be most appropriate?
- **A. Bupivacaine 0.5% with 1:200,000 epinephrine**
- **B. Mepivacaine 3%**
- **C. Lidocaine 2% with 1:100,000 epinephrine**
- **D. All of the above**

5. Which of the following is the sequence of signs of local anesthetic toxicity?
- **A. CNS depression, CNS stimulation, respiratory depression**
- **B. CNS stimulation, CNS depression, respiratory depression**
- **C. Respiratory stimulation, CNS stimulation, CNS depression**
- **D. Respiration depression, CNS depression, CNS stimulation**

References

Armitage, G. (1999). Development of a classification system for periodontal diseases and conditions. *Ann. Periodontol.* 4: 1–6.

Boyce, R.A., Kirpalani, T., and Mohan, N. (2016). Updates of topical and local anesthetic agents. *Dent. Clin. N. Am.* 60: 445–471.

Fayans, E.P., Stuart, H.R., Carsten, D. et al. (2010). Local anesthetic use in the pregnant and postpartum patient. *Dent. Clin. N. Am.* 54: 697–713.

Hersh, E.V. and Giannakopoulos, H. (2010). Beta-adrenergic blocking agents and dental vasoconstrictors. *Dent. Clin. N. Am.* 54: 687–696.

Hersh, E.V., Pinto, M., Saleh, N. et al. (2016). Double-masked, randomized, placebo-controlled study to evaluate the efficacy and tolerability of intranasal K305 (3% tetracaine plus 0.05% oxymetazoline) in anesthetizing maxillary teeth. *J Am Dent Assoc* 147 (4): 278–287.

Moore, P.A. and Hersh, E.V. (2010). Local anesthetics: pharmacology and toxicity. *Dent. Clin. N. Am.* 54: 587–599.

Additional Resources

Malamed, S.F. (2013). *Handbook of Local Anesthesia*, 6e. St. Louis, MO.: Elsevier.

Answers to Self-Study Questions

1. D
2. C
3. C
4. B
5. B

Case 3

Pain and Anxiety Control: Nitrous Oxide

CASE STORY

A 72-year-old female patient presented with pain of three days duration associated with her mandibular left fixed bridge.

PROBLEM-BASED LEARNING GOALS AND OBJECTIVES

- Understand the properties of nitrous oxide
- Describe the appropriate use of nitrous oxide-oxygen
- Understand the safety features of contemporary nitrous oxide-oxygen systems

Medical History

The patient's medical history was significant for hypertension and anxiety. Current medications included hydrochlorothiazide 25 mg and alprazolam 0.25 mg.

Review of Systems

- Vital signs
  - Blood pressure: 128/70 mmHg
  - Pulse rate: 62 beats/min
  - Respiration: 12 breaths/min

Dental History

The patient has seen the same dentist regularly twice a year for over 30 years. Approximately 22 years ago the patient had complex prosthetic treatment completed, including a maxillary full arch fixed reconstruction and a mandibular left five-unit fixed bridge extending from the mesial root of tooth #17 to tooth #21. The patient reports that she brushes twice a day and does not floss.

Social History

The patient does not smoke or drink alcohol.

Extraoral and Intraoral Examination

There were no significant extraoral findings, no swelling, or masses detected. Intraoral examination revealed fair oral hygiene with generalized mild gingival inflammation. Caries was noted under the distal margin of bridge retainer #18.

Radiographic Examination

Radiographic examination revealed distal caries #18 and an associated periapical radiolucency (see Figure 5.3.1).

Diagnosis

Dental caries, symptomatic apical periodontitis #18.

Treatment Plan

The treatment plan for the patient involved sectioning the mandibular left fixed bridge at the distal aspect of retainer #20 and extracting teeth #17 and #18. Dental implants were placed in sites #18 and #19. The surgical treatment was accomplished under local anesthesia supplemented by nitrous oxide-oxygen analgesia due to the patient's anxiety.

Discussion

Nitrous oxide is an inorganic, nonirritating, colorless, slightly sweet smelling, inhalation analgesic gas. It is nonflammable, but will support combustion. While usually described in the category of anesthetic gases, nitrous oxide cannot achieve true anesthesia. The potency of anesthetic gases is described in terms of minimum alveolar concentration (MAC), which is defined as the alveolar concentration of anesthetic gas at which 50% of patients fail to respond to a surgical stimulus. Nitrous oxide has a MAC of 104%, which is

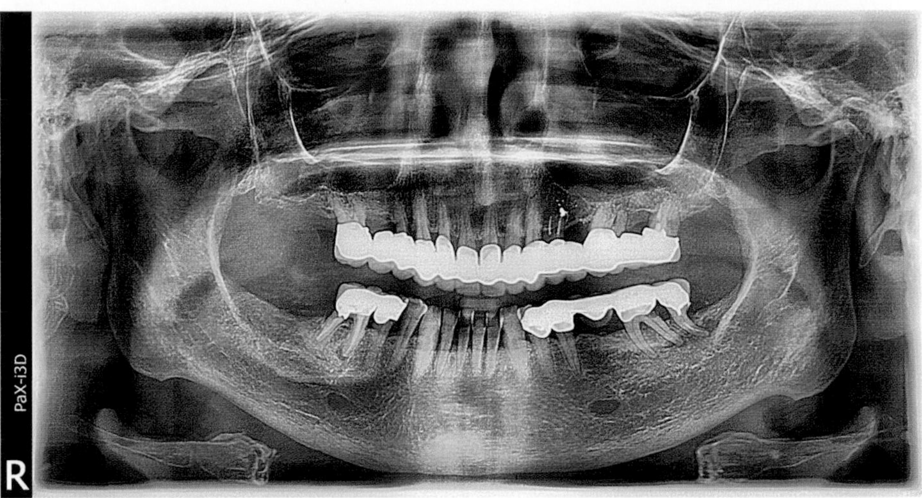

Figure 5.3.1: Panoramic radiograph.

only achievable in a hyperbaric chamber. Typical nitrous oxide concentrations utilized in the dental setting range from 20 to 60%, which does not represent the true concentrations delivered from the unit to the patient due to mouth breathing and mask leakage. For these reasons true anesthesia, defined as nonresponsive CNS depression, cannot be achieved with nitrous oxide. Nitrous oxide is poorly soluble in blood. As a result, a state of equilibrium of the nitrous oxide concentrations in the lung alveoli and blood is achieved quickly, leading a rapid onset of sedation and analgesia and a rapid resolution when nitrous oxide administration is discontinued. The exact mechanism of action of nitrous oxide's analgesic and sedative properties is unknown. Theories include the stimulated release of enkephalins to bind to opioid receptors, activation of benzodiazepine receptors, and the inhibition of excitatory amino acid receptors (Jackson and Johnson 2002; Becker and Rosenberg 2008).

Nitrous oxide has properties that aid the clinician in the delivery of dental treatment (see Table 5.3.1). In addition to its analgesic and sedative properties, nitrous oxide reduces anxiety and provides an amnesic effect. These properties may make the dental experience less stressful for patients who are fearful or anxious, those who are cognitively, physically, or medically compromised, those with certain medical conditions (hypertension, cardiac conditions, asthma, cerebral palsy), or those with a severe gag reflex (see Table 5.3.2). Nitrous oxide-oxygen should not be used in patients with chronic obstructive pulmonary disease (COPD), as the high concentrations of oxygen would block the hypoxic drive those patients use as the stimulant for respiration (see Table 5.3.3). Nitrous oxide should also be avoided in patients with an upper respiratory obstruction, such as stuffy nose, nasal polyps, upper respiratory infection, or blocked Eustachian tubes. Nitrous oxide has been associated with an increase in miscarriages and should not be used on patients in the first trimester of pregnancy or around pregnant dental team members. Gas volume and pressure can become dangerously high in a patient with bowel obstruction. It would also be inappropriate to use nitrous oxide-oxygen in an individual with severe

Table 5.3.1: Properties of nitrous oxide.

Analgesia
Mild sedation
Anxiolysis
Amnesia

Table 5.3.2: Indications for nitrous oxide use.

Fearful, anxious patient
Cognitively, physically, or medically compromised patient
Gag reflex interfering with oral health care
Profound local anesthesia cannot be obtained
Cardiac conditions, hypertension, asthma, cerebral palsy

Table 5.3.3: Contraindications to nitrous oxide use.

Chronic obstructive pulmonary disease (COPD)
Upper respiratory obstruction
Blocked Eustachian tubes
First trimester pregnancy
Bowel obstruction
Lack of consent

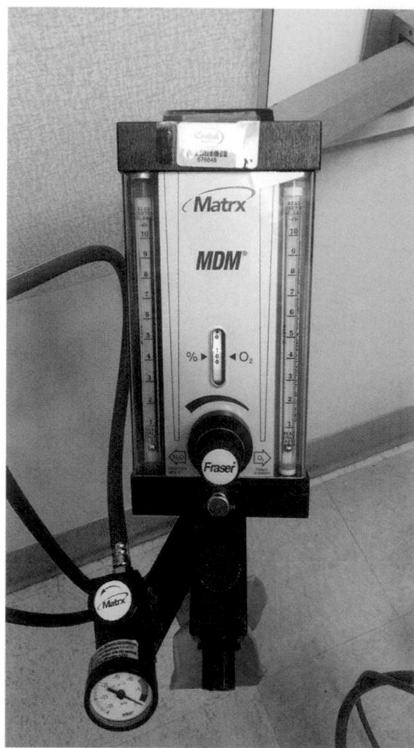

Figure 5.3.2: Contemporary nitrous oxide-oxygen unit.

cognitive impairment or in a patient who does not consent to its use (Becker and Rosenberg 2008; Weinberg et al. 2013).

Typical utilization of nitrous oxide-oxygen involves titration of the dose of gases. Pure oxygen (100%) is administered for the first two to three minutes and then nitrous oxide is added incrementally up to the desired concentrations. The nitrous oxide-oxygen is commonly dosed at its highest level (40/60–50/50) to allow for the delivery of local anesthesia, and is then lowered to working dosage of 20/80–30/70 to allow for comfort during the dental procedure. At the completion of treatment 100% oxygen is delivered for five minutes. Theoretically, diffusion hypoxia may occur when insufficient oxygen is delivered, although this may not be of clinical significance. Contemporary nitrous oxide-oxygen units (see Figure 5.3.2) are designed so that the concentration of oxygen cannot drop below 30%, which is higher than that which exists in ambient air. Nausea and vomiting are the most side effects of nitrous oxide administration.

Nitrous oxide-oxygen analgesia is safe and effective when used as directed. It does not cause respiratory depression, bronchodilation, cardiac arrhythmias, or hypotension. Despite its long history of safe use in dentistry, there is the risk of an untoward event if safety

Table 5.3.4: Safety features of contemporary nitrous oxide-oxygen units.

Color coded tanks and tubing (blue: nitrous oxide, green: oxygen)
Noninterchangable diameter indexed connection systems
Minimum oxygen percentage
Minimum oxygen liter flow
Oxygen fail-safe system
Scavenger systems
Alarms
Reservoir bag

protocols are not followed. The greatest concern is the prevention of hypoxia. Contemporary nitrous oxide-oxygen units have several design features intended to allow for safe use of the system (see Table 5.3.4). The gas supply tanks and associated tubing are color coded for ease of identification prior to attachment to the unit. In the United States, nitrous oxide tanks and tubing are coded blue; oxygen tanks and tubing are coded green. Connections of the gas supply to the unit have noninterchangable diameter indexed systems that do not allow the attachment of a gas to an improper inlet on the unit. The units are designed to supply a preset minimum oxygen concentration (30%) and a minimum oxygen liter flow (2.5–3 liters per minute). The oxygen fail-safe system will completely shut down all gas supply to the patient and allow the patient to breathe room air when oxygen delivery is compromised or depleted. The low-oxygen pressure alarm will sound or flash when the pressure in the oxygen line falls below 38 psi. The reservoir bag is easier for the patient to breathe from compared to the continuous flow of gases. The scavenger system vents expired gases to the office vacuum systems and reduces the occupational exposure of nitrous oxide by dental team members (Donaldson et al. 2012). Ignition of the nasal hood delivering nitrous oxide to a patient has been reported, which led to severe facial burns. The source of ignition was heat that originated during the preparation of a titanium post from a high-speed carbide bur with irrigation. Other sources of ignition could include electrosurgical units, lasers, and sparks from preparing other dental materials (Bosack et al. 2016).

Take-Home Hints

1. The anxiolytic properties of nitrous oxide-oxygen can effectively relax fearful, hypertensive, and cardiac patients, allowing the clinician to complete the proposed procedure. Patients with COPD utilize

low-oxygen concentrations in the blood as the driving force for respiration. High concentrations of oxygen can stop the respiratory drive in COPD patients. Use of nitrous oxide-oxygen would be inappropriate in COPD patients.

2. The use of color coded gas tanks and tubing identifies the gas product and reduces the risk of inappropriate gas supply attachment to the unit. The oxygen fail-safe system protects the patient by shutting down the flow of gases when the oxygen delivery is depleted or compromised. Scavenger systems protect the dental staff members from occupational exposure to expired nitrous oxide.
3. Asthmatic patients use a carbon dioxide drive for respiration, not a low oxygen drive. Nitrous oxide-oxygen does not cause hypotension. It can be safely used with the selective beta blocker metoprolol. Nitrous oxide-oxygen has no effect on the antiplatelet effects of aspirin and may be used for these patients.

Self-Study Questions

1. Which of the following patients would be an inappropriate candidate for nitrous oxide-oxygen therapy?
- **A. Fearful patient**
- **B. Hypertensive patient**
- **C. COPD patient**
- **D. Cardiac patient**

2. Which of the following safety features of contemporary nitrous oxide-oxygen units is intended to reduce occupational nitrous oxide exposure to dental team members?
- **A. Color coded tanks and tubing**
- **B. Oxygen fail-safe system**
- **C. Scavenger systems**
- **D. None of the above**

3. A 68-year-old male presents for scaling and root planning therapy. Review of medical history reveals that the patient is asthmatic, hypertensive, and had a coronary artery stent placed three years ago. Current medications include aspirin 81 mg, metoprolol 50 mg, and an albuterol inhaler that he uses approximately once a month. Which of the following statements regarding the use of nitrous oxide-oxygen in this patient is correct?
- **A. Use of nitrous oxide-oxygen should be avoided due to concerns of suppressing the patient's hypoxic drive.**
- **B. Use of nitrous oxide-oxygen should be avoided as the combination with metoprolol may lead to hypotension.**
- **C. Use of nitrous oxide-oxygen should be avoided as it may counteract the antiplatelet effects of aspirin, theoretically increasing the risk of thrombus formation in the cardiac stent.**
- **D. Nitrous oxide-oxygen use is appropriate in this patient.**

References

Becker, D.E. and Rosenberg, M. (2008). Nitrous oxide and the inhalation anesthetics. *Anesth. Prog.* 55: 124–131.

Bosack, R.C., Bruley, M.E., VanCleave, A.M., and Weaver, J.M. (2016). Patient fire during dental care. *J Am Dent Assoc* 147 (8): 661–666.

Donaldson, M., Donaldson, D., and Quarnstrom, F.C. (2012). Nitrous oxide-oxygen administration. When safety features no longer are safe. *J. Am. Dent. Assoc.* 143 (2): 134–143.

Jackson, D.J. and Johnson, B.S. (2002). Inhalational and enteral conscious sedation for the adult dental patient. *Dent. Clin. N. Am.* 46: 781–802.

Weinberg, M.A., Theile, C.M., and Fine, J.B. (2013). Sedation and general anesthetics. In: *Oral Pharmacology for the Dental Hygienist*, 2e, 73–86. Upper Saddle River, NJ: Pearson.

Additional Resources

Malamed, S.F. (2009). *Sedation. A Guide to Patient Management*, 5e. St. Louis, MO: Elsevier.

Answers to Self-Study Questions

1. C

2. C

3. D

Case 4

Topical Drug Delivery (Local Drug Delivery, Oral Rinses, and Irrigation)

CASE STORY

An 82-year-old Caucasian male presented for his regularly scheduled periodontal maintenance therapy appointment with a complaint of localized bleeding and gingival discomfort around his maxillary right first molar.

PROBLEM-BASED LEARNING GOALS AND OBJECTIVES

- Understand the therapeutic goals and limitations of localized delivery of antimicrobials in the treatment of periodontal diseases
- Understand the therapeutic goals and limitations of oral antimicrobial rinses and irrigation with oral antimicrobial rinses in the treatment of periodontal diseases

Medical History

The patient's medical history was significant for hypertension and hyperlipidemia. Current medications included Verapamil 240 mg, Diovan HCT 160 mg/12.5 mg, Toprol XL 25 mg, and Lipitor 10 mg.

Review of Systems

- Vital signs
  - Blood pressure: 124/68 mmHg
  - Pulse: 70 beats/min
  - Respiration: 14 breaths/min

Dental History

The patient had been treated for generalized moderate to severe chronic periodontitis 22 years earlier. Active treatment had entailed home care education, scaling and root planing therapy, pocket reduction periodontal surgery, and implant therapy in the upper left (UL) sextant. The patient was highly compliant with a regular schedule of three-month periodontal maintenance therapy and demonstrated fair oral hygiene. The patient reported brushing twice a day, flossing three times a week, and rinsing with Listerine Rinse.

Social History

The patient was a former smoker, having smoked a pack a day for 36 years. The patient quit smoking 21 years ago.

Extraoral and Intraoral Examination

There were no significant extraoral findings, no swellings or masses detected. Intraoral examination revealed no overt swellings, masses, or ulcers. Periodontal probing depths generally ranged from 2 to 3 mm, with a localized 5 mm probing depth mesial site #03. Generalized recession of 2–5 mm was noted. Generalized mild bleeding upon probing was noted, with localized moderate bleeding upon probing mesial of tooth #3 (see Figures 5.4.1 and 5.4.2).

Diagnosis

Localized moderate chronic periodontitis in tooth #3, generalized gingivitis on a reduced periodontium.

Treatment Plan

The treatment plan for the patient included home care reinforcement and periodontal maintenance therapy, with special attention to the mesial of tooth #3. Arestin, a localized chemotherapeutic antimicrobial agent, was placed in the mesial pocket of tooth #3. Arestin contains the tetracycline derivative minocycline. Subgingival delivery of Arestin into a periodontal pocket is intended

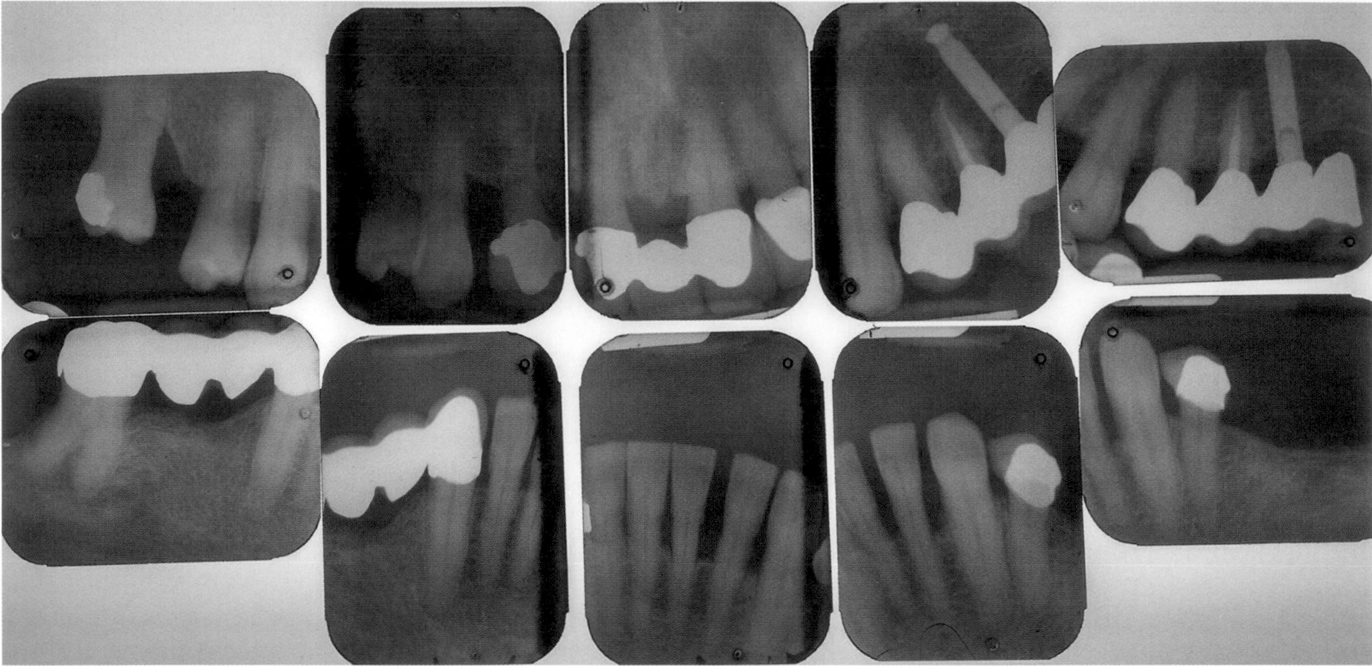

Figure 5.4.1: Full mouth series.

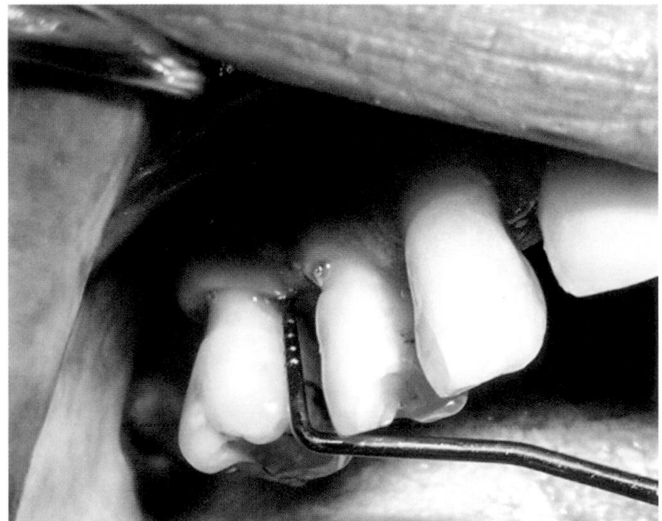

Figure 5.4.2: Deep probing depth mesial #3.

to reduce the subgingival biofilm load, with a resultant reduction in bleeding and probing pocket depth. The patient was advised to continue his home regimen of brushing, flossing, and rinsing with Listerine.

Discussion

Periodontal diseases are complex phenomena that are initiated by the body's host response to pathogenic subgingival biofilm. The infectious bacteria stimulate a cascade of inflammatory responses that result in the progressive destruction of the connective tissue attachment and supporting bone around teeth. The resultant periodontal pocket formation and alveolar bone loss contribute to patient discomfort, tooth mobility, decrease in chewing efficiency, and tooth loss. There is an overall decrease in the patient's quality of life.

Effective treatment of periodontal diseases involves addressing the etiologic factors of the subgingival biofilm mass and the patient's host response to the biofilm mass. Primary efforts are directed towards disrupting the plaque biofilm mass, which in turn will alter the host response. The disease gingivitis is treated biomechanically through a combination of meticulous supragingival and subgingival scaling, supragingival polishing, and patient home care education. The disease periodontitis is treated through a combination of meticulous supragingival scaling, subgingival scaling and root planning, patient home care education, and various types of periodontal surgical therapies when necessary. These treatments are highly effective and are considered the "gold standard" of periodontal therapy.

There may be instances where the goal of effectively disrupting the biofilm load may not be achieved. Patient compliance with home care procedures may be suboptimal. Anatomic variables (root proximity, root grooves or furcations, enamel pearls, deep periodontal pockets, etc.) may make mechanical debridement by the dental professional challenging. The patient's

Table 5.4.1: Requirements for a chemotherapeutic agent for use in periodontitis.

Criterion	Rinse	Irrigation	Localized Delivery
Reach site of action	Poor	Poor	Good
Adequate drug concentration	Good	Good	Good
Adequate duration of therapy	Poor	Poor	Good

medical status or economic factors may make advanced periodontal surgical procedures impractical. In those instances, a clinician may consider alternate methods to affect the biofilm load. Pharmacotherapeutic agents used as adjuncts to mechanical disruption of plaque include oral rinses, supragingival and subgingival irrigation with oral rinse solutions, and localized drug delivery of chemotherapeutics formulated for direct placement into the subgingival periodontal pocket. These agents have narrow, defined parameters in the treatment of periodontal diseases. It is imperative that both the dental professional and the patient be aware of the goals and the limitations of the products, so that unrealistic expectations of efficacy and patient outcomes can be avoided.

For any pharmacotherapeutic agent to be effective in treating a disease process, it must meet specific criteria (see Table 5.4.1). The drug product must reach the intended site of action, it must achieve an adequate drug concentration at that site of action, and it must maintain adequate drug concentration at the site of action for a minimum duration of time to affect the desired outcome.

Applying these criteria to oral rinse products, it has been shown that oral rinses do not enter the gingival sulcus to the depth of the periodontal inflammatory lesion at the base of the pocket. As such, oral rinses are not effective in treating the disease periodontitis. Oral rinses are available at adequate concentrations to affect plaque biofilm mass, but most products are of very limited duration of action with the effects decreasing rapidly after expectoration. Therefore, oral rinse products can be considered appropriate adjunctive therapy to biomechanical plaque removal in the treatment of gingivitis, but not in the treatment of periodontitis.

There are three major oral rinse products available in the United States that are effective antiplaque and antigingivitis agents (see Table 5.4.2). Chlorhexidine gluconate is a cationic bisbiguanide agent that ruptures bacterial cell walls. It is available as the products Peridex, PerioGard, and Paroex (alcohol free) a 0.12% prescription only oral rinse intended to reduce plaque and gingivitis. It is the only oral rinse product that demonstrates substantivity, the ability to adhere to oral tissues for an extended period after expectoration, and subsequently has a longer duration of antimicrobial activity compared with other oral rinse products. Its unintended side effects include alteration of taste, increase in calculus deposition, and brown staining of teeth and dental restorations. It is usually intended for short-term use, with the appropriate directions of rinsing with 15 ml twice a day. It should not be used immediately after tooth brushing, as the sodium lauryl sulfate component of most toothpastes will impede its effectiveness (Drisko 2001; Hill and Moore 2004).

Table 5.4.2: Oral antimicrobial rinses.

Product	Active Ingredient	Rx/OTC	Substantivity
Peridex	Chlorohexidine	Rx	Yes
Listerine	Essential oils	OTC	No
Crest ProHealth	Cetylpyridium chloride	OTC	No

Phenolic compound or essential oils antiseptic rinse is an effective nonprescription antiplaque and antigingivitis agent that disrupts bacterial cell walls. It is available as the product Listerine, and contains the ingredients menthol, thymol, eucalyptol, and methylsalicylate in a very high concentration (21.6–26.9%) alcohol solution. It is recommended for twice a day rinsing after brushing. It does not demonstrate substantivity, has a lower plaque-reduction effect, and a shorter duration of action than chlorhexidine. Its high alcohol concentration can lead to drying or burning of oral soft tissues and there are concerns about its use by patients in recovery from alcohol abuse (Drisko 2001; Hill and Moore 2004).

Cetylpyridium chloride is a quaternary ammonium compound cationic agent that ruptures bacterial cell walls. It is the antiplaque and antigingivitis agent in the nonprescription products Crest ProHealth Rinse, an alcohol free product containing 0.07% cetylpyridium chloride and Scope, a product containing 0.045% cetylpyridium chloride and 15% alcohol. Both products lack substantivity and have lower plaque reduction effects and duration of action than chlorhexidine or essential oils rinses (Hill and Moore 2004).

Supragingival and subgingival irrigation with water or a pharmacotherapeutic medicament has been evaluated

Table 5.4.3: Local chemotherapeutics agents.

Product	Active Ingredient	Sites Treated per Unit of Product
Periochip	2.5 mg Chlorhexidine gelatin chip	One
Atridox	10% Doxycycline gel	Several
Arestin	2% Minocycline microspheres	One

in several studies. Supragingival irrigation has been shown to enhance the gingival inflammation reduction effect of toothbrushing in patients with suboptimal plaque control. The addition of a medicament did not show any additional benefit than that achieved by irrigation with water. Subgingival irrigation with water or an oral rinse product did not result in a reduction of gingival inflammation, probing pocket depth, or gain in clinical attachment level beyond that achieved by scaling and root planing (Greenstein 2000). Subgingival irrigation does not extend to the site of the periodontal inflammatory lesion at the base of the pocket due to the presence of subgingival calculus and the continuous outward flow of gingival crevicular fluid.

Localized chemotherapeutic agents or site-specific antimicrobial agents are meant to be delivered directly into the subgingival periodontal pocket (see Table 5.4.3). They are controlled release products that contain a high concentration of antimicrobial impregnated within a delivery vehicle. After placement in the periodontal pocket, the active ingredient is slowly released in the pocket. Localized chemotherapeutic agents meet all three criteria for use in periodontitis. They reach the intended site of action, they achieve adequate drug concentration, and they maintain adequate drug concentration over a period of time. They also have the advantage of being resorbable and do not require removal by the dental clinician. There are three localized chemotherapeutic agents available in the United States: Periochip, Atridox, and Arestin.

Periochip contains 2.5 mg of chlorhexidine gluconate in a gelatin chip vehicle. It is intended as an adjunct to scaling and root planing therapy to reduce bleeding and periodontal probing depths. It is placed into the periodontal pocket and elicits antimicrobial effects over a seven to ten day period. Each unit of product treats one periodontal pocket; therefore multiple units would be required to treat multiple periodontal pockets. Studies comparing scaling and root planing alone to scaling and root planing combined with Periochip show small statistical improvements in probing depths and clinical attachment levels with the combination therapy, although the changes may not be clinically relevant (Greenstein and Polson 1998; Greenstein 2000).

Atridox contains 10% doxycycline hyclate, a tetracycline derivative, in a gel polymer formulation indicated as an adjunct to scaling and root planing therapy. The final delivery product is unstable, and requires mixing of the active doxycycline powder and the gel vehicle in a two-syringe system. Once mixed, one unit of product is sufficient to treat several periodontal pockets. Studies have shown that treatment with Atridox alone was equivalent, but not superior, to scaling and root planing in probing depth reduction. As doxycycline is a tetracycline derivative, review of the patient's medical history is necessary to confirm that the patient is not allergic to the tetracycline family of antibiotics. Additionally, use in female patients of child bearing age is a concern, as tetracyclines are known to stain the teeth of a developing fetus or nursing infant (Greenstein and Polson 1998; Drisko 2001; Hill and Moore 2004).

Arestin contains 1 mg of the tetracycline derivative minocycline microencapsulated in a bioresorbable polymer. It is indicated as an adjunct to scaling and root planing therapy. Each unit of product treats one periodontal pocket. Once delivered Arestin maintains therapeutic drug concentrations for 14 days. Studies have shown statistical benefits favoring the combination of Arestin with scaling and root planing compared with scaling and root planing alone (Hill and Moore 2004). As with the use of Atridox, consideration of treatment with Arestin necessitates the review of the patient's medical history to rule out allergy to tetracyclines. Use of Arestin in women of child bearing age is a concern due to potential effects on the developing fetus or nursing infant (Hill and Moore 2004).

Localized delivery of antimicrobials in the treatment of periodontitis has narrow, defined parameters. None of the currently available products have shown superiority over scaling and root planing as a monotherapy. Most studies of the combined therapy of a local antimicrobial agent with scaling and root planing have shown small benefits of statistical significance and questionable clinical significance (less than 1 mm). It is up to the individual clinician to determine when and if the use of an agent is in the patient's best interest. Considerations would include the patient's level of home care, the response to traditional therapy (scaling and root planing, surgery), the patient's medical status, and the number of symptomatic sites. The cost of the use of the products should be considered compared with alternate therapies (surgical therapy, increase in the frequency of maintenance therapy).

Take-Home Hints

1. For any product to be recommended for use in patient care, the professional must be aware of the disease process being treated, and the effectiveness of the product in treating that specific disease process. In the disease process periodontitis, the site of the inflammatory infectious lesion is at the base of the periodontal pocket. For a chemotherapeutic agent to be effective against the disease process periodontitis it would have to reach the base of the periodontal pocket. While oral rinse products are effective against bacterial plaque, they are unable to enter the periodontal pocket and reach the site of the lesion at the base of the pocket. Oral rinses are not effective in the treatment of the disease periodontitis. Oral rinse products are effective against the disease gingivitis, as they can reach the site of the gingivitis lesion.
2. Localized chemotherapeutic agents reduce the subgingival biofilm load, but they have narrow, defined parameters of appropriate use. A suboptimally controlled diabetic patient with generalized deep periodontal pockets following initial therapy would be better treated by reinforcement of homecare practices, stricter diabetic control by his physician, frequent maintenance therapy, and possibly periodontal surgical therapy. Localized drug delivery agents are never a substitute for scaling and root planing therapy. A smoker with generalized mild chronic periodontitis would be treated with smoking cessation counseling, home care education, and scaling and root planing. A patient with pregnancy associated gingivitis would be treated with home care education, scaling, and polishing. A well-maintained patient after comprehensive therapy for moderate chronic periodontitis, with an isolated deep inflamed periodontal pocket would be an appropriate candidate for localized delivery of a chemotherapeutic agent as an adjunct to scaling and root planing.
3. Prior to treating any patient, the dental therapist has a professional obligation to be aware of the patient's current medical history and be aware the effects of dental therapy on the patient's medical status. Knowledge of a patient's drug allergy is essential. If a patient has a known allergy to the tetracycline class of antibiotics, Atridox should be avoided as it contains the tetracycline derivative doxycycline. Periochip contains the active ingredient chlorhexidine. Crest ProHealth Rinse contains cetylpyridium chloride.
4. Irrigation with water or with any oral rinse has not demonstrated superiority above scaling and root planning. Scaling and root planning remains the standard against which all other therapies for periodontitis are measured. Calculus cannot be dissolved by any oral rinse product. Subgingival irrigation with water or any oral rinse product does not reach the base of the periodontal pocket due to the continuous flow of gingival crevicular fluid and the presence of subgingival calculus.

Self-Study Questions

1. Which of the following rinse products is effective against plaque and periodontitis?
- **A. Peridex**
- **B. Listerine**
- **C. Crest ProHealth Rinse**
- **D. None of the above**

2. The use of a localized chemotherapeutic agent to alter the subgingival biofilm would be most appropriate in which of the following clinical situations?
- **A. A type 2 diabetic patient with an HbA1c of 8.6% and generalized periodontal probing depths of 6–8 mm after initial therapy for severe chronic periodontitis.**
- **B. A patient with an isolated, bleeding, 6 mm periodontal pocket during the maintenance phase after comprehensive periodontal therapy for moderate chronic periodontitis.**
- **C. As a substitute for scaling and root planning in a patient with mild chronic periodontitis and a one pack per day smoking habit.**
- **D. As an adjunctive therapy to oral hygiene reinforcement in a patient with pregnancy associated gingivitis.**

3. Which of the following products should be avoided in a patient with a medically confirmed allergy to the tetracycline family of medications?
- **A. Periochip**
- **B. Crest ProHealth Rinse**
- **C. Atridox**
- **D. All of the above**

4. Which of the following statements is true regarding the use of irrigation in periodontal therapy?
- **A. Subgingival irrigation with chlorhexidine rinse is superior to scaling and root planing in disrupting the biofilm load.**
- **B. Subgingival irrigation with essential oils rinse has been demonstrated to dissolve calculus.**
- **C. Subgingival irrigation with cetylpyridium rinse has been demonstrated to extend to the base of the periodontal pocket.**
- **D. None of the above**

References

Drisko, C.H. (2001). Nonsurgical periodontal therapy. *Periodontol 2000* 25: 77–88.

Greenstein, G. (2000). Nonsurgical periodontal therapy in 2000: a literature review. *J. Am. Dent. Assoc.* 131 (11): 1580–1592.

Greenstein, G. and Polson, A. (1998). The role of local drug delivery in the management of periodontal diseases: a comprehensive review. *J. Periodontal.* 69 (5): 507–520.

Hill, M.H. and Moore, R.L. (2004). Locally acting oral chemotherapeutic agents. In: *Periodontics: Medicine, Surgery, and Implants* (ed. L.F. Rose, B.L. Mealy, R.J. Genco and D.W. Cohne), 276–287. St. Louis, MO: Mosby.

Additional Resources

Da Rocha, H.A., Silva, C.F., Santiago, F.L. et al. (2015). Local drug delivery systems in the treatment of periodontitis: a literature review. *J. Int. Acad. Periodontol.* 17 (3): 82–90.

Hanes, P.J. and Purvis, J.P. (2003). Local anti-infective therapy: pharmacological agents. A systemic review. *Ann. Periodontol.* 8 (1): 79–98.

Answers to Self-Study Questions

1. D

2. B

3. C

4. D

Case 5

Systemic Antibiotics and Enzyme Suppression Therapy

CASE STORY
A 48-year-old female patient presented with complaint of pain and swelling of five days duration associated with her mandibular left first molar.

PROBLEM-BASED LEARNING GOALS AND OBJECTIVES
Understand the appropriate use of antibiotics in patients with periodontitis
Understand the goals and limitations of enzyme suppression/host modulation therapy in periodontics

Medical History

The patient reported that she had been diagnosed with type II diabetes three weeks prior to presenting for dental care. Her physician initiated a regimen of metformin 500 mg twice a day and advised her to return in six weeks for reassessment. Review of the patient's family medical history revealed that both her mother and her mother's sister are type II diabetics. The patient does not have a relationship with her father and is unaware of his medical history.

Review of Systems

- Vital signs
  - Blood pressure: 126/76 mmHg
  - Pulse rate: 73 beats/min
  - Respiration: 15 breaths/min

Dental History

The patient reports that she has not seen a dentist in about eight years and that she only sees a dentist when she is in pain. The patient reports brushing twice a day and states that she has never flossed.

Social History

The patient reports that she has smoked a pack of cigarettes per day since age 15 (33 pack years), uses marijuana three times a week, and drinks alcohol occasionally.

Extraoral and Intraoral Examination

There were no significant extraoral findings, no swellings, or masses detected. Limited intraoral examination revealed a fluctuant buccal swelling associated with tooth #19. Periodontal probing of tooth #19 revealed deep probing depths (5–9 mm), a deep Class II (possibly Class III) furcation defect with a 9 mm vertical component. Probing of the buccal furcation region elicited a mixed purulent serosanguinous discharge. Uneven marginal ridges and an open proximal contact between teeth #19 and #20 were noted. Radiographic examination revealed previous endodontic therapy #19 and restoration with a ceramometal crown. Large periapical radiolucencies were associated with both roots of tooth #19 (see Figures 5.5.1 through 5.5.4).

Diagnosis

Periodontal abscess #19, combined periodontic-endodontic lesion #19 (Armitage 1999).

Treatment Plan

As tooth #19 was deemed to have a poor prognosis, extraction was recommended. The patient did not consent to extraction that day, but did consent to drainage of the infection. After inferior alveolar block anesthesia with one carpule 2% lidocaine with 1 : 100,000 epinephrine, drainage was established through the furcation with combined ultrasonic and

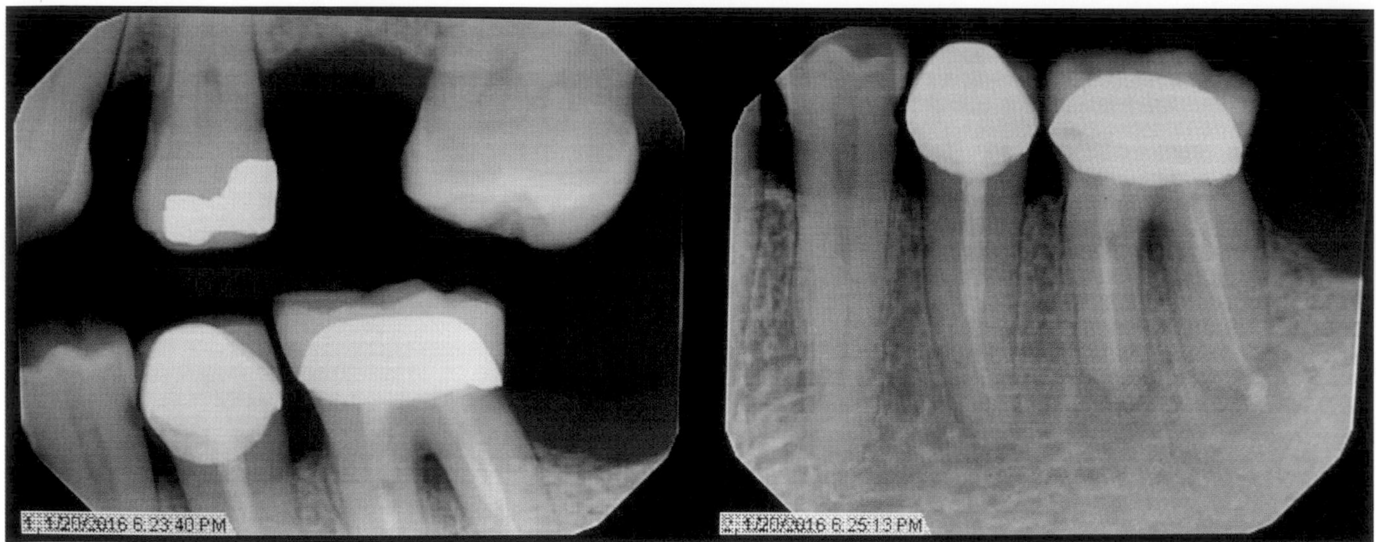

Figure 5.5.1: Radiographs of tooth #19.

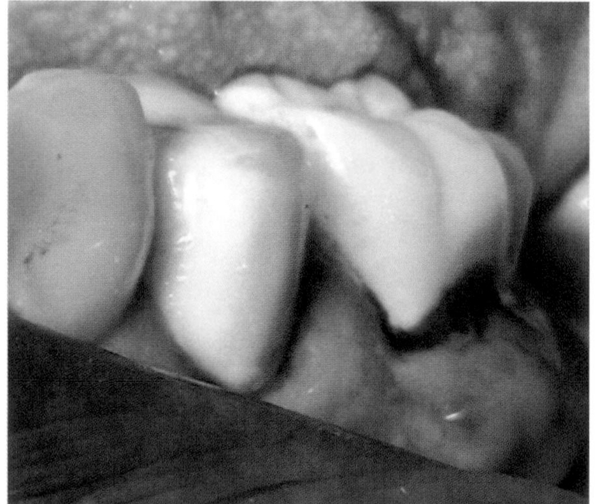

Figure 5.5.2: Periodontal abscess #19.

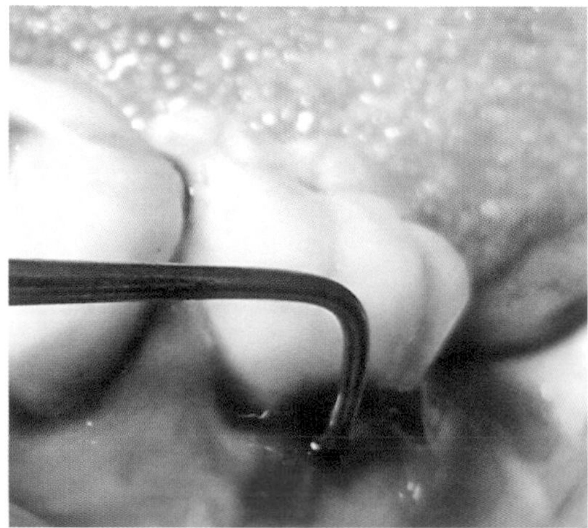

Figure 5.5.4: Horizontal component of defect.

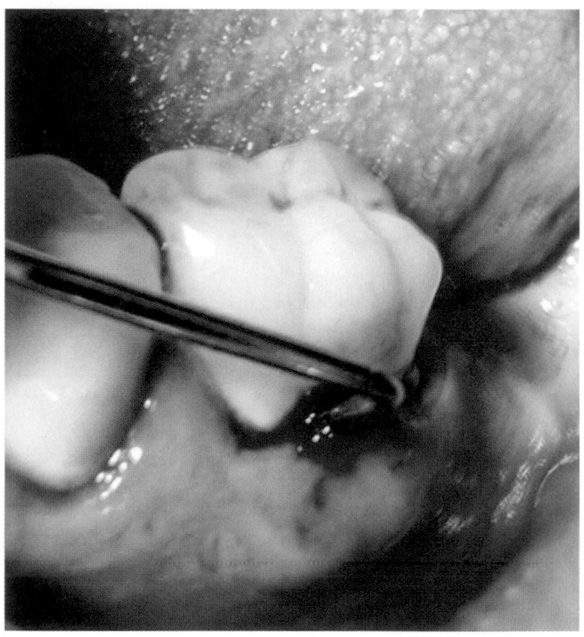

Figure 5.5.3: 9 mm vertical component of defect.

curette instrumentation. Antibiotics (amoxicillin 500 mg TID for seven days) were prescribed and the patient was advised to return in one week for extraction of #19 and for a comprehensive oral evaluation. The patient did not return and has been lost to follow up.

Discussion

Periodontitis is a bacterially initiated series of inflammatory processes that result in the destruction of periodontal connective tissue attachment and supporting bone. Traditional therapy focuses on disruption of the subgingival biofilm mass by mechanical methods such as intensive home care, scaling and root planing, and surgical debridement. Biofilm removal is a difficult task and ultimately incomplete. Most patients demonstrate a favorable clinical response, while some subpopulations of patients respond poorly.

Attempts have been made to address the subgingival biofilm mass through the use of systemic antibiotics with the intention of removing the residual biofilm remaining after mechanical therapy. Multiple clinical studies have been performed to evaluate the potential benefits of adjunctive use of systemic antibiotics in the treatment of chronic periodontitis, aggressive periodontitis, and periodontitis unresponsive to conventional therapy, previously referred to as refractory periodontitis (The American Academy of Periodontology 1989). Variations in research methodology, including study design, antibiotics utilized, dosages, and duration of therapy make comparisons between studies difficult. A recent systematic review of the use of systemic antibiotics in periodontics could not establish definitive conclusions or treatment recommendations (Garcia Canas et al. 2015). Individual clinicians will need to decide if and when antibiotic therapy is appropriate. If antibiotics are to be used, scaling and root planing therapy with intense home care education should be provided first to lower the biofilm load (Jorgenson and Slots 2000). Antibiotic use is generally considered during instances of acute infection (abscesses), and possibly in patients with aggressive periodontitis.

Prior to using systemic antibiotics, the clinician has the obligation to consider multiple patient factors (see Table 5.5.1). A comprehensive review of the patient's history is necessary with regard to allergies, comorbid medical conditions, current medication profile, and scheduled medical tests or procedures. Possible adverse drug reactions (side effects) of the antibiotics should be considered, as well as potential drug interactions with the patient's other medications. Most antibiotics can cause nausea and diarrhea, with resultant dehydration raising the blood levels of other medications. Indiscriminate antibiotic use may contribute to the development of bacterial resistance to antimicrobials. Patient compliance with the drug regimen and the economic cost should be considered. Finally, as with all medications, one must consider whether the use of the medication is expected to alter the overall clinical outcome of the disease.

Amoxicillin is a broad-spectrum penicillin that is bactericidal to both gram-positive and gram-negative bacteria (see Table 5.5.2). It is well absorbed orally and can be taken irrespective of meals. It is usually dosed at 500 mg every eight hours. As there is a great overuse of penicillin globally, there is potential for both bacterial resistance and allergic responses. It is susceptible to the bacterial enzyme beta-lactamase, which renders it ineffective. For that reason, a product has been developed that combines amoxicillin with a beta-lactamase inhibitor called clavulanic acid. The amoxicillin-clavulanic acid combination is marketed as the product Augmentin with recommended dosage 500 mg every 12 hours (Ciancio and Mariotti 2014).

Doxycycline is a tetracycline derivative that is bacteriostatic against gram-positive, gram-negative, spirochetes, and motile rods. The usual dose is 100 mg daily, but a dose of 100 mg twice a day for the first day

Table 5.5.1: Considerations prior to initiating antibiotic therapy.

Patient's medical history (allergies, comorbidities)
Potential drug interactions with patient's other medications
Side effects of the proposed antibiotic therapy
Patient's compliance with the antibiotic regimen
Risk of contributing to the development of bacterial resistance to antibiotics
Risk of alterations of the normal flora
Will the drug therapy alter the overall clinical outcome of the disease?
Economic issues

Table 5.5.2: Antibiotics used to treat periodontal diseases.

Class	Drug	Dosage
Penicillin	Amoxicillin	500 mg Q8H × 8 days
Penicillin + beta-lactamase inhibitor	Amoxicillin + clavulanic acid	500 mg Q12H × 8 days
Tetracycline	Doxycycline	100 mg once a day
Nitroimidazole	Metronidazole	500 mg Q8H × 8 days
Lincomycin	Clindamycin	300 mg Q8H × 10 days
Fluoroquinolone	Ciprofloxacin	500 mg Q12H × 8 days
Macrolide	Azithromycin	500 mg once a day for 4–7 days
Penicillin/Nitroimidazole Combination Therapy	Amoxicillin+ Metronidazole	250 mg of each Q8H × 8 days

Table 5.5.3: Unique adverse drug reactions (ADRs) of antibiotics.

Drug	ADR
Tetracyclines	Photosensitivity, staining of developing teeth of children and fetuses
Clindamycin	Pseudomembranous enterocolitis
Fluoroquinolones	Photosensitivity
Metronidazole	Disulfiram type reaction (severe vomiting when used with alcohol)

Table 5.5.4: Features of subantimicrobial dose doxycycline (SDD).

Does not have antimicrobial properties
Lowers matrix metalloprotease (MMP) levels
Long-term use does not lead to changes in antimicrobial susceptibility
Long-term use exerts no antibacterial effect on the subgingival microflora
Long-term use has no effect on the microflora of the GI tract, the GU tract, or the skin

and then 100 mg daily is not uncommon. Known side effects are photosensitivity and staining of the developing teeth of fetuses and nursing infants, leading to concerns about use in women of child bearing age (Slots and Ting 2002; Ciancio and Mariotti 2014).

Metronidazole is a nitroimidizole compound that is bactericidal to anaerobes, including spirochetes. It has been used to treat patients with necrotizing ulcerative gingivitis who present with systemic symptoms. It is usually dosed at 500 mg every eight hours. To increase its effectiveness against Aggregatibacter actinomycetemcomitans, it may be combined with amoxicillin at a dose of 250–500 mg of both agents every eight hours (Jorgenson and Slots 2000; Slots and Ting 2002). It has the unique side effect of a disulfiram reaction, in that it may induce severe vomiting when used with alcohol (See Table 5.5.3).

Clindamycin is a lincomycin derivative commonly used in patients with allergies to penicillin. It is bacteriostatic against anaerobes. A common dosage when used in periodontics is 300 mg every eight hours. A potentially fatal side effect of pseudomembranous colitis due to the overgrowth of Clostridium difficile is associated with clindamycin, although the condition may also occur with the use of other antibiotics (Jorgenson and Slots 2000). Clindamycin should not be used in patients with colitis.

Ciprofloxacin is a fluoroquinolone antibiotic effective against anaerobes. It is the only product effective against all strains of A. actinomycetemcomitans. Its usual dose when used in periodontics is 500 mg every 12 hours (Ciancio and Mariotti 2014). It may cause photosensitivity.

Azithromycin is a macrolide effective against anaerobes and gram-negative bacilli. The usual dose is 500 mg once a day (Ciancio and Mariotti 2014).

While systemic antibiotics are used with the intent of altering the subgingival biofilm mass, a reduced dose of the tetracycline derivative doxycycline, referred to as subantimicrobial dose doxycycline (SDD), is used with the intent of modifying the patient's host response to the biofilm challenge (see Table 5.5.4). Doxycycline is an effective inhibitor of the matrix metalloprotease enzymes (MMPs) that are responsible for the degradation of collagen, which leads the loss of periodontal connective tissue attachment and bone loss. At a dose of 20 mg twice a day, subantimicrobial dose doxycycline has demonstrated statistically significant and some minor clinically significant effects on periodontal probing depths and clinical attachment levels in selected patients with generalized severe chronic periodontitis (Caton et al. 2000). Less impressive effects are seen in patients with mild or moderate chronic periodontitis. The effects on probing depths and clinical attachment levels were not to the extent that would alter clinical decision making. Available as the prescription product Periostat, it is meant to be used for a minimum of 90 days.

At the recommended dose of 20 mg twice a day, doxycycline demonstrates no antimicrobial properties, and as such does not lead to any changes in the normal flora of the oral cavity, gastrointestinal tract, genitourinary tract, or skin. It does not lead to changes in bacterial sensitivity or resistance to tetracyclines. Since it is tetracycline derivative, there are concerns about its use in women of child bearing age due to its potential for staining of teeth in developing fetuses or nursing infants. It may cause photosensitivity.

Take-Home Hints

1. Prior to considering prescribing any medication, the responsible clinician would have reviewed the patient's medical history and would be aware of the potential for an adverse drug reaction (including allergic reaction) or drug interaction. Clindamycin is

from the lincomycin class of drugs. Doxycycline is from the tetracycline class of drugs. Metronidazole is from the nitroimidazole class of drugs. Amoxicillin is from the penicillin class of drugs and should be avoided in a patient with known allergy to penicillin.

2. Most periodontal conditions are effectively treated without the use of systemic antimicrobials. Generalized mild chronic periodontitis is treated with a combination of home care education and scaling and root planing. Medication associated gingival overgrowth is treated with a combination of home care education, scaling (or scaling and root planing if attachment loss is present), and possible periodontal surgery. Consultation with the patient's physician, with a possible change in drug therapy, may be appropriate. Herpetic gingivostomatitis is self-limiting and is usually treated with palliative care and occasional antivirals. A periodontal abscess is usually treated with definitive care: extraction if the tooth is nonmaintainable, or drainage of the infection. In those cases where definitive care is not possible or if the patient presents with uncontrolled risk factors (diabetes, smoking, immunosuppression, etc.) use of an antimicrobial may be appropriate.
3. The concept behind the use of subantimicrobial dose doxycycline is that the product can block the matrix metalloprotease enzyme collagenase without antimicrobial effects. Doxycycline at a dose of 20 mg twice a day demonstrates no antimicrobial properties. At doses of 50 mg or greater, doxycycline acts as an antimicrobial.
4. Even with long-term use, a subantimicrobial dose of doxycycline does not contribute to bacterial resistance as the product does not have any antimicrobial properties. Doxycycline is from the tetracycline class of medications and should not be used in patient allergic to tetracycline. The mechanism of action of low dose doxycycline is the inhibition of the matrix metalloprotease enzyme collagenase, not the reduction of Streptococcus mutans. There are concerns about the use of the product in women of child bearing age because tetracyclines are known to cause staining of the teeth of a developing fetus.

Self-Study Questions

1. Which of the following antibiotics would be inappropriate to prescribe to a patient with a medically confirmed allergy to penicillin?
- **A. Clindamycin**
- **B. Doxycycline**
- **C. Metronidazole**
- **D. Amoxicillin**

2. The use of a systemic antimicrobial agent may be considered appropriate in which of the following diagnoses?
- **A. Generalized mild chronic periodontitis**
- **B. Medication associated gingival overgrowth**
- **C. Periodontal abscess**
- **D. Herpetic gingivostomatitis**

3. Which of the following is the correct dosing regimen for a subantimicrobial dose of doxycycline?
- **A. 100 mg once a day**
- **B. 300 mg every eight hours**
- **C. 20 mg twice a day**
- **D. 500 mg every eight hours**

4. Which of the following statements is true regarding the use of a subantimicrobial dose of doxycycline?
- **A. Use of the product greater than 60 days is discouraged due to the risk of developing bacterial resistance.**
- **B. It can be used without concern in women of childbearing age.**
- **C. It should not be used in patients with a medically confirmed allergy to tetracycline.**
- **D. Its intended mechanism of action is to reduce salivary levels of Streptococcus mutans.**

References

Armitage, G. (1999). Development of a classification system for periodontal diseases and conditions. *Ann. Periodontol.* 4: 1–6.

Caton, J.G., Ciancio, S.G., and Blieden, T.M. (2000). Treatment with subantimicrobial dose doxycycline improves the efficacy of scaling and root planing in patients with adult periodontitis. *J. Periodontol.* 71 (4): 521–532.

Ciancio, S. and Mariotti, A. (2014). Anti-infective therapy. In: *Carranza's Clinical Periodontology*, 12e (ed. M.G. Newman, H.H. Takei, et al.), 515–524. St. Louis, MO: Elsevier.

Garcia Canas, P., Khouly, I., Sanz, J., and Loomer, P.M. (2015). Effectiveness of systemic antimicrobial therapy in combination with scaling and root planing in the treatment of periodontitis: a systemic review. *J. Am. Dent. Assoc.* 146 (3): 150–163.

Jorgenson, M.G. and Slots, J. (2000). Practical antimicrobial periodontal therapy. *Compend. Contin. Educ. Dent.* 21 (2): 111–114.

Slots, J. and Ting, M. (2002). Systemic antibiotics in the treatment of periodontal disease. *Periodontol 2000* 28: 106–176.

The American Academy of Periodontology. (1989). Proceedings of the World Workshop in Clinical Periodontics. Chicago, IL

Additional Resources

van Winkelhoff, A.J., Rams, T., and Slots, J. (1996). Systemic antibiotic therapy in periodontics. *Periodontol 2000* 10: 45–78.

Answers to Self-Study Questions

1. D

2. C

3. C

4. C

6

Surgical Periodontal Procedures

With thanks extended to Angelita L. Leon and Yung Cheng Paul Yu

Clinical Cases in Dental Hygiene, First Edition. Edited by Cheryl M. Westphal Theile, Mea A. Weinberg and Stuart L. Segelnick.

Case 1

Surgical Support Services

CASE STORY

An 87-year-old African American female presented with a chief complaint of "My gums bleed every time I brush."

PROBLEM-BASED LEARNING GOALS AND OBJECTIVES

- Understand when surgery is necessary to facilitate oral health
- Understand post-operative care

Medical History

Patient has hypertension and hypercholesterolemia. She takes the following medications: Toprol, Benicar, HCTZ, Norvasc, and Crestor. Her vital signs on her initial examination: blood pressure 135/74 mmHg and pulse 60 beats/min.

Social History

Patient does not consume alcohol or report the use of recreational drugs or tobacco.

Extraoral Examination

No significant findings were found. There were no abnormalities identified while palpating the various landmarks. The temporomandibular joint (TMJ) was within normal limits and the patient did not report any pain.

Intraoral Examination

Patient had thick fibrotic gingival tissue and generalized plaque and calculus deposits.

Periodontal Examination

A periodontal chart was completed during the visit.

- Localized plaque deposits and generalized BOP was noted.
- The pocket depths ranged from 2 to 4 mm, except for the premolars and molars where pockets of 6 and 7 mm were found
- Furcation involvement was found on all molars
- There was little to no mobility on all teeth

Occlusion

The patient presents with a Class I occlusion.
The patient also has an overbite of 2 mm and over jet of 1 mm.

Radiographic Examination

A full-mouth series of x-rays were taken. Upon radiographic examination:

- generalized horizontal bone loss
- radiographic calculus
- endodontically treated teeth

Diagnosis

Generalized moderate to severe chronic periodontitis.

Treatment Plan

Oral hygiene instructions, initial phase therapy consisting of supra-and subgingival scaling with polishing and re-evaluation at six weeks were performed. After re-evaluation osseous surgery was completed. Postoperative instructions were given and home care instructions reviewed. Recall every three months for periodontal maintenance.

Discussion

Without regular removal, dental plaque undergoes a process of maturation that results in development of pathogenic bacterial flora. The primary etiologic factor for periodontitis is bacteria versus the host response. Chronic periodontitis is defined as an inflammatory disease of the supporting tissues of the teeth caused by groups of specific microorganisms, resulting in progressive destruction of the periodontal ligament and alveolar bone with pocket formation, recession, or both. Chronic periodontitis affects most of the adult population and may be further classified on the basis of extent and severity. It has been reported that 47.2% of the US population has periodontitis; 64% of adults aged 65 years and older have periodontitis (Eke et al. 2012). Furthermore, chronic periodontitis may be associated with modifying factors such as systemic diseases, cigarette smoking, and local factors (Heitz-Mayfield et al. 2002).

Osseous resective surgery has been demonstrated to be more effective at reducing pocket depth when compared to nonsurgical treatment or open-flap debridement (Kaldahl et al. 1988; Serino et al. 2001). Osseous surgery is a procedure to modify bone support that has been altered by periodontal disease. The surgery is completed by either reshaping the alveolar process to create physiologic form or by removing bone to change the position of the crestal bone (Schluger 1949).

Osteoplasty is the removal of nonsupporting bone and is completed to facilitate flap adaptation. Ostectomy is the removal of supporting bone and is aimed for pocket elimination (Figure 6.1.1). Osteoplasty and ostectomy are utilized to establish positive architecture. Physiologic form is classified as positive architecture where the interproximal bone is coronal to the mid-buccal or mid-lingual bone. Negative architecture would be considered the opposite as the interproximal bone is more apical.

A full-thickness flap should be raised to examine the bony architecture. The least amount of trauma to the bone is desirable to allow for improved healing and less damage. The mean height of bone removed is between 0.06–1.2 mm (Carnevale and Kaldahl 2000).

Indications for osseous surgery include:

- reduce pocket depths >5 mm
- access for thorough debridement
- preserve teeth
- reduce bleeding on probing
- allow for better plaque control
- create positive architecture of the alveolar process.

Contraindications for osseous surgery include:

- shallow pockets
- pockets in visible esthetic areas
- three wall boney defects where regeneration is indicated
- medically contraindicated
- advanced bone loss (Figure 6.1.2)

(A)

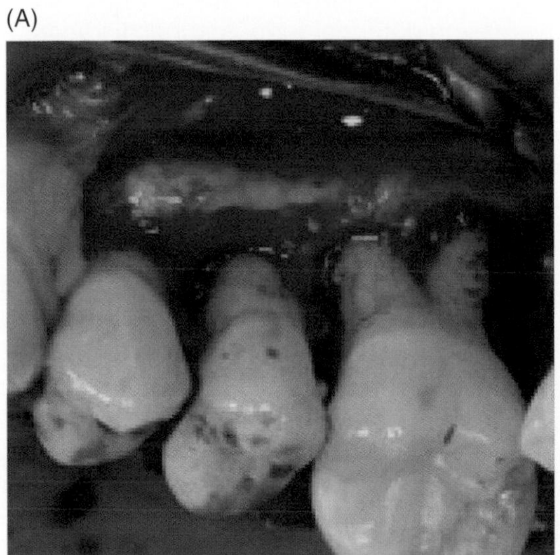

(B)

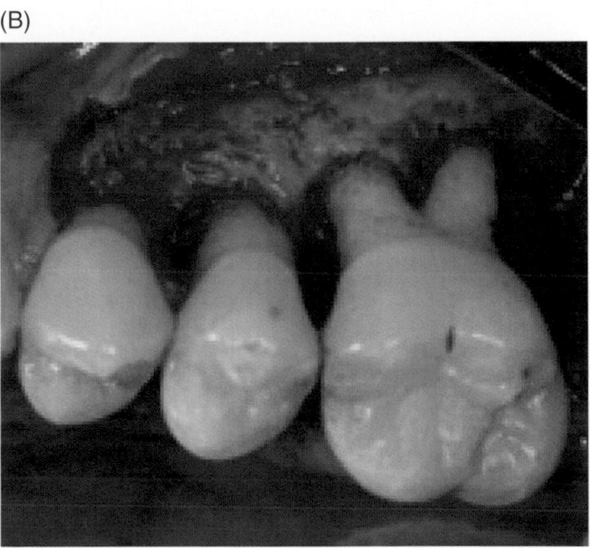

Figure 6.1.1: Before osseous surgery (A), notice the spacing between the bone to the tooth that created a crater defect. After osseous recontouring (B), the bony craters have been removed this will allow for better flap adaptation and pocket reduction.

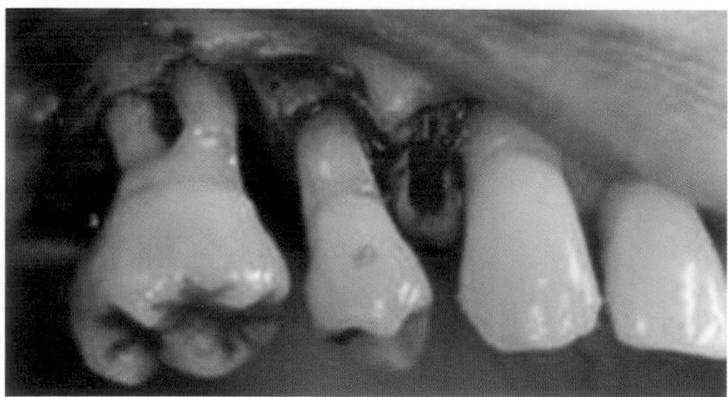

Figure 6.1.2: Negative architecture too severe to allow for osseous surgery.

- inadequate oral hygiene
- future periodontal maintenance not possible.

Proper instructions for self-oral care may help the affected patients to maintain good oral health in the postoperative period. Vallerand et al. (1994) showed that providing postoperative instructions both verbal and written improved compliance of the instructions given by the professional after molar removal. Although several variables could interfere with the adherence to postoperative guidelines, adapting the instructions to the needs of each patient or case, especially with regard to the limitations of understanding certain terms or language is necessary. A complete and detailed postoperative course and instructions not only reduces the anxiety that a patient might experience but also encourages adherence to them indirectly. The adherence and understanding to postoperative care instructions are components that impact the healing process after a surgical procedure.

Postoperative Instructions

- Explain and provide a written copy of postoperative care instructions to the patient that includes an emergency contact telephone number.
- Provide patient with prescription for an analgesics.
- Discuss with the patient instructions for taking the medications, and provide these instructions in writing.
- Ensure that the patient has someone to drive him or her home, depending on the type of anesthesia, and medications administered.
- Give the patient an ice pack to help reduce swelling immediately after surgery.
- Inform the patient to not brush or floss their teeth in the surgical area for a week.
- Bleeding is normal after surgery and there may be blood in the saliva for up to 24 hours.
- Care of periodontal dressing.
- Eat room temperature foods and avoid foods such as nuts, seeds, and popcorn that can irritate the surgical site.
- Smoking is an irritant to the surgical area, advise the patient to refrain from smoking for as long as possible.
- Schedule a postoperative appointment approximately one week after surgery.

Periodontal Dressing

The use of periodontal dressing arose from the desire to:

- Protect surgical sites from trauma
- Increase patient comfort
- Prevent wound contamination by oral debris
- Stabilize periodontal flaps (maintain blood clot)
- Tooth desensitization
- Tooth splinting
- Attempts to prevent excessive proliferation of granulation tissues.

Suture

A suture is a strand of material used to ligate blood vessels and approximate tissue. Sutures are necessary in many oral surgical procedures when a surgical wound must be closed, a flap positioned, or tissue grafted. Through time, a wide range of suture materials has been used, including silk, cotton, linen, synthetic, and animal tendons, and intestines. Today's suture materials are designed for specific procedures, thus decreasing potential for postsurgical infections while providing patient comfort and convenience (Daniel et al. 2008).

Resorbable sutures include plain gut, chromic gut, Polyglycolic Acid (PGA). Gut sutures are absorbed by enzymatic degradation. Plain gut is absorbed in five to seven days and chromic gut is absorbed in 10 to 15 days. PGA is a multifilament suture that is absorbed by hydrolysis and can last from two to four weeks.

Nonresorbale sutures include nylon, dPTFE, ePTFE, and silk. Silk sutures have the ability to collect bacteria, which makes them undesirable in sites where a graft has been placed.

Suture Removal

Most sutures are removed 7 to 10 days after placement. The steps of suture removal are (Daniel et al. 2008):

- Carefully remove any periodontal dressing to ensure that the healing gingival tissues are not disrupted.

- Carefully lift suture knots, and cut the sutures stand close to the gingival tissue.
- When removing continuous sutures, cut each section individually to prevent the dragging of lengthy, contaminated sutures through the healing tissue.
- Secure and gently pull each knot away from the surgical area, allowing short segments of suture to be guided from the surgical site with minimal discomfort to the patient.
- Place each knot on the gauze as it is removed.
- Count all knots to secure complete removal of the suture material.
- Record on the patient file the appearance of the tissue, healing characteristics, and number of knots removed.
- Check and gently remove any plaque and calculus in the area, especially around adjacent teeth.

With the knowledge of wound healing and dental materials, the dental hygienist is in a position to provide patients with an understanding of expectations after surgery and to assess surgical sites when dressings and sutures are removed (Daniel et al. 2008).

Surgery for treatment of diseases and correction of defects of the periodontal tissues is categorized specifically as periodontal surgery. Within the scope of periodontal surgery are Pocket Reduction Procedures, Periodontal Plastic Procedures, Periodontal Regenerative Procedures, and placing dental implants (Wilkens 2009).

Take-Home Hints

1. Chronic periodontitis is an inflammatory process that affects the supportive and protective tissues around the teeth. The characteristic feature of chronic periodontitis is its slow progression rate (Slim 2010). Chronic periodontitis can be localized or generalized and the severity is based on clinical attachment loss of mild (1–2 mm), moderate (3–4 mm), or severe (>5 mm).
2. Aggressive periodontitis is a specific type of periodontitis with clearly identifiable clinical and laboratory findings that make it sufficiently different from chronic periodontitis. It is a group of periodontal diseases characterized by localized or generalized loss of alveolar bone. Localized aggressive periodontitis has interproximal attachment loss on at least two permanent first molars and incisors, with attachment loss on no more than two teeth other than first molars and incisors. Generalized aggressive periodontitis has interproximal attachment loss on at least three teeth that are not first molars and incisors (Califano 2003).
3. Patients with a history of chronic periodontal infections are strong candidates for developing peri-implant disease and possible bone loss. It is important to control periodontal disease before placing dental implants (Donos et al. 2012). The reduction of oral bacterial count can aid in the preparation of the surgery; making postsurgical infection less likely or less severe (Peterson 1990). Reduction of inflammation of the gingiva and tissue tone improvement can be achieved by:
   - Removal of calculus deposits
   - Instructing in pre-surgical personal oral care procedures
   - Instructing in the use of foods
   - Interpretation of the dentist's directions
   - Motivating the patient who will have remaining teeth

Self-Study Questions

1. All of the following are indications for osseous surgery except:
- **A. Pocket reduction**
- **B. Debridement**
- **C. Advanced bone loss**
- **D. Create positive architecture**

2. Which suture material is nonresorbable?
- **A. Vicryl**
- **B. Plain gut**
- **C. Chromic Gut**
- **D. Silk**

3. All of the following are advantages of surgical dressing except:
- **A. Increased comfort**
- **B. Plaque retention**
- **C. Stabilizes the flap**
- **D. Retains the graft material**

References

Califano, J.V. (2003). Research, science, and therapy committee of the American Academy of Peridonotology. Position paper: periodontal disease of children and adolescnets. *J. Periodontol.* 74: 1696–1704.

Carnevale, G. and Kaldahl, W.B. (2000). Osseous resective surgery. *Periodontol* 2000 (22): 59–87.

Daniel, S., Harfst, S., and Wilder, R. (2008). *Mosby's Dental Hygiene, Concepts, Cases, and Competencies*. Mosby Inc.

Donos, N., Laurell, L., and Mardas, N. (2012). Heirarchical decisions on teeth vs. implants in the periodontitis-susceptible patient: the modern dilemma. *Periodontol* 2000 (59): 89–110.

Eke, P.I., Dye, B.A., Wei, L. et al. (2012). Prevalence of periodontitis in adults in the United States: 2009 and 2010. *J. Dent. Res.* 91: 914–920.

Heitz-Mayfield, L.J., Trombelli, L., Heitz, F. et al. (2002). A systematic review of the effect of surgical debridement vs. non-surgical debridement for the treatment of chronic periodontitis. *J. Clin. Periodontol.* 29 (Suppl. 3): 92–102.

Kaldahl, W.E.B., Kalkwarf, K.L., Patil, K.D. et al. (1988). Evaluation of four modalities of periodontal therapy. Mean probing depth, probing attachment level and recession changes. *J. Periodontol.* 59: 783–789.

Peterson, L.J. (1990). Antibiotic prophylaxis against wound infections in oral and maxillofacial surgery. *J. Oral Maxillofac. Surg.* 48: 617–620.

Schluger, S. (1949). Osseous resection: a basic principle in periodontal surgery. *Oral Surg. Oral Med. Oral Pathol.* 2: 316–325.

Serino, G., Rosling, B., Ramberg, P. et al. (2001). Initial outcome and long term effect of surgical and non-surgical treatment of advanced periodontal disease. *J. Clin. Periodontol.* 28: 910–916.

Lynne H. Slim. 2010 Chronic vs Aggressive Periodontitis [Online]. Available at: https://www.rdhmag.com/articles/print/volume-30/issue-8/columns/chronic-vs-aggressive.html (May 21, 2018).

Vallerand, W.P., Vallerand, A.H., and Heft, M. (1994). The effects of postoperative preparatory information on the clinical course following third molar extraction. *J. Oral Maxillofac. Surg.* 52: 1165–1170.

Wilkens, E.M. (2009). *Clinical Practice of the Dental Hygienist*, 10e. Philadelphia: Wolters Kluwer Health/Lippincott Williams & Wilkins.

Answers to Self-Study Questions

1. C
2. D
3. B

Case 2

Implant Procedures and Maintenance

CASE STORY

A 63-year-old African American female presented with the chief complaint of "I am due for a cleaning."

PROBLEM-BASED LEARNING GOALS AND OBJECTIVES

- To identify the signs and symptoms of peri-implant disease
- Understand implant maintenance

Medical History

Patient has hypertension and hypercholesterolemia. Current medications include Lipitor, Losartan, and 81 mg Aspirin. Patient states allergy to clindamycin. On maintenance visit blood pressure was 132/80 mmHg, pulse 74 beats/min.

Social History

Patient drinks socially and does not report the use of recreational drugs or tobacco.

Dental History

The patient's maxillary arch is restored with seven implants and has a history or periodontal disease.

Extra-Oral Examination

No significant findings were found. No abnormalities were identified and the TMJ was within normal limits.

Intraoral Examination

Generalized gingival inflammation was found due to plaque accumulation. The gingival tissue around implant #13 was erythematous and edematous. Upon palpation, suppuration was present. The platform margin of implant #12 was visible (Figure 6.2.1A).

Radiographic Examination

A radiograph revealed a saucer shaped defect with bone loss up to and around the fourth thread of implant #13 (Figure 6.2.1B).

Diagnosis

After reviewing the history and both the clinical and radiographic examinations, a clinical diagnosis of peri-implantitis was rendered (Figures 6.2.2 and 6.2.3).

Peri-implant diseases are inflammatory reactions in the tissues surrounding an implant. Peri-implant mucositis is confined to the mucosa without signs of loss of supporting bone. Peri-implantitis includes inflammation of the mucosa and loss of supporting bone (Zitzmann and Berglundh 2008). If left untreated, peri-implantitis may progress and lead to implant loss. It has been reported that peri-implantitis occurs between 28–56% of patients treated with implants, and peri-implant mucositis in 80% of patients (Lindhe and Meyle 2008).

Treatment Plan

The patient first completed an initial debridement of the area using hand instrumentation with titanium curettes and irrigation with chlorhexidine. This initial therapy was completed to reduce the amount of bacteria in the area and to improve the tissue consistency prior to surgical therapy. Six weeks after this initial treatment, the inflammation of the gingival tissue had reduced, but erythema was still present. Surgical therapy was initiated to restore the bony architecture that had been lost. The implant crowns were removed to gain access to the area of the defect. Once all the granulation tissue was removed, a detoxification of the implant was

(A)

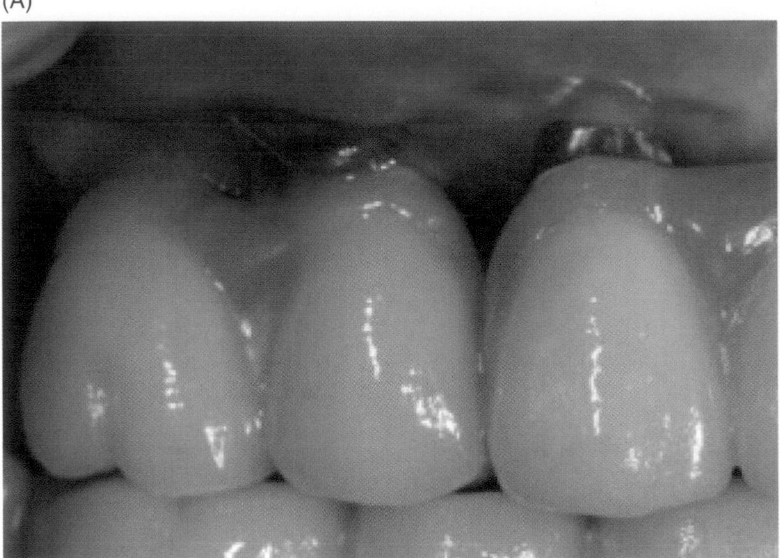

(B)

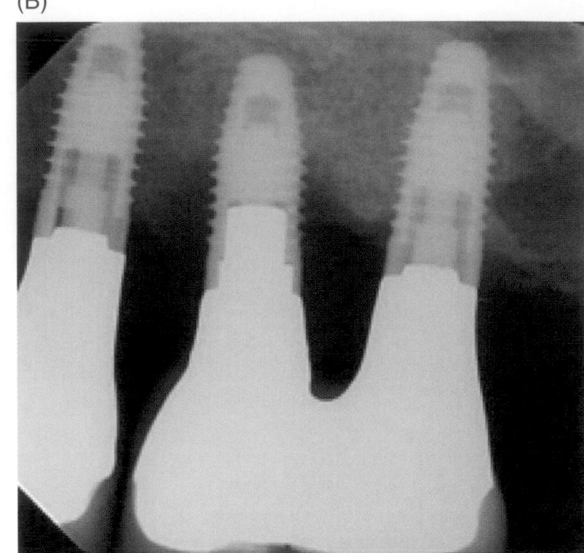

Figure 6.2.1: Clinical (A) and radiographic (B) images of implant #13 with peri-implantitis. Note the erythema and edema in the peri-implant mucosa (A) and the crater formed destruction around the implant (B).

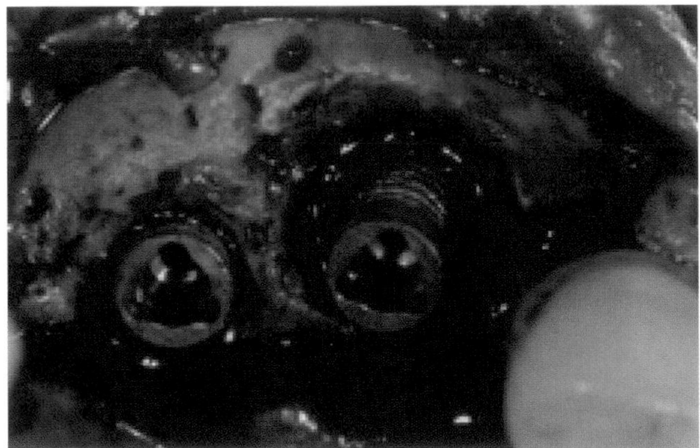

Figure 6.2.2: After crown removal and reflection of the gingival flap, the extent of the bone loss is observed.

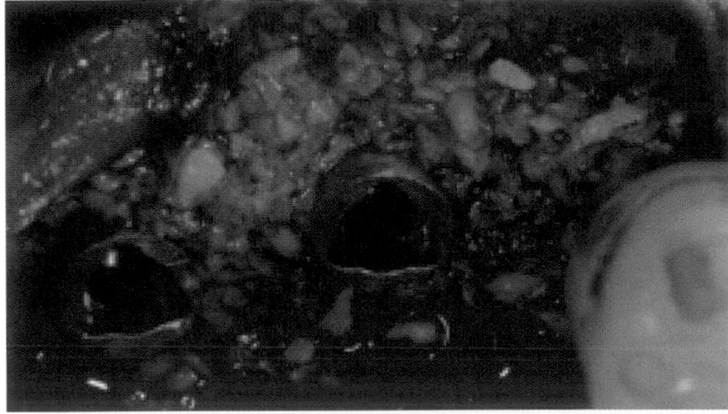

Figure 6.2.3: Bone graft placed to restore defect.

completed by chemical treatment of 35% phosphoric acid etching gel (Strooker et al. 1998) and implantoplasty using a fine diamond bur (Schwarz et al. 2011). A bone graft was placed to resolve the defect with an acellular dermal matrix to increase the soft tissue.

Discussion

There are many factors that can lead to peri-implant disease including (El Chaar 2009):

- history of periodontitis
- tobacco smoking
- bone quality
- excess cement
- lack of compliance and limited oral hygiene
- systemic diseases
- soft tissue defects or lack of keratinized gingiva
- implant malpositioning
- overcontouring the restoration.

The development of peri-implant disease appears to be accompanied by an increase in the bacterial species that have similarly been found to increase in periodontitis such as *Porphyromonas gingivalis*, *Tannerella forsythia*, and *Aggregatibacter actinomycetemcomitans* (Leonhardt et al. 1999).

The diagnostic parameters for peri-implant disease are probing, bleeding on probing, suppuration, implant mobility, and radiographic bone loss (Salvi and Lang 2004). Probing around an implant is used for bone sounding, as the epithelial and connective tissue around an implant differs from that of a natural tooth. Due the fibrotic nature of the gingival tissue around an implant, the connective tissue attachment is loosely arranged and not as tightly bound when compared to a natural tooth. Therefore, probing depth measurements at implants and teeth yield different information (Shou et al. 2002).

Treatment for peri-implant mucositis would be a nonsurgical intervention.

Nonsurgical treatment includes:

- Hand instrumentation using titanium or plastic curettes
- Prophy jet
- Laser
- Local antiseptic medication
- Oral hygiene instructions.

Treatment for peri-implantitis would be a surgical intervention.

Surgical therapy includes:

- Open flap debridement
- Regenerative procedures – such as bone grafting and guided tissue regeneration
- Resective procedures – implantoplasty
- Implant removal.

Assessment

At each maintenance visit, record:

- any sign of inflammation or changes in color, contour, or consistency of the gingiva
- if the gingiva around the implant is keratinized or nonkeratinized
- bleeding on probing
- probing depth
- mobility
- if suppuration is present
- review radiographs if any changes in bone level or crater like defect present (Wingrove 2013)
- if patient reports any discomfort around the implant.

For radiographs, if one to four implants: take vertical bitewing or periapical (PA) of each implant. Five or more implants: panoramic x-ray or individual PAs of all implants. The panoramic radiograph will not be able to assess peri-implant bone loss as well as individual PAs, but can be used to examine multiple implants at once. Radiographs should be present for time of implant placement, restoration, and one year for comparison. Radiographs should be taken yearly for implant sites (Wingrove 2013). Report all findings to the dentist.

Instrumentation

The key to proper instrumentation is the removal of plaque and any other deposits without scratching the surface of the implant or prosthesis. Instrument tip designs should provide the clinician with adequate options to address the patient's individual implant abutment and prosthetic components' needs. The instrument should offer some of the same basic features as a metal scaler or curette, while being made for an implant-friendly/compatible material. Some qualities to assess are: familiar design, ergonomic handles, rigidity to withstand scaling pressure without the risk of fracture or breakage, the ability of the instrument not to leave any residue behind, blade dimensions that allow easy and atraumatic access to implant abutment angulations and tissue tightness, and lightweight to avoid hand and wrist fatigue (http://www.rdhmag.com/articles/print/volume-32/volume-12/features/more-than-maintenance.html).

Implant Scalers Selection

Safe instrumentation on titanium implant surfaces should be performed with an implant scaler that is biocompatible, "titanium on titanium," to prevent instrument debris from becoming lodged on the surface, as it can harbor bacteria and increase the risk for peri-implantitis. They are thinner than plastic or graphite implant scalers, yet provide more strength to dislodge calculus and residue cement, which makes them more effective (Karring et al. 2005). Some implant instruments have been shown to achieve optimal implant maintenance results while preserving abutment and prosthesis surfaces without altering or scratching (Rentsch-Kollar et al. 2010). Polishing with a rubber cup and nonabrasive toothpaste, fine prophy paste, and tin oxide have all been shown not to alter titanium implant surfaces (http://www.rdhmag.com/articles/print/volume-32/volume-12/features/more-than-maintenance.html).

Take-Home Hints

1. The formation of plaque biofilm is considered the primary etiological factor in peri-implant disease initiation, and it is essential for the development of typical peri-implant infections (Mombelli and Lang 1994; Salvi et al. 2012).
2. Peri-implant mucositis is confined to the soft tissue with no signs of bone loss and can be treated nonsurgically. Peri-implantitis affects the soft tissue and displays bone loss. Peri-implantitis can be treated by nonsurgical and/or surgical therapy.

3. Early diagnosis of peri-implant diseases is important to ensure that the pathological processes can be arrested before the stability of the implant is compromised. After completion of dental implant treatment, the patient must be put on a tightly monitored maintenance schedule. Dental hygienists who perform these maintenance treatments play important roles in detecting the initial signs of peri-implant diseases.
4. Implant maintenance is a corner stone in the prevention of peri-implant diseases.
   Maintaining an implant patient is very similar to maintaining a patient with treated periodontitis. The maintenance recall interval is based on the patient's past history, susceptibility to periodontitis, and ability to control local factors at home. A maintenance visit should consist of a thorough visual examination of peri-implant soft tissues, tissue response upon external pressure by a periodontal probe, presence of suppuration, and periodical radiographs (El Chaar 2016). At home recommendations for patients with fixed implant-borne restorations include patient education regarding brushing and use of oral hygiene aids (Kumarswamy 2015).
5. Medical grade titanium scalers are recommended because they are biocompatible and thinner than plastic implant scalers. They also provide the needed strength to dislodge calculus and even residue cement.
6. Professional preventive measures need to be personalized to the individual patient, based upon clinical findings and lifestyle factors. This requires diagnosis to stratify subjects into:
   i. periodontally healthy, (ii) gingivitis (peri-implant mucositis), and (iii) periodontitis (peri-implantitis) as well as risk assessment for future status. Validated periodontal screening methods are now a fundamental requirement for all patients, given the high prevalence of periodontal and peri-implant conditions and should be applied universally (Tonetti et al. 2015).

Self-Study Questions

1. What is a risk factor for peri-implantitis and mucositis?
- **A. Excess cement**
- **B. Smoking**
- **C. Implant malposition**
- **D. All of the above**

2. Which of the following is surgical therapy for peri-implantitis?
- **A. Hand instrumentation**
- **B. Local antiseptic medical**
- **C. Implant removal**
- **D. Laser**

3. What type of implant scaler is used for implants?
- **A. Titanium**
- **B. Gracey currette**
- **C. Plastic**
- **D. Both A and C**

References

El Chaar, E. (2009). *J de Parodontologie et d'Implantologie Orale* 28 (3): 225–236.

El Chaar, E. (2016). *Ch 31–33 Horizontal Alveolar Ridge Augmentation in Implant Dentistry: A Surgical Manual.* Wiley Pub.

Karring, E.S., Stavropoulos, A., Ellegaard, B., and Karring, T. (2005). Treatment of periimplantitis by the Vectors system. A pilot study. *Clin. Oral Implants Res.* 16: 288–293.

Kumarswamy, A. (2015). Trends in prevention of Peri-implantitis. *Dimensions of Dental Hygiene* [Online] Available at: http://www.dimensionsofdentalhygiene.com/2016/05_May/Features/Trends_in_the_Prevention_Of_Peri-Implant_Diseases.aspx (May 21, 2018).

Leonhardt, A., Renvert, S., and Dahlen, G. (1999). Microbial findings at failing implants. *Clin. Oral Implants Res.* 10: 339–345.

Lindhe, J. and Meyle, J. (2008). Group D of European workshop on periodontology. Peri-implant dis-ease:

consensus report of the sixth european workshop on periodontology. *J. Clin. Periodontol.* 35 (8 suppl): 282–285.

Mombelli, A. and Lang, N.P. (1994). Clinical parameters for evaluation of dental implants. *Periodontol.* 4: 81–86.

Rentsch-Kollar, A., Huber, S., and Mericske-Stern, R. (2010). Mandibular implant overdentures followed for over 10 years: patient compliance and prosthetic maintenance. *Int. J. Prosthodont.* 23: 91–98.

Salvi, G.E. and Lang, N.P. (2004). Diagnostic parameters for monitoring peri-implant conditions. *Int. J. Oral Maxillofac. Implants* 19: 116–127.

Salvi, G.E., Aglietta, M., Eick, S. et al. (2012). Reversibility of experimental peri-implant mucositis compared with experimental gingivitis in humans. *Clin. Oral Implants Res.* 23: 182–190.

Schwarz, F., Sahm, N., Iglhaut, G., and Becker, J. (2011). Impact of the method of surface debridement and decontamination on the clinical outcome following combined surgical therapy of peri-implan-titis: a randomized controlled clinical study. *J. Clin. Periodontol.* 38: 276–284.

Shou, S., Holmstrup, P., Stolze, K. et al. (2002). Probing around implants and teeth with healthy or inflamed marginal tissues. A histologic comparison in cynomolgus monkeys. *Clin. Oral Implants Res.* 23: 313–323.

Strooker, H., Rohn, S., and Van Winkelhoff, A.J. (1998). Clinical and microbiological effects of chemical versus mechanical cleansing in professional supportive implant therapy. *Int. J. Oral Maxillofac. Implants* 13: 845–850.

Tonetti, S.M., Chapple, I., Jepsein, S., and Sanz, M. (2015). Primary and secondary prevention of periodontal and peri-implant diseases. *J. Clin. Periodontol.* 42: S1–S4.

Wingrove, S.S. (2013). *Peri-Implant Therapy for the Dental Hygienist: Clinical Guide to Mainte-Nance and Disease Complications (1).* Somerset, US: Wiley-Blackwell ProQuest library. Web. 16 May 2016.

Zitzmann, N.U. and Berglundh, T. (2008). *J. Clin. Periodontol.* 35 (Suppl. 8): 286–291. 6th European Workshop on Periodontology.

Answers to Self-Study Questions

1. D
2. C
3. A

7

Preventive Therapies

Clinical Cases in Dental Hygiene, First Edition. Edited by Cheryl M. Westphal Theile, Mea A. Weinberg and Stuart L. Segelnick.

Case 1

Plaque Removal; Individualized Patient Education

CASE STORY

The patient is Mrs. A., a 58-year-old Caucasian female with a history of periodontal disease, and who has been under periodontal maintenance for the past six years. At her dental hygiene appointment, the patient provided the following information summarizing the purpose of her visit: "I am concerned because recently my gums are sore on my lower jaw. Every time I brush there, it bleeds, and I think my breath has been bad lately. I used to be better at cleaning under my bridges but getting floss under those areas has become too difficult lately, my hands are not as good as they used to be. Plus, I have been traveling so I am overdue for my cleaning appointments."

PROBLEM-BASED LEARNING GOALS AND OBJECTIVES

- Customize oral hygiene instruction for plaque removal
- Identify specific patient needs and advise for appropriate oral self-care for implants, crowns, and bridges
- Techniques for behavioral modifications

Medical History

Mrs. A has a history of mild hypertension that is under dietary control. Drug allergies include sulfa and tetracycline. Due to menopause, the patient has been experiencing symptoms of xerostomia and insomnia. She has been taking a low dose 0.25 mg of Alprazolam to help with sleep when needed.

Dental History

Mrs. A has had the following dental treatments on her existing dentition: extractions, amalgam and composite resin restorations, endodontic therapy, implant placement, crowns, and in-office teeth whitening. She received nonsurgical periodontal therapy six years ago with recommended periodontal maintenance appointments every three months, which she continued until approximately 14 months ago. She is pleased with her smile and is interested in keeping her natural teeth as long as possible. She has not had any dental treatments in over 14 months due to her professional and personal schedule (see Figure 7.1.1).

Review of Systems

- Vital signs
- Blood pressure: 128/85 mmHg
- Pulse: 72 beats/min
- Respiration: 16 breaths/min

Social History

Mrs. A is married and is excited to be a new grandma. She is also planning to retire this year from her stressful job as the CFO of a large finance firm. Her friends and family are a big part of her life. She enjoys golf, working out, and traveling. Mrs. A consumes alcohol on a social basis of approximately two to four drinks per week. She admits to taking more Alprazolam during the workweek to help with the stress of her job. She does not smoke or have a history of recreational drugs use.

Extraoral/Intraoral Examination

Details shown in Figure 7.1.2.

Extraoral Findings

Mrs. A's face is moderately symmetrical, and there were no palpable nodes. The muscles of mastication

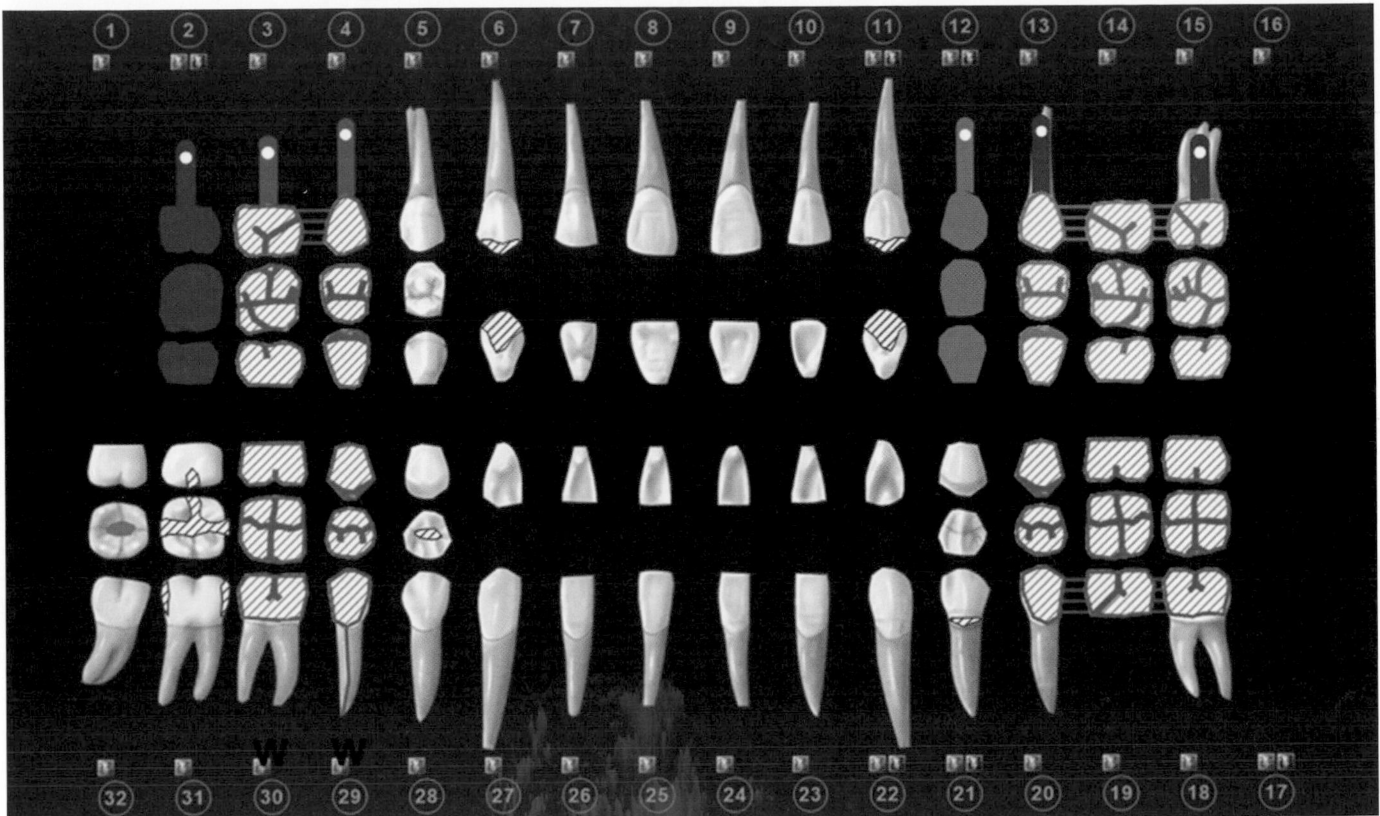

Figure 7.1.1: Odontogram of Mrs. A's current oral restoration status. Green color indicated "Existing Other," restorations completed by patients previous Doctor of Dental Surgery (DDS), blue color indicated existing restorations completed with current DDS. W indicated "watches."

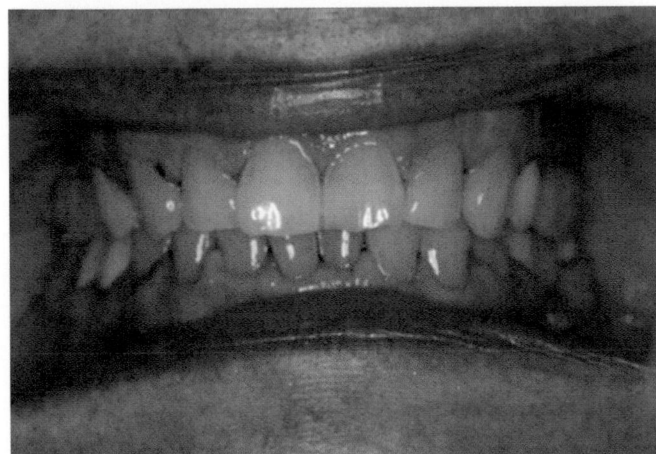

Figure 7.1.2: Oral photo using cheek retractors. Note uneven anterior wear from bruxism, #9 thinning enamel near the cervical third of tooth. Gingival color and texture are visible in the photo.

and facial expressions were asymptomatic. Mandibular range of motion was within normal limits, and the temporomandibular joints were asymptomatic.

Intraoral Findings

Soft tissue examination of the lips, tongue, oral mucosa, and pharyngeal tissues was within normal limits. Salivary glands were not swollen, and salivary ducts flowed freely. No swelling or irritation to the tonsillar area was apparent. Present were moderate inflammation and bleeding upon probing with a range of 4–6 mm pocket depth in the posterior aspects, and Class II embrasure spaces in the posterior region. Examination of the hard tissues confirmed light dental calculus and moderate dental biofilm subgingivally. Moderate dental biofilm was detected supragingivally around the gingival margins of the posterior lingual aspects. Clinical gingival characteristics included: gingiva color was uniformly pale pink, anterior consistency was firm while posterior consistency was soft, spongy, and dented slightly with the probe. Attrition of the anterior teeth was apparent.

Radiographic Examination

Updated vertical bitewings revealed vertical bone loss (see Figure 7.1.3).

Periodontal Charting

Confirmed Periodontitis, Stage III (Severe Periodontitis with potential for additional tooth loss) generalized, Grade A (slow rate of progression) with gingival inflammation and bleeding upon probing localized to sextant one, four, and six (see Figure 7.1.4).

Dental Hygiene Diagnosis

Problems	Related to Risks and Etiology
Periodontitis	Recurring periodontal pockets/dental neglect
Peri-implantitis	Dental biofilm invading implant site
Generalized alveolar bone loss	Chronic periodontal disease/dental neglect
Bleeding upon probing	Pathogenic microorganisms found in biofilm
Anterior abrasion	Parafunctional bruxism

Dental Hygiene Treatment Plan

Dental Hygiene Planned Interventions

Clinical	*Education/Counseling*	*Oral Hygiene Instruction*
Selective nonsurgical periodontal therapy with local infiltration anesthesia to selected quadrants and tooth numbers. LRQ: #28, 29, 30 and LLQ: #20,18 Removal of dental calculus and soft plaque deposits on all tooth and root surfaces. Implant scalers (plastic or titanium) used to scale and debride implant sites. Chemotherapeutics delivered to #18M, 18D, 31M, 30M. Fabrication of occlusal appliance (night guard) to help with bruxism. Periodontal re-evaluation four to eight weeks. Periodontal maintenance appointments every three months.	Educate and motivate about: The importance of regular dental visits including three-month periodontal maintenance appointments with chemotherapeutic agents if needed to reduce the risk of recurrence of periodontal pockets and advancement of alveolar bone loss. The importance of daily mechanical removal of biofilm around implants and bridges to maintain the longevity of restorations and maintain periodontal health. Hands-on demonstration using plaque removal aids that are appropriate to help heal the periodontium and manage self-care maintenance. Compliance and hygiene maintenance for occlusal guard	Patient education of oral self-care hygiene instructions included reinforcing brushing techniques to *Bass Sulcular* for posterior lingual aspects along with interproximal brushes for interdental care and a water irrigator for implants, crowns, and bridges. Recommended the use of a floss threader or tufted floss when traveling or when the patient does not have access to her water irrigator to cleanse under abutments and around implants properly. Recommended antimicrobial cleaning tablets for maintenance of occlusal appliance. The patient should be bringing the occlusal guard appliance in at all recare appointments to evaluate and professionally clean the appliance in the ultrasonic bath.

Discussion

There are myriad options to consider when selecting appropriate oral hygiene aids for patient self-care programs. The availability of self-care aids can be overwhelming; therefore it may be useful to limit the number of suggestions and choose an aid, (or aids) that can address multiple conditions. The hygienist should include with their recommendations: why the selected aids are necessary, how to use them correctly, the times and frequency with which they should be used, benefit factors, and expected outcomes. Individualized patient education can be motivational and increase the chances of the patient being responsive to the suggested behavioral modifications as part of their self-care regimen. Patient education should also include a discussion of the risks factors involved if neglecting to follow the individualized self-care program. Keep in mind that creating changes in behavior is neither quick nor easy. Research shows that the formation of a new habit can take considerable time and that the patient has to develop intrinsic motivation before new oral hygiene behaviors are likely to become a habit. The road to habit formation starts with unawareness and moves through six steps to finally the habit. Esther M. Wilkins, RDH, DMD describes the six steps of habit formation as follows:

I. **Unawareness** – many patients have little concept of the new information about dental and periodontal infections and how they are prevented or controlled.

II. **Awareness** – patient may have a food knowledge of the scientific facts, but they do not apply the facts to personal action.

III. **Self-interest** – realization of the application of facts/knowledge to the well-being of the individual is an initial motivation.

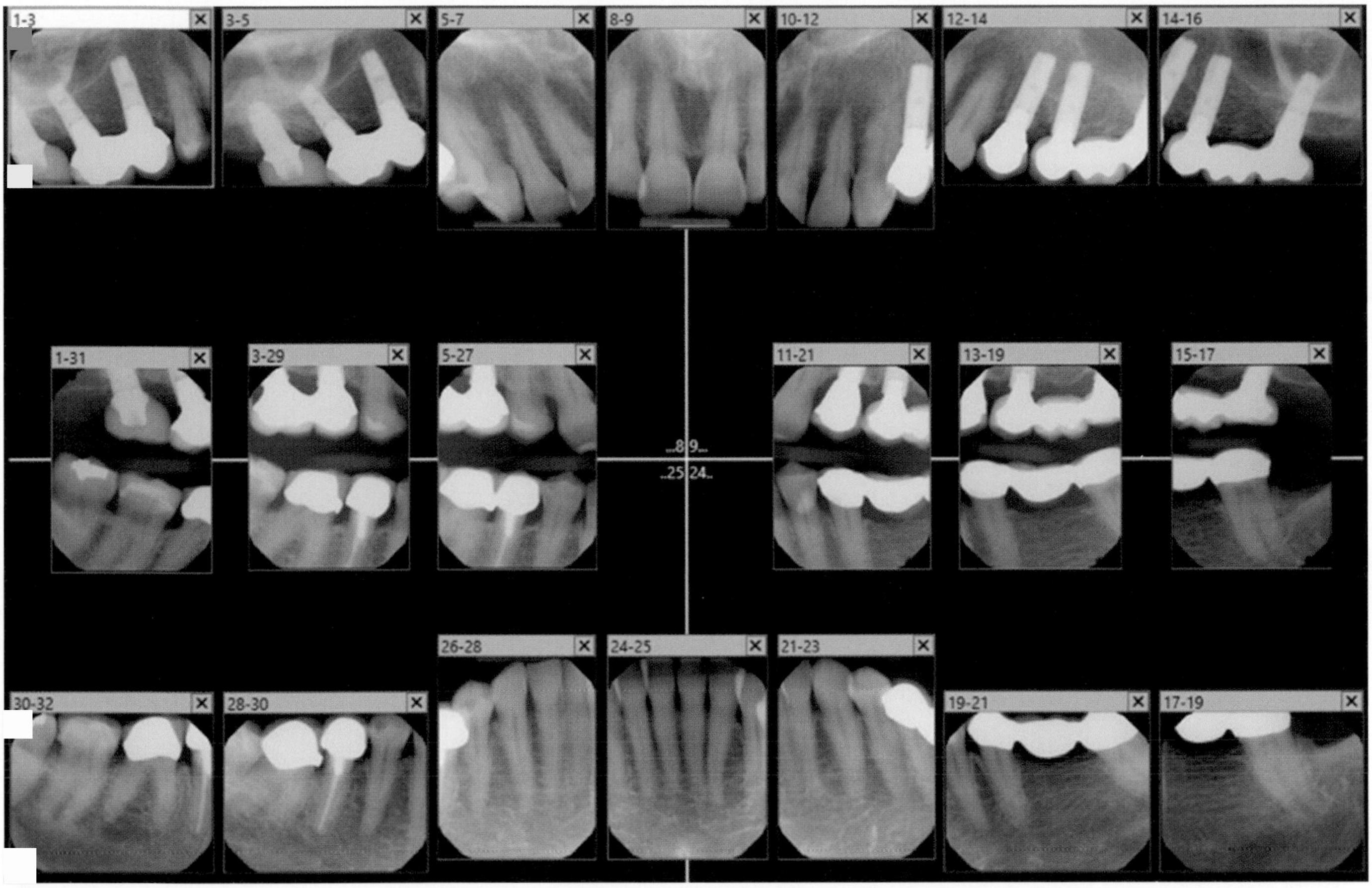

Figure 7.1.3: Full mouth series radiographs, updated vertical bitewings to reveal bone loss.

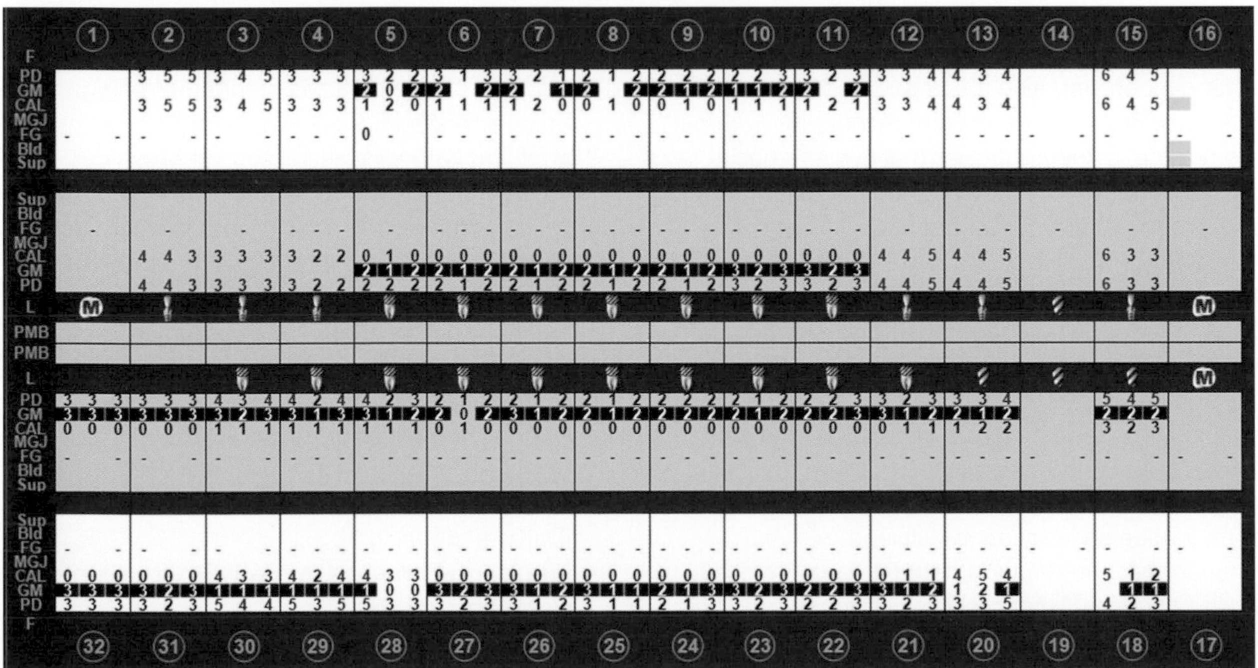

Figure 7.1.4: Periodontal charting indicated chronic periodontitis.

IV. **Involvement** – with awareness and application to self, the response to action is forthcoming when attitude is influenced.

V. **Action** – testing new knowledge and beginning of change in behavior may lead to an increased awareness that a real health goal is possible to attain.

VI. **Habit** – self-satisfaction in the comfort and value of sound teeth and healthy periodontal tissues helps to make certain practices become part of a daily routine. Ultimate motivation is finally reached.

In the situation with Mrs. A, she starts with the second stage of habit formation – *awareness*. She has prior dental knowledge of her periodontal history. Therefore, the best way to help her form a new self-care habit is to educate her about her current specific stage of oral health. It is helpful to show Mrs. A her most current periodontal charting record, radiographs, and intraoral photos of the areas that need attention. The information presented to Mrs. A is a comprehensive way to describe her individual needs by explaining the concerns regarding her current oral state, and the reasons why new recommendations for a customized plaque removal regime, are taking place. It is important to be clear with instructions, use demonstrations, and to take the time to answer all questions. Mrs. A will be more aware of her oral condition thereby creating self-interest that will hopefully encourage involvement in new oral self-care habits.

Mrs. A's next dental hygiene periodontal maintenance appointment is an excellent time to revisit the past individualized patient education recommendations, and also it is a good opportunity to continue to motivate and or modify techniques with her self-care regime. Creating proper oral hygiene habits take constant motivation and continuous education plus support from the entire dental team.

The goal for Mrs. A. is to prevent the progression and recurrence of periodontal disease and peri-implantitis. Patients who have nonsurgical periodontal treatment, and/or restorative treatment including implants and bridges need thorough and customized oral hygiene instructions to keep the tissue, and dental restorations maintained to achieve optimum oral health.

Periodontitis is reactive to plaque-induced factors. Therefore, plaque accumulation will lead to inflammation that can result in negative outcomes such as alveolar bone loss. This is why daily removal of biofilm is critical for Mrs. A. Data indicates that plaque control is a major contributor when improving gingival health by reducing inflammation (Chapple et al. 2015; Wilkins 2013). The removal of dental plaque by the forces of mechanical interdental cleaning will remove the primary etiological factor for periodontal or gingival diseases (Johnson et al. 2015). Toothbrushing with an acceptable dentifrice is the standard recommended self-care practice for cleaning the lingual, facial, and occlusal surfaces of all the teeth (Darby and Walsh 2015), but toothbrushing alone does not reach the interproximal surfaces effectively. Dental floss or other interproximal self-care aids are a helpful tool for plaque removal within the interproximal space and col area. However, the patient's dexterity and the likelihood of compliance is a consideration when recommending specific aids.

Assessments for Mrs. A include vitals, extraoral and intraoral exams, FMX (full mouth x-rays), periodontal charting, plaque index, calculus detection, following up today's reports of bleeding upon probing around the upper right implant bridge, the lower left three-unit bridge, and the lower right molars with Class II embrasure spaces around porcelain fused to metal crowns. Mrs. A's assessment results are an immediate concern to the dental hygienist to avoid peri-implantitis and the advancement of periodontitis.

Individualized patient education was created for Mrs. A to help restore her to gingival health and prevent further periodontal destruction. Mrs. A was instructed with regards to the following:

- **Toothbrushing twice a day for at least two minutes**
  Toothbrushing was recommended for the patient twice per day, morning and night after meals, for a duration of two minutes (minimum) using the Bass Sulcular method. Clinical evidence shows that brushing with a mechanical toothbrush can be more efficient than using a manual toothbrush (Lyle 2015; Yaacob et al. 2014), so with that in mind, and considering the moderate loss of dexterity she reported, Mrs. A was encouraged to use a mechanical brush. She was instructed focus on the lingual surfaces because she has higher rates of plaque and inflammation in these areas. To address Mrs. A's complaint of malodor, she was instructed to brush her tongue each time she brushes her teeth to reduce the bacteria that inhabit the dorsal surface (Darby and Walsh 2015).
- **Interdental brushes for daily interproximal cleaning**
  Interdental brushes were recommended for the patient over dental floss because they will be easier for her to use with her appliances, and evidence

suggests that interdental brushes are the most efficient method for interproximal plaque control (Chapple et al. 2015; Lyle 2015). Interdental brushes come in a variety of sizes for a range of embrasure spaces, including type II and III and recently even small or slim sizes are available for tight interproximal spaces. It is important to demonstrate the use of interdental brushes: if used incorrectly there is a chance that the patient can cause harm to the papilla or dental restoration. Interdental brushes for cleaning around implants should have a coated wire to avoid scratching the titanium or implant material (Johnson et al. 2015). Mrs. A was instructed how to determine the appropriate size and shape of interdental brush for her embrasure spaces, implants, bridges, and crowns. The dental hygienist demonstrated how to insert the brush into the embrasure space at a 90° angle while moving the brush in and out from facial to lingual. The wire should not bend when inserting into the embrasure space; this will be an indicator that the brush size is too big. Insertion should be easy, yet the brush bristles should be slightly larger than embrasure space to be able to reach both interproximal tooth surfaces.

- **Water irrigation at least once per day**
  Daily water irrigation can help reduce the levels of biofilm and inflammation. A water irrigator is helpful to remove plaque and food debris around and implants and under pontic teeth. Irrigation is beneficial to implants, crowns, and bridges due to the hydrokinetic activity, which produces a pulsating stream of fluid subgingivally where toothbrushes and interdental aids cannot reach (Darby and Walsh 2015; Jahn 2010; Johnson et al. 2015). The water stream of the irrigator can reach deeper than any other self-care aid. Multiple studies have shown that adding a dental water irrigator to self-care regimes can help reduce periodontal pathogens, bleeding, pocket depth, and inflammatory mediators (Jahn 2010; Lyle 2015). Oral irrigators should be used with caution because incorrect use around implants can cause damage to the junctional epithelium (Johnson et al. 2015). Mrs. A was instructed to use a low setting and to hold the irrigator tip horizontally while the nozzle tip is directed toward the interproximal area along the implant to avoid excessive water pressure and to help flush the aspects under the pontic teeth. Chlorhexidine gluconate or phenol compounds can be added to the water irrigators' reservoir to aid in the reduction of bacteria (Ernst et al. 2004; Jahn 2010; Johnson et al. 2015).
- **Floss threader or tufted/braided floss**
  Mrs. A has a two unit implant bridge on the upper right quadrant (URQ) tooth #3–4, a three unit implant bridge in the upper left quadrant (ULQ) tooth #'s 13–15, and a three unit bridge in the lower left quadrant (LLQ) tooth #'s 18–20. Dental tape or tufted/braided dental floss can clean around the abutments and crown margins. Some tufted or braided floss comes with a rigid needle attached to the floss acting as a floss threader to help with insertion into the abutment interproximal space. Gently guide the floss facial to lingual to cleanse interproximal space and then swept under pontic to the next interproximal space to remove and disturb biofilm accumulation. The tufted or braided floss can be wrapped around the implant to help clean the sulcular areas (Darby and Walsh 2015; Wilkins 2013).
  Include follow-up discussions with Mrs. A. regarding her self-care regime at every dental or dental hygiene appointment. Other self-care aid options can help Mrs. A. achieve optimum oral health if these above aids do not produce expected outcomes, and/or cause a lack of compliance (see Table 7.1.1).

Table 7.1.1: Self-care aid options and their use.

Self-care device	Description	Indication
Rubber tip stimulator	Rubber tapered cone tip on the top of a metal or plastic handle	Use light pressure to massage gingival margin and sulcus areas. Best for type II and III embrasures
Wooden wedge	Triangular toothpick	Use light pressure to remove plaque and food debris from type II or III embrasure (mild in and out motions)
End-tuft brush	Small brush head with a few tufted bristles on a handle.	Mimics vibration movements of Bass toothbrushing method for posterior areas and around dental restorations
Floss holder	Reusable plastic handles with floss attachments on the end in a Y or C shape.	Thread floss attachments and hold handle to cleanse interproximal spaces. Suitable for users with limited dexterity.

Take-Home Hints

1. Interviewing the patient during recare appointments is critical to determine if the suggested self-care aids are being used or helpful, or if modifications are needed.
2. Document what specific oral hygiene self-care recommendations are for each patient with proper education, demonstration, and include the risks and benefits in a legal record.
3. It is important when discussing recommendations to have samples devices or literature to help educate the patient on the purpose of the aid. They can then take the literature or sample to the store to purchase the new product.
4. Demonstrations are critical for increasing patient compliance. The patient has a better chance recalling the instruction when they were able to observe what they were taught by the dental hygienist.
5. Many individuals are noncompliant with traditional flossing techniques they do not know when traditional floss is required and its limitations (Segelnick 2004).
6. It is important to stay updated with which oral self-care aids consumers have access to, know which device is adequate for each condition, and recommend modifications if needed.

Self-Study Questions

1. The interdental brush needs to be ________ the embrasure space.

A. The same size of
B. Smaller than
C. Not bend into
D. Slightly larger

2. Which self-care aid uses hydrokinetic activity to help with biofilm reduction?

A. Power toothbrush
B. Rubber tip stimulator
C. Dental water irrigator
D. Floss holder

3. Self-care instructions should consider the patient's

A. Size of interproximal embrasures
B. Types of dental restorations present
C. Level of dexterity
D. Cost, safety, and effectiveness
E. All of the above

4. Which provides self-care aid can reach into the periodontal pocket further than any other device?

A. Extra-soft toothbrush
B. Tufted floss
C. Dental water irrigator
D. Rubber tip stimulator

5. Creating new habits or change in behavior

A. Starts with an old habit
B. Takes only one visit
C. Starts with unawareness
D. Starts with involvement

References

Chapple, I.L.C., Weijden, F.V.D., Doerfer, C. et al. (2015). Primary prevention of periodontitis: managing gingivitis. *J. Clin. Periodontol.* 42: 71–76. doi: 10.1111/jcpe.12366.

Darby, M.L. and Walsh, M.M. (2015). *Dental Hygiene: Theory and Practice*, 4e. Philadelphia: Saunders.

Ernst, C.-P., Pittrof, M., Fürstenfelder, S., and Willershausen, B. (2004). Does professional preventive care benefit from additional subgingival irrigation? *Clin. Oral Investig.* 8: 211–218. doi: 10.1007/s00784-004-0266-3.

Jahn, C.A. (2010). The dental water jet: a historical review of the literature. *J. Dent. Hyg.* 84 (3): 114–120.

Johnson, T.M., Worthington, H.V., Clarkson, J.E. et al. (2015). Mechanical interdental cleaning for preventing and controlling periodontal diseases and dental caries. Cochrane Database Syst. Rev. 1–15. doi: 10.1002/14651858.cd012018.

Lyle, D. (2015). Current evidence on primary prevention of periodontitis: self-care management of gingivitis. *Int. J. Evid. Based Pract. Dent. Hyg.* 1: 86–91. doi: 10.11607/ebh.23.

Wilkins, E.M. (ed.) (2013). *Clinical Practice of the Dental Hygienist*, 364–434. United States: Wolters Kluwer.

Yaacob, M., Worthington, H.V., Deacon, S.A. et al. (2014). Powered versus manual toothbrushing for oral health. Cochrane Database Syst. Rev. doi: 10.1002/14651858.cd002281.pub3.

Additional Resources

Crocombe, L.A., Brennan, D.S., Slade, G.D., and Loc, D.O. (2011). Is self interdental cleaning associated with dental plaque levels, dental calculus, gingivitis and periodontal disease? *J. Periodontal Res.* 47: 188–197. doi: 10.1111/j.1600-0765.2011.01420.x.

Dawson, T. (2013). An overview of interdental cleaning aids. *Dent. Nurs.* 9: 580–583. doi: 10.12968/denn.2013.9.10.580.

Gulati, M., Govila, V., Anand, V., and Anand, B. (2014). Implant maintenance: a clinical update. *Int. Sch. Res. Notices* 2014: 1–8. doi: 10.1155/2014/908534.

Manresa, C., Sanz, E., Bravo, M., and Echeverría, J.J. (2011). Interventions for the maintenance of the dentition in patients treated for periodontal disease. Cochrane Database Syst. Rev. doi: 10.1002/14651858.cd009376.

Sambunjak, D., Nickerson, J.W., Poklepovic, T. et al. (2011). Flossing for the management of periodontal diseases and dental caries in adults. Cochrane Database Syst. Rev. doi: 10.1002/14651858.cd008829.pub2.

Segelnick, S.L. (2004). A survey of floss frequency, habit, and technique in a hospital dental clinic and private periodontal practice. *N. Y. State Dent. J.* 70 (5): 28–33.

Saltmarsh, H. and Frantsve-Hawley, J. (2015). Evidence on the efficacy of dental floss, interdental brushes, wood sticks, and oral irrigation on reduction of plaque and gingivitis. Int. J. Evid. Based Pract. Dent. Hyg. 42–44. doi: 10.11607/ebh.001508.

Salvi, G.E. and Ramseier, C.A. (2015). Efficacy of patient-administered mechanical and/or chemical plaque control protocols in the management of peri-implant mucositis. A systematic review. *J. Clin. Periodontol.* 42: doi: 10.1111/jcpe.12321.

Answers to Self-Study Questions

1. D

2. C

3. E

4. C

5. C

Case 2

Fluoride – Systemic and Topical

CASE STORY

A 20-year-old female presents for dental examination after a three year hiatus from dental care. The patient has been away at college and has not been home for dental care for three years. At the dental examination just prior to leaving for college the third molars were removed and she was free from all dental disease, had received sealants on her molars, and had excellent oral hygiene.

Current clinical examination reveals eight intact sealants, previously extracted third, and no history of dental caries or restorations.

See Figures 7.2.1 to 7.2.3 for further details.

C0000, Caries
- C0001, Demineralized (Initial) Active
- C0002, Cavitated (Moderate) Active
- C0003, Cavitated (Extensive) Active
- C0004, Root Cavitated Active
- C0005, Root Demineralized Active
- C0006, Demineralized (Initial) Active
- C0007, Cavitated (Moderate) Inactive
- C0008, Cavitated (Extensive) Inactive
- C0009, Root Cavitated Inactive
- C0010, Root Demineralized Inactive
- C0011, E1 - Outer 1/2 Enamel Initial
- C0012, E2 - Inner 1/2 Enamel Initial
- C0013, D1 - Outer 1/3 Dentin Moderate
- C0014, D2 - Middle 1/3 Dentin Moderate
- C0015, D3 - Inner 1/3 Dentin Extensive
- C0016, RC - Caries in Pulp

Figure 7.2.1: Dental charting options for caries depth and activity in axiUm™ electronic health record.

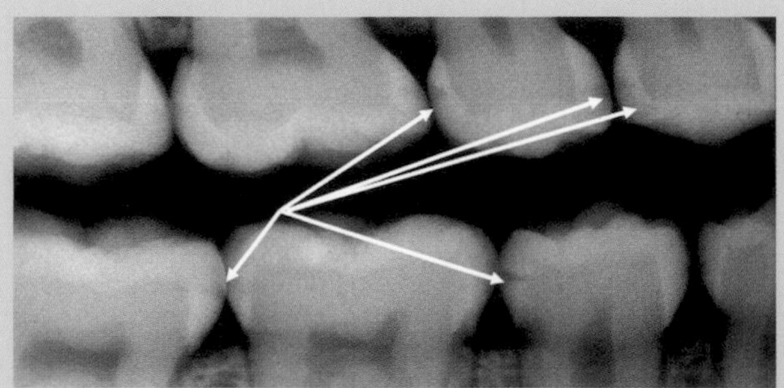

Figure 7.2.2: Bitewing radiograph displaying approximal caries of varied severity (E1, E2, and D1).

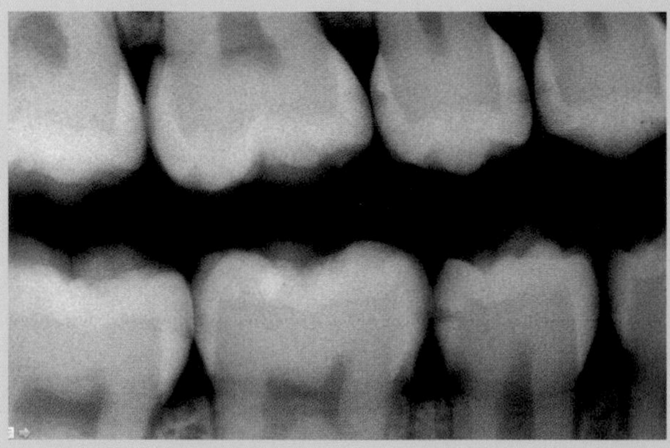

Figure 7.2.3: Bitewing radiograph.

PROBLEM-BASED LEARNING GOALS AND OBJECTIVES

- Identify the risk factors associated with development of dental caries
- Identify the fluoride based prevention/remineralization strategies available to manage early dental caries and recommend the appropriate therapies

Medical History, Review of Systems, Social History, Extra/Intraoral Examination, Occlusion, and Radiographic Examination

The patient is healthy in all aspects. She uses oral contraceptives and occasional antihistamines for seasonal allergies. Her past medical history and her review of systems are unremarkable. Her social history is positive for social intake of alcohol and patient denies use of recreational drugs or tobacco. The patient's extra/intraoral examinations are within normal limits and current clinical examination of teeth reveals no evidence of caries and excellent occlusion without evidence of excessive wear or physical damage. Radiographic examination is positive for initial to moderate approximal caries as highlighted below

Though caries penetration to the dentoenamel junction is only obvious on the lower second premolar, early caries is noted on the approximal surfaces of both first molars and the maxillary premolars.

Diagnosis

Dental caries and high caries risk.

Treatment Plan

Nonsurgical Caries Management

- Improvement in oral hygiene including twice per day brushing with fluoride toothpaste (1000 ppm).
- Diet counseling to reduce the frequency of sugar containing foods and drinks (particularly drinks).
- High-concentration fluoride paste (5000 ppm) just prior to bedtime.
- Dental recall with professionally applied fluoride varnish three to four times per year.

Discussion

This patient presents with early active dental caries. In order to determine the proper therapeutic approach to treat these lesions, it is first necessary to classify the lesions by depth and activity of the disease (Ismail et al. 2013a). It is recognized that caries is a bidirectional disease with demineralization resulting in cavitation and remineralization resulting in lesion arrest or reversal (Pitts 2004). Cavitation is a continuum of a disease that starts with simple demineralization and if left untreated continues to deep cavitation and eventual loss of the tooth. Initial demineralization lesions penetrating as deep as one third the distance into the dentin (radiographically) may still have an intact outer enamel surface, have no bacterial penetration, and may be remineralizable (Ekstrand 1995; Ekstrand et al. 2007). The approximal lesions are classified by depth of penetration through the enamel. The decay is active as it did not exist three years ago (Ismail et al. 2013a). The causation of dental caries can be due to many factors. Changes in oral hygiene, diet, and systemic factors (particularly as they relate to salivary flow) are conditions most frequently associated with increased caries risk (Hara and Zero 2010). As there have been no changes in this patient's medical history and there is no clinical evidence of xerostomia on examination, changes in diet and oral hygiene are the most likely cause. The patient's social history indicates a significant change in living conditions, associated with living at college. Marsh and others demonstrated that stresses on the previously stable dental plaque ecoenvironment can result in a shift in that biofilm from healthy to one that is acid producing and, in this case, likely to cause caries (Marsh 2010; Marsh and Bradshaw 1995). Further demonstrated is that change in homecare can result in shifting the biofilm to a more acid forming, cariogenic, biofilm. In this case, the young dentally healthy female leaving home where diet and homecare had permitted a healthy ecosystem to thrive, allowed a shift in the ecosystem toward acid production. Minor changes in the patient's diet can result in significant acid production thereby creating an environment likely to produce caries (Newbrun 1979, 1982). Inquiry as to homecare patterns and diet with the patient is appropriate to confirm why the shift in ecosystem has occurred. The college experience is replete in habit changes including sleep, hygiene, and eating. The frequently discussed "freshman 15" weight gain is an example of a shift in dietary habits, whereby college students in their first-year gain 15 lbs. The changes in oral hygiene associated with changes in the student schedule are legendary (Levitsky et al. 2004).

Management of these initial caries lesions has shifted from surgical intervention to a medical management (Wolff and Larson 2009). Fluoride therapies represent the most common intervention for remineralization of initial lesions. Fluoride therapies can be divided into two categories, preventive and remineralization, with the therapeutic mechanisms often overlapping. Public water fluoridation is the mainstay of public health caries prevention therapies (Newbrun 1989; O'Mullane et al. 1988; Rozier 1995; Rugg-Gunn and Do 2012). Though highly effective in reducing new caries, fluoridated public water is unlikely to remineralize early lesions (particularly with changes in the local environment with improved hygiene and reduced carbohydrate consumption). Fluoride containing toothpastes (900–1500 ppm fluoride) are also very effective caries preventive methodologies with increased frequency of utilization demonstrated to prevent caries (Marinho et al. 2003, 2004; Twetman et al. 2003). Remineralization of initial lesions requires the reduction of plaque, reduction of the frequency of fermentable carbohydrate consumption, and the use of higher concentration fluorides. These high concentration fluoride products are being utilized as active therapeutics (not preventives) that are expected to reverse the active disease damage by remineralizing the initial lesions with calcium, phosphate, and fluoride. The most common therapies recommended for remineralization are 5000 ppm pastes for daily homecare and high concentration varnish products three to four times per year (Bailey et al. 2009; Ismail et al. 2013a, 2015; Marinho et al. 2013; Tellez and Wolff 2016). The products must be utilized for six months to multiple years after the initial caries is discovered. The lesions can be expected to reverse, arrest, or (at worst) stay the same (Featherstone 1996, 2009; Lynch and Baysan 2001). This program requires patient education, patient participation, and professional persistence with the remineralization program.

Take-Home Hints

1. Dental caries is preventable.
2. Dental caries is frequently treatable without a drill.
3. The dental team is integral in controlling this disease.
4. High-concentration fluoride (particularly varnish) frequently applied is a critical portion of nonsurgical caries management.

Self-Study Questions

1. Dental caries is a multifactorial disease that may be caused by all of the following except:

A. Diseases or medications that cause dry-mouth
B. Plaque accumulation
C. Excess consumption of acidic beverages
D. Frequent consumption of sugar containing beverages

2. Dental caries is a reversible condition in its initial phases

A. True
B. False

3. Management of dental caries requires:

A. Patient participation
B. Utilization of high concentration fluorides
C. Utilization of high concentration home fluorides
D. Use of antibiotics

References

Bailey, D.L., Adams, G.G., Tsao, C.E. et al. (2009). Regression of post-orthodontic lesions by a remineralizing cream. *J. Dent. Res.* 88: 1148–1153.

Ekstrand, K., Kuzmina, I., Bjorndal, L., and Thylstrup, A. (1995). Relationship between external and histological features of progressive stages in caries in the occlusal fossa. *Caries Res.* 29: 243–250.

Ekstrand, K.R., Martignon, S., Ricketts, D.J.N., and Qvist, V. (2007). Detection and activity assessment of primary coronal caries lesions: a methodologic study. *Oper. Dent.* 32: 225–235.

Featherstone, J. (1996). Clinical implications: new strategy for caries prevention. In: *Early Detection of Dental Caries* (ed. G. Stooky). Indiana: Indiana University.

Featherstone, J.D.B. (2009). Remineralization, the natural caries repair process–the need for new approaches. *Adv. Dent. Res.* 21: 4–7.

Hara, A.T. and Zero, D.T. (2010). The caries environment: saliva, pellicle, diet, and hard tissue ultrastructure. *Dent. Clin. N. Am.* 54: 455–467.

Ismail, A.I., Tellez, M., Pitts, N.B. et al. (2013a). Caries management pathways preserve dental tissues and promote oral health. *Community Dent. Oral Epidemiol.* 41: e12–e40.

Ismail, A.I., Pitts, N.B., Tellez, M. et al. (2015). The international caries classification and management system (ICCMS) an example of a caries management pathway. *BMC Oral Health* 15 (Suppl 1): S9.

Levitsky, D.A., Halbmaier, C.A., and Mrdjenovic, G. (2004 Nov). The freshman weight gain: a model for the study of the epidemic of obesity. *Int. J. Obes. Relat. Metab. Disord.* 28 (11): 1435–1442.

Lynch, E. and Baysan, A. (2001). Reversal of primary root caries using a dentifrice with a high fluoride content. *Caries Res.* 35 (Suppl 1): 60–64.

Marinho, V.C., Higgins, J.P., Sheiham, A., and Logan, S. (2003). Fluoride toothpastes for preventing dental caries in children and adolescents. *Cochrane Database Syst. Rev.* 7: CD002278.

Marinho, V.C., Higgins, J.P., Sheiham, A., and Logan, S. (2004). Combinations of topical fluoride (toothpastes, mouthrinses, gels, varnishes) versus single topical fluoride for preventing dental caries in children and adolescents. Cochrane Database Syst. Rev. (1): CD002781.

Marinho, V.C., Worthington, H.V., Walsh, T., and Clarkson, J.E. (2013). Fluoride varnishes for preventing dental caries in children and adolescents. *Cochrane Database Syst. Rev.* 7: CD002279.

Marsh, P.D. (2010). Microbiology of dental plaque biofilms and their role in oral health and caries. *Dent. Clin. N. Am.* 54: 441–454.

Marsh, P.D. and Bradshaw, D.J. (1995). Dental plaque as a biofilm. *J. Ind. Microbiol.* 15: 169–175.

Newbrun, E. (1979). Dietary carbohydrates: their role in cariogenicity. *Med. Clin. N. Am.* 63: 1069–1086.

Newbrun, E. (1982). Sucrose in the dynamics of the carious process. *Int. Dent. J.* 32: 13–23.

Newbrun, E. (1989). Effectiveness of water fluoridation. *J. Public Health Dent.* 49: 279–289.

O'|Mullane, D.M., Clarkson, J., Holland, T. et al. (1988). Effectiveness of water fluoridation in the prevention of dental caries in Irish children. *Community Dent. Health* 5: 331–344.

Pitts, N. (2004). Modern concepts in caries measurement. *J. Dent. Res.* 83: C43–C47.

Radike, A.W. (1968). Criteria for diagnosis of dental caries. Proceedings of the Conference on the Clinical Testing of Cariostatics Agents. *American Dental Association, Abstract* 18: 87–88.

Rozier, R.G. (1995). The effectiveness of community water fluoridation: beyond dummy variables for fluoride exposure. *J. Public Health Dent.* 55: 195.

Rugg-Gunn, A.J. and Do, L. (2012). Effectiveness of water fluoridation in caries prevention. *Community Dent. Oral Epidemiol.* 40 (Suppl 2): 55–64.

Twetman, S., Axelsson, S., Dahlgren, H. et al. (2003). Caries-preventive effect of fluoride toothpaste: a systematic review. *Acta Odontol. Scand.* 61: 347–355.

Tellez, M. and Wolff, M.S. (2016). The public health reach of high fluoride vehicles: examples of innovative approaches. *Caries Res.* 50 (Suppl 1): 61–67.

Wolff, M.S. and Larson, C. (2009). The cariogenic dental biofilm: good, bad or just something to control? *Braz. Oral Res.* 23 (Suppl 1): 31–38.

Additional Resources

Ismail, A.I., Tellez, M., Pitts, N.B. et al. (2013b). Caries management pathways preserve dental tissues and promote oral health. *Community Dent. Oral Epidemiol.* 41: e12–e40.

Young, D.A., Fontana, M., and Wolff, M.S. (eds.) (2010 Jul). Current concepts in cariology. *Preface. Dent. Clin. N. Am.* 54 (3): xiii–xv. UI: 20630186.

Answers to Self-Study Questions

1. C

2. A

3. D

Case 3

Pit and Fissure Sealants

CASE STORY

A 25-year-old male presents for dental examination after a seven-year hiatus from dental care. The patient has been away at college, started working and has not been examined for dental care during that time. His past dental history includes:

- Continuing ongoing dental preventive care at six month intervals prior to the hiatus;
- Has never had any sealants;
- Has lived in a fluoridated water community;
- Has brushed twice per day with a fluoride toothpaste;
- Had dentist applied fluoride treatment two times per year between ages 3 and 18;
- Has never had approximal caries;
- Has had his third molars removed;
- Has been free from all dental disease.

Current clinical examination reveals no caries but a number of early occlusal lesions, previously extracted third molars, and no history of dental caries or restorations. Patient demonstrates no gingival inflammation and only slight calculus formation (especially for a seven-year hiatus from care).

PROBLEM-BASED LEARNING GOALS AND OBJECTIVES

- Identify the indications and contraindications for sealant placement in children and adults
- Identify the strategies for appropriate identification and classification of caries lesions

Medical History, Review of Systems, Social History, Extra/Intraoral Examination, Occlusion, and Radiographic Examination

The patient is healthy in all aspects, eats a normal diet, exercises, and utilizes occasional antihistamines for seasonal allergies. His past medical history and his review of systems are unremarkable. His social history is positive for daily beer or wine consumption and he denies use of recreational drugs or tobacco. He exercises regularly and periodically runs marathons. During marathon training he utilizes sports drinks for rehydration. The patient's extra/intraoral examinations are within normal limits and the current clinical examination of teeth reveals no evidence of caries, except where noted, and excellent occlusion without evidence of excessive wear or physical damage (Figure 7.3.1). Radiographic examination is negative for approximal caries and occlusal radiographic findings are discussed later (Figure 7.3.2).

Though caries penetration to the dentoenamel junction is only obvious on the lower first molar radiographically and initial caries is noted on the occlusal surface of several molars clinically.

Diagnosis

Initial and moderate dental caries on occlusal surface and high caries risk for "occlusal caries" ONLY. Low caries risk for smooth surface caries.

Treatment Plan

Nonsurgical Caries Management

No change in oral hygiene, as the patient has low smooth surface caries risk and no periodontal disease. He should continue brushing twice per day with fluoride toothpaste (1000 ppm) and performing current interproximal care regime as it has been successful in preventing all disease.

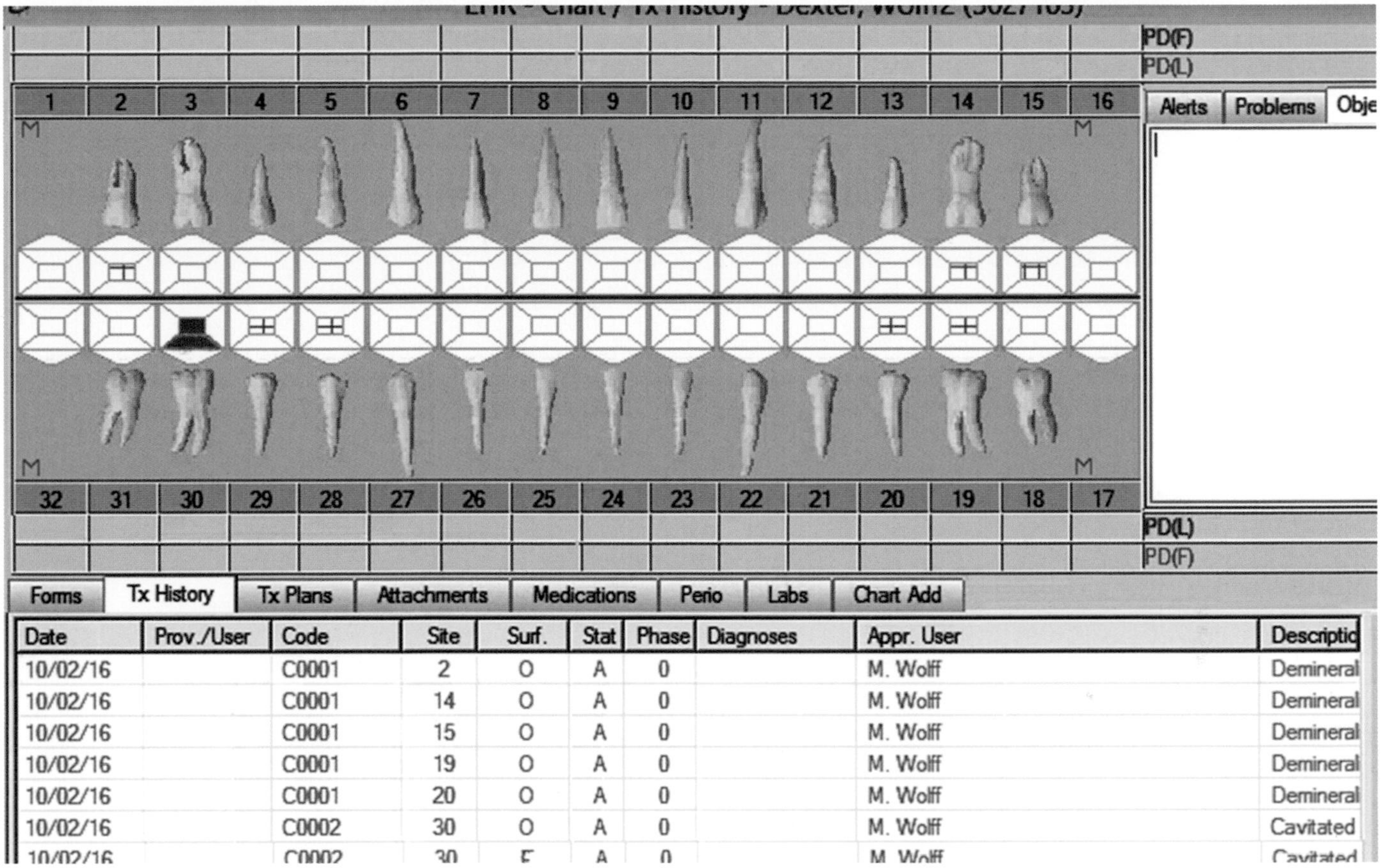

PD(F)
PD(L)

1	2	3	4	5	6	7	8	9	10	11	12	13	14	15	16
32	31	30	29	28	27	26	25	24	23	22	21	20	19	18	17

Alerts | Problems | Obje

PD(L)
PD(F)

Forms | Tx History | Tx Plans | Attachments | Medications | Perio | Labs | Chart Add

Date	Prov./User	Code	Site	Surf.	Stat	Phase	Diagnoses	Appr. User	Descriptio
10/02/16		C0001	2	O	A	0		M. Wolff	Demineral
10/02/16		C0001	14	O	A	0		M. Wolff	Demineral
10/02/16		C0001	15	O	A	0		M. Wolff	Demineral
10/02/16		C0001	19	O	A	0		M. Wolff	Demineral
10/02/16		C0001	20	O	A	0		M. Wolff	Demineral
10/02/16		C0002	30	O	A	0		M. Wolff	Cavitated
10/02/16		C0002	30	F	A	0		M. Wolff	Cavitated

Figure 7.3.1: Dental charting.

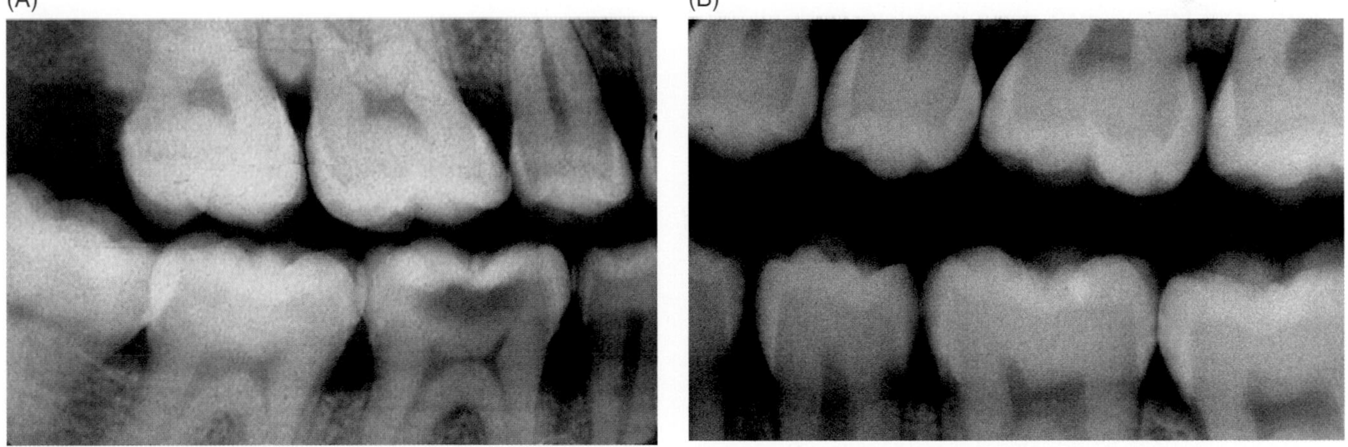

Figure 7.3.2: Bitewing radiograph.

No change in diet except diet counseling as to the risk of sports drinks for erosion and as a sugar source for caries and dried fruits as "sticky" sugar source.

Sealant placement on molars with initial lesions, do not seal teeth that do not have evidence of disease activity.

Dental recall once per year with bitewing dental radiographs every 24 months unless risk changes.

Surgical Caries Management

The patient requires surgical management of the caries defect on the occlusal of tooth #30. The tenets of minimal intervention require that: the caries be removed to obtain clean margins at the enamel interface; the caries is excavated, without exposure of the pulp; and the tooth restored. No surgical extension of the preparation through the sound enamel, rather sealant is applied to any susceptible fissures, preventing future disease rather than destroying sound tooth structure (Ismail et al. 2015; Ripa and Wolff 1992; Wolff et al. 2007).

Discussion

The diagnosis of the caries on the occlusal surface is no longer performed utilizing a sharpened explorer pressed into the fissure and looking for "tug back." Caries detection starts prior to the physical examination of the patient with a comprehensive history. Like any of the healing arts, listening to what the patient tells the practitioner about the nature of the conditions afflicting them is important … in this case the patient is 26 years old and has never had evidence of occlusal caries, which indicates that the anatomy was not highly susceptible to caries because over 20 years these surfaces would have developed caries. The current clinical findings, active demineralization, and the deep lesion associated with fissures, indicates that the prior environment has obviously changed.

Visual and Visual/Tactile Detection

The physical detection of caries starts with a process of careful examination. The utilization of the sharp explorer to locate carious teeth was described by Taft in his text *A Practical Treatise to Operative Dentistry* in 1859 and later editions 1888, but there was no mention of the utilization of any pressure in the examination (Taft 1883). Radike (1968) enhanced Black's original diagnostic criteria by describing areas as carious when the explorer catches with moderate to firm pressure in the pits and fissures, as well as, translucency around the fissures. Visual/tactile examination utilizing an explorer with moderate pressure, as recommended by Black and Radike, has fallen into significant disfavor. Ekstrand et al. (1987) demonstrated that use of a sharp explorer in a compressive fashion when examining the occlusal surface of teeth produced irreversible traumatic defects in the occlusal fissures that actually favored lesion progression (Ekstrand et al. 1987). Further, in a study of 34 dentists examining 61 teeth for occlusal caries revealed that there was no difference in diagnostic accuracy between those that utilized the traditional explorer and those that utilized visual only examinations. The explorer did not add to the accuracy of the examination. The percentage of "clinically" correct treatment decisions was about 73% for both techniques with examinations utilizing explorers having higher incidence of "over treatment" and examinations utilizing visual only having a higher incidence of "under treatment" (Lussi 1991). Teeth classified in the "under treatment" category utilizing the visual only examination technique probably should be recommended for sealant therapy, rendering this "under" diagnosis probably nonclinically significant (Beauchamp et al. 2008; Griffin et al. 2008). The finding of "over treatment" with the explorer were reported earlier by Bergman and Linden (1969). In addition, their experiments indicated that the explorer can convert a white-spot lesion into actual cavitation. Ekstrand et al. (2007) demonstrated that the use of a periodontal probe lightly moved across the lesion to detect roughness improved a practitioner's ability to determine lesion activity (Ekstrand et al. 2007). Roughness detected when lightly stroking the periodontal probe across the enamel in question is a sign of the current acid activity on the enamel surface and is classified as active disease. By 2001 the NIH Consensus Development Conference on Dental Caries Diagnosis and Management Throughout Life concluded that "the use of sharp explorers in the detection of primary occlusal caries appears to add little diagnostic information to other modalities and may be detrimental" (2001). The utilization of the explorer in a compressive force mode does not add diagnostic reliability if proper visual and radiographic examinations are conducted first. In fact, the use of the explorer AFTER visual and radiographic examination is minimally likely to locate undiagnosed lesions, rather more likely to inappropriately diagnose as carious lesions that at best should be sealed (see Figure 7.3.2). Avoiding damage created by explorers is important as Ismail (2004) emphasized that the "disease process may reverse or stop, resulting in complete healing of the demineralized dental tissue or in preservation of minutely damaged tissue" (Ismail 2004).

This patient presents with both initial dental caries with deep fissures on distal losing anatomy. In order to determine the proper therapeutic approach to treat these lesions, it is necessary to classify the lesions not only by depth and but also by activity (Ismail et al. 2013). The concept of caries activity recognizes that caries is a bidirectional disease with continued demineralization resulting in cavitation and continued remineralization resulting in lesion arrest or reversal (Pitts 2004). Cavitation is a continuum of a disease that starts with simple demineralization and if left untreated continues to deep cavitation and eventual loss of the tooth.

Caries examination of the occlusal fissure requires bright light, clean surfaces, compressed air, and a blunt ended explorer or periodontal probe. Quadrants should be isolated from saliva, surfaces cleaned so that fissures can be visualized, careful examination while the tooth is wet and then after thorough drying with compressed air. The periodontal probe/blunt probe is lightly scratched over the surface of the fissure to determine integrity AND to feel for surface roughness. The visualization is to determine whether the tooth appears glossy and smooth, white and frosted or whether there is a dark shadow beneath the fissure. Further visualization is performed to determine whether the fissure has lost integrity visually to or beyond the dentoenamel junction (DEJ). The fissure is evaluated for caries visually and tactilely as being: (i) Sound-perfect dental anatomy with an intact fissure (Figure 7.3.3A and B); (ii) Initial caries-loss of fissure anatomy (even if stained) that does not reach the DEJ (Figure 7.3.4A and 7.3.3B); (iii) Moderate caries, caries obviously penetrating beyond the DEJ (Figure 7.3.5A); and Extensive caries, caries penetrating deeply into the dentin approaching the pulp (Ismail et al. 2015) (Figure 7.3.6). The activity is assessed visually wet and dry with rough, chalky/white, nonreflective, and darkly colored sub-surfaces all indicate that the decay is active (Ekstrand et al. 2007). Comprehensive examination of the occlusal surface requires diagnostic bitewing radiographs. The bitewing radiograph must be examined to confirm that no occult caries is present at or below the dentoenamel junction that indicates occult caries (Figure 7.3.5B). Teeth may have regions of many levels of caries with fissures ranging from sound to moderate or severe, in scoring the surface is always scored at the worst level.

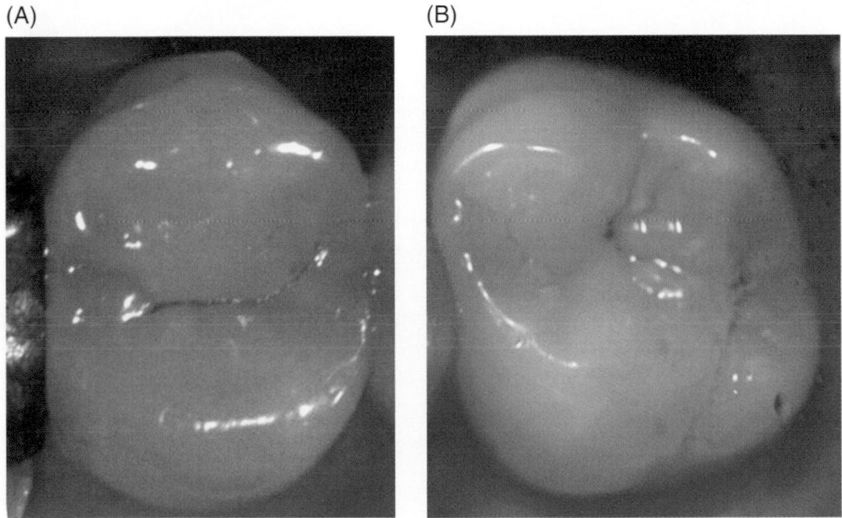

Figure 7.3.3: (A) Sound enamel (note the smooth shiny surface). (B) Sound enamel (note the smooth shiny surface).

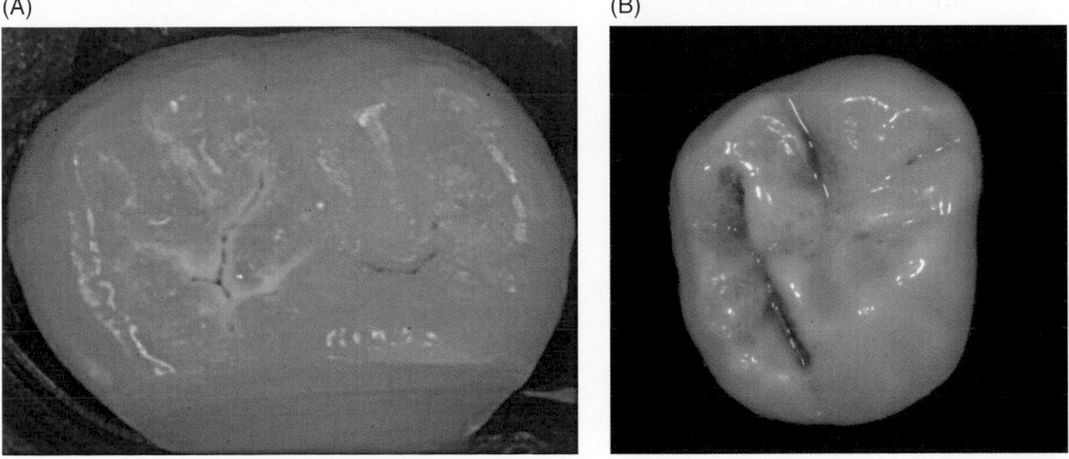

Figure 7.3.4: (A) Initial caries with active demineralization. (B) Initial caries with no demineralization.

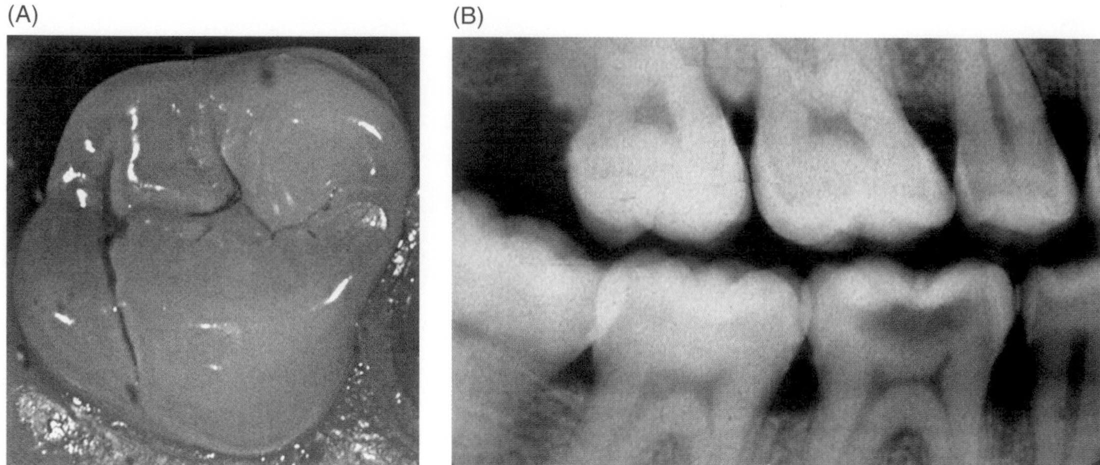

Figure 7.3.5: (A) Moderate caries (visible caries on distal). (B) Bitewing radiograph to confirm that occult caries is present at or below the dentoenamel junction.

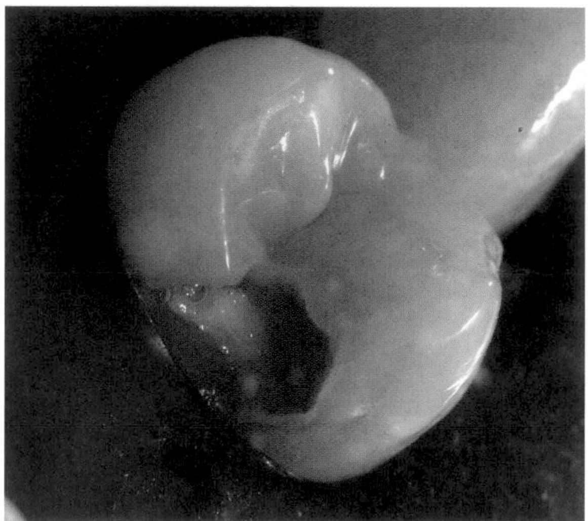

Figure 7.3.6: Extensive caries.

Caries in the Pits and Fissures ... It Is Different ... Why?

After completion of a comprehensive examination it is necessary to decide on appropriate treatment. It is necessary to understand the unique environment of the fissure that makes treatment modalities different. Fissures are created during tooth formation by the coalescing of independent lobes of the tooth. The fissure formed may be totally coalesced (creating little likelihood of capturing food and developing caries), partially coalesced leaving periodic gaps or noncoalesced leaving a gap to the dentin (Figure 7.3.7) (Ripa and Wolff 1992). In the partially or noncoalesced, an ecologic environment is developed that retains bacteria, retains sugars, and restricts the ability of saliva or oral hygiene to reach the food/bacteria source. This allows the sugar-fed bacteria resident in the fissure to produce acids for longer periods of time with little access to saliva to remove the acids or to buffer the acids (Wolff and Larson 2009). Changes in oral hygiene, diet, and systemic factors (particularly as they relate to salivary flow) are conditions most frequently associated with increased caries risk (Hara and Zero 2010). As there have been no changes in this patient's medical history and there is no clinical evidence of xerostomia on examination, changes in diet and oral hygiene may be

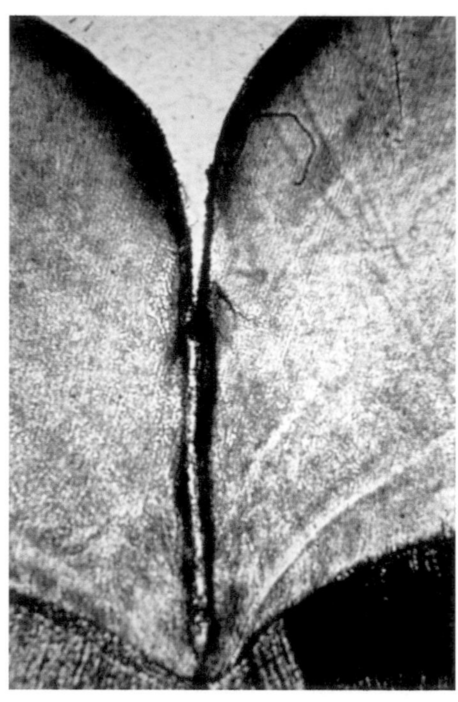

Figure 7.3.7: Noncoalesced leaving a gap to the dentin (Ripa and Wolff 1992).

the likely cause. Hygiene on the occlusal surface is often made difficult by the anatomy of the fissure, which may be narrower than the diameter of the toothbrush bristle, thereby allowing food debris to remain in the fissure. In this case, the young dentally healthy male, leaving home where diet and homecare had permitted a healthy ecosystem to thrive, allowed a shift in the ecosystem toward acid production. Minor changes in the patient's diet can result in significant acid production thereby creating an environment likely to produce caries (Newbrun 1979, 1982).

Management of Occlusal Caries

Management of occlusal initial caries lesions has shifted from surgical intervention to a medical management (Wolff and Larson 2009). Remineralization of initial lesions requires the reduction of plaque and reduction of the frequency of fermentable carbohydrate consumption (particularly sticky foods when speaking about occlusal surfaces). Unfortunately, due to the narrowness of the occlusal fissure, it is often difficult to remove the plaque better and equally difficult to prevent fermentable carbohydrate from penetrating deeply into the fissures (Figure 7.3.7).

Dental sealants protect the fissure from further demineralization by blocking the pits and fissures from caries causing bacteria and introduction of fermentable carbohydrate. This is done by blocking plaque accumulation. Sealants are highly successful in preventing caries (Beauchamp et al. 2008; Griffin et al. 2008; Oong et al. 2008) Sealing noncavitated active lesions had better outcomes than unsealed early lesions. Active initial lesions should be considered for immediate sealants and inactive initial lesions may be monitored for changes in activity (Ismail et al. 2013, 2015). The sealants resulted in caries reductions of 71% five years after placement (Griffin et al. 2008). It has even been demonstrated that sealing lesions with active caries results in the arresting of caries and prevents the lesions from advancing (Mertz-Fairhurst et al. 1986; Mertz-Fairhurst et al. 1998). The outcomes of all of this research indicate that the evidence-based treatment decision for prevention and treatment of early lesions should be sealant placement whenever frank cavitation is not present (and in some cases even when it is present). When in doubt SEAL-IT! Teeth #s 2, 14, 15, 19, 20, 28, and 29 will receive carefully applied resin-based sealants. The lower-right molar (tooth #30) will be treated with a lesion specific bonded composite restoration preserving the maximal amount of tooth structure, not the "old" extension for prevention. These guiding principles mean the preparation removes necessary caries, provides sound margins, and selects the restorative material utilizing the principle of the best evidence-based material. Tooth destruction is kept to a minimum and form and function re-established (Ismail et al. 2015; Ripa and Wolff 1992; Wolff et al. 2007).

Take-Home Hints

1. Dental occlusal caries requires a different diagnosis than present or not.
2. Dental caries is diagnosed without a sharp explorer.
3. Bitewing radiographs may demonstrate occult caries.
4. When the extent and activity are questionable, the occlusal surface should be sealed rather than restored.

Self-Study Questions

1. Dental caries in the fissure may be caused by or likelihood increased by:
- **A. Incomplete coalesced fissure**
- **B. Inability to physically clean the fissure**
- **C. The stickiness of the food**
- **D. All of the above**

2. Initial dental caries in the fissure should be sealed as soon as possible:
- **A. True**
- **B. False**

3. Management of dental early caries requires:
- **A. Better oral hygiene**
- **B. Sealant placement**
- **C. Surgical restoration before caries becomes worse**

4. When the status of the fissure is unknown, caries requiring surgery or not, sealant should be placed because sealants have been demonstrated to arrest caries:
- **A. True**
- **B. False**

References

Beauchamp, J., Caufield, P.W., Crall, J.J. et al. (2008). Evidence-based clinical recommendations for the use of pit-and-fissure sealants: a report of the American dental association council on scientific affairs. *J. Am. Dent. Assoc.* 139: 257–268.

Bergman, G. and Linden, L.A. (1969). The action of the explorer on incipient caries. *Sven. Tandlak. Tidskr.* 62: 629–634.

Ekstrand, K.R., Martignon, S., Ricketts, D.J.N., and Qvist, V. (2007). Detection and activity assessment of primary coronal caries lesions: a methodologic study. *Oper. Dent.* 32: 225–235.

Ekstrand, K.R., Qvist, V., and Thylstrup, A. (1987). Light microscope study of the effect of probing in occlusal surfaces. *Caries Res.* 21: 368–374.

Griffin, S.O., Oong, E., Kohn, W. et al. (2008). The effectiveness of sealants in managing caries lesions. *J. Dent. Res.* 87: 169–174.

Hara, A.T. and Zero, D.T. (2010). The caries environment: saliva, pellicle, diet, and hard tissue ultrastructure. *Dent. Clin. N. Am.* 54: 455–467.

Ismail, A.I. (2004). Visual and Visula-tactile detection of dental caries. *J. Dent. Res.* 83: C56–C66.

Ismail, A.I., Pitts, N.B., Tellez, M. et al. (2015). The international caries classification and management system (ICCMS) an example of a caries management pathway. *BMC Oral Health* 15 (Suppl 1): S9.

Ismail, A.I., Tellez, M., Pitts, N.B. et al. (2013). Caries management pathways preserve dental tissues and promote oral health. *Community Dent. Oral Epidemiol.* 41: e12–e40.

Lussi, A. (1991). Validity of diagnostic and treatment decisions of fissure caries. *Caries Res.* 25: 296–303.

Mertz-Fairhurst, E.J., Curtis, J.W. Jr., Ergle, J.W. et al. (1998). Ultraconservative and cariostatic sealed restorations: results at year 10. *J. Am. Dent. Assoc.* 129: 55–66.

Mertz-Fairhurst, E.J., Schuster, G.S., and Fairhurst, C.W. (1986). Arresting caries by sealants: results of a clinical study. *J. Am. Dent. Assoc.* 112: 194–197.

National Institute of Health Consensus Development Panel (2001). Diagnosis and management of dental caries throughout life. National Institutes of Health consensus development conference statement, march 26–28, 2001. *J. Dent. Educ.* 65: 1162–1168.

Newbrun, E. (1979). Dietary carbohydrates: their role in cariogenicity. *Med. Clin. N. Am.* 63: 1069–1086.

Newbrun, E. (1982). Sucrose in the dynamics of the carious process. *Int. Dent. J.* 32: 13–23.

Oong, E.M., Griffin, S.O., Kohn, W.G. et al. (2008). The effect of dental sealants on bacteria levels in caries lesions: a review of the evidence. *J. Am. Dent. Assoc.* 139: 271–278. quiz 357-8.

Pitts, N. (2004). Modern concepts in caries measurement. *J. Dent. Res.* 83: C43–C47.

Ripa, L.W. and Wolff, M.S. (1992). Preventive resin restorations: indications, technique, and success. *Quintessence Int.* 23: 307–315.

Taft, J. (1883). *A Practical Treatise on Operative Dentistry.* Philadelphia: P. Blakiston, Son and Co.

Wolff, M.S. and Larson, C. (2009). The cariogenic dental biofilm: good, bad or just something to control? *Braz. Oral Res.* 23 (Suppl 1): 31–38.

Wolff, M.S., Allen, K., and Kaim, J. (2007). A 100-year journey from GV black to minimal surgical intervention. *Compend. Contin. Educ. Dent.* 28: 130–134. quiz 135, 152.

Additional Resources

Fontana, M. and Wolff, M. (2011 Oct). Translating the caries management paradigm into practice: challenges and opportunities. *J. Calif. Dent. Assoc.* 39 (10): 702–709. UI:22132581.

Ripa, L.W. and Wolff, M.S. (1992). Preventive resin restorations: indications, technique, and success. *Quintessence Int.* 23 (5): 307–315.

Young, D.A., Fontana, M., and Wolff, M.S. (eds.) (2010 Jul). Current concepts in cariology. Preface. *Dent. Clin. N. Am.* 54 (3): xiii–xv. UI: 20630186.

Answers to Self-Study Questions

1. D

2. A

3. B

4. A

8

Introduction to Biomaterials

Clinical Cases in Dental Hygiene, First Edition. Edited by Cheryl M. Westphal Theile, Mea A. Weinberg and Stuart L. Segelnick.

Simply stated, biocompatibility is the ability of material to be in contact with living tissues and not produce an adverse effect (Anusavice et al. 2013). Ideally, materials used in the oral cavity should be harmless to oral tissues – gingiva, mucosa, pulp, and bone (Anusavice et al. 2013). Furthermore, a material should contain no toxins, nor should it be a diffusible substance that can be absorbed into the bloodstream causing systemic toxic responses, including teratogenic or carcinogenic effects (Anusavice et al. 2013). The material should also be free of agents that could elicit sensitization or allergic response in a patient (Anusavice et al. 2013). Placement of material in the body creates an interface that must exhibit both biological and structural stability during the lifetime of the implanted device (Anusavice et al. 2013). These interfaces are dynamic, and their transitional functionality is dependent on the quality of the junction and the biocompatibility of the material (Anusavice et al. 2013). The dynamics of the interfacial interaction affect the material's biocompatibility and its acceptance by the body, which depend on the shape, size, and location of the material, its physical properties, its composition, and the stresses that develop during the function (Anusavice et al. 2013).

Three major factors are linked to the success of dental materials: (i) material properties, (ii) the design of the dental device, and (iii) the biocompatibility of basic materials (Anusavice et al. 2013). The biocompatibility of dental restorative materials, for instance, is evaluated using compositional analysis, surface degradation tests, cell culture tests, clinical testing in humans, and animal model tests (Anusavice et al. 2013). The biocompatibility of a material depends on multiple factors. These include:

1. the chemical nature of its components;
2. the physical character of the components;
3. the types and locations of patient tissues that will be exposed to the device;
4. the duration of the exposure;
5. the surface characteristics of the material; and
6. the amount and nature of substances eluted from the material.

(Anusavice et al. 2013)

The primary purpose of biocompatibility tests is to protect dental patients who will be treated with the materials and anyone in the dental setting who will be handling these materials (Anusavice et al. 2013). Since no dental biomaterial is entirely free from the potential risk of adverse reactions, the testing of biocompatibility is related to risk assessment (Anusavice et al. 2013). Thus, the challenge for the users of dental biomaterials is to select those products for which the known benefits far outweigh the known risks (Anusavice et al. 2013).

Case 1

Biomaterials: Dental Implants and Peri-implantitis

CASE STORY

Mr. X is a 34-year-old male who will be relocating after obtaining a position as an illustrator in Los Angeles. Recently he has noticed a dental implant he had placed when he was in his mid-20s "feels weird and seems loose." He would like to "make sure all is ok" before moving and beginning his new position.

Review of Symptoms

- Vital signs
  - Blood pressure: 120/75 mmHg
  - Pulse: 60 beats/min
  - Respiration: 14 breaths/min

Medical History

The medical history reveals no significant findings. The patient is not on any medications and takes an over-the-counter (OTC) multivitamin daily.

Social History

The patient smoked marijuana occasionally in his late teens but does not smoke anymore. He has never used tobacco. He drinks two to three beers on the weekend and drinks one cup of coffee daily.

Extraoral Examination

No significant findings

Intraoral Examination

The intraoral exam reveals maxillary third molars have been extracted. Tooth #20 is congenitally missing. The patient had an implant placed to replace tooth #20 at age 24.

Occlusion

Class I occlusion.

The patient had orthodontic treatment from age 13–15 to correct an underbite.

Radiographic Examination

Four bitewings and one periapical were recommended of tooth #20. A cone beam computed tomography (CBCT) scan was obtained from the patient's previous oral health-care provider.

Diagnosis and Prognosis

The patient's general oral health is good. He brushes twice daily, and flosses at least three times a week. No other auxiliary aids are used. Light plaque accumulation is present with localized inflammation around teeth #17, #30, #31, and #32. The gingiva around the implant replacing tooth #20 is inflamed and the implant is mobile. Prognosis for tooth #20 is poor (see Figure 8.1.1).

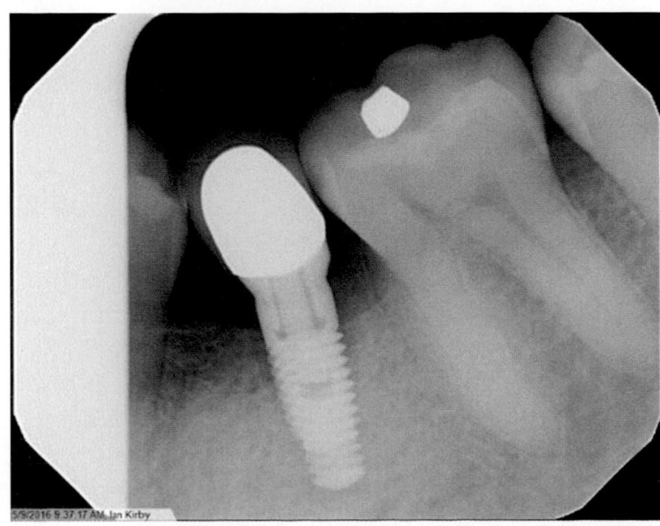

Figure 8.1.1: Tooth #20, implant with peri-implantitis.

Dental Hygiene Diagnosis/Treatment Plan

Problems	Related to risks and etiology
Bleeding upon probing, teeth #s 17, 30, 31, and 32	Localized periodontal disease, difficulty removing biofilm in mandibular molar areas
4mm periodontal pocket on distal of #17 and 4mm periodontal pockets on mesial of #30 and #31, 5mm periodontal pocket on distal of #32	Localized periodontal disease, difficulty removing biofilm in mandibular molar areas
Peri-implantitis, implant tooth #20	Poor bone quality, loss of integration

Planned Interventions

Clinical	Educational/counseling	Oral Hygiene Instructions
Evaluate soft and hard tissue Dental prophylaxis with selective SRP on #s 17, 30, 31, 32 with 4 to 8week periodontal re-evaluation, After completion of localized scaling and root planing (SRP) Refer to Doctor of Dental Surgery (DDS) for extraction of #20, bone grafting, implant replacement	Encourage brushing daily and flossing daily Stress importance of maintaining recare visits, continued flossing, increase to daily, and brushing twice daily Stress importance of full mouth plaque control to reduce transfer of microorganisms to implant site where periodontal pathogens can colonize	Soft bristle brush/ modified Bass technique Emphasize importance of flossing and accessing third molar areas when brushing and flossing Use of soft toothbrush with end rounded filaments, spongy filament floss, and end tufted brush with soft filaments

See Figures 8.1.2–8.1.5.

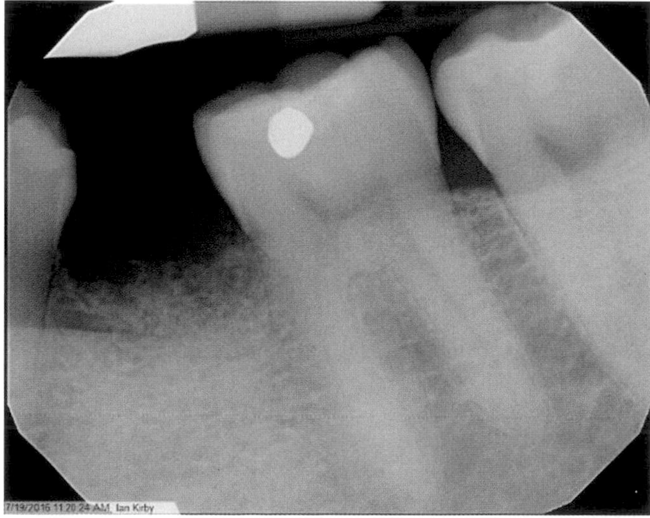

Figure 8.1.2: Bone grafting: allograft (cortical/cancelous) with collagen membrane.

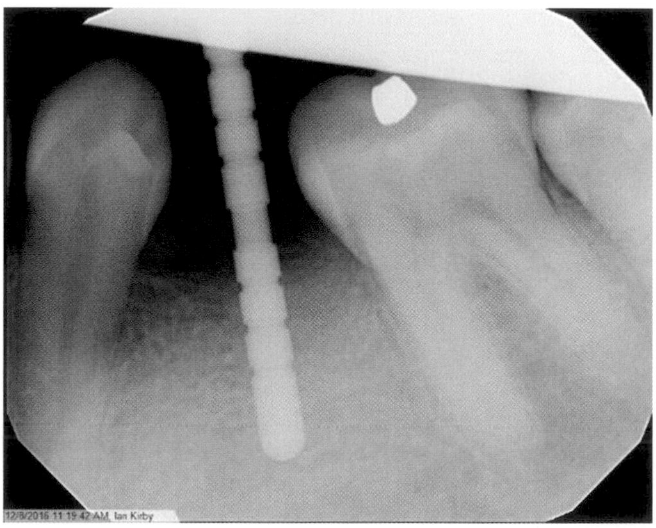

Figure 8.1.3: Implant guidance.

Discussion

The design and selection of a biomaterial depends on the specific application in order to be useful and assure its properties as long as required, without rejection. In order to be considered a biomaterial it should, besides not inducing inflammation, toxic reactions, and allergenic symptoms in the body, be biocompatible, biofunctional, bioactive, bioinert, and sterilizable. The biomaterial surface being directly exposed to the living organism plays a crucial role in regards to biocompatibility. When this issue is considered, the physical, morphological, and biologic characteristics can be adapted to promote improvement in the interaction of biomaterial and tissue. In recent years the concept of biocompatibility has changed. At first it was believed that a material was biocompatible by being completely inert to the human body without any response from the biological medium to its presence. The idea of a totally inert material was abandoned when it could be observed that the presence of any kind of material

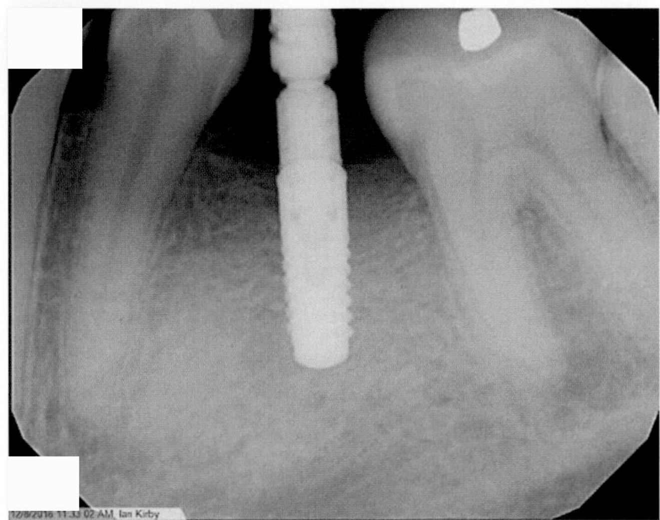

Figure 8.1.4: Implant placement.

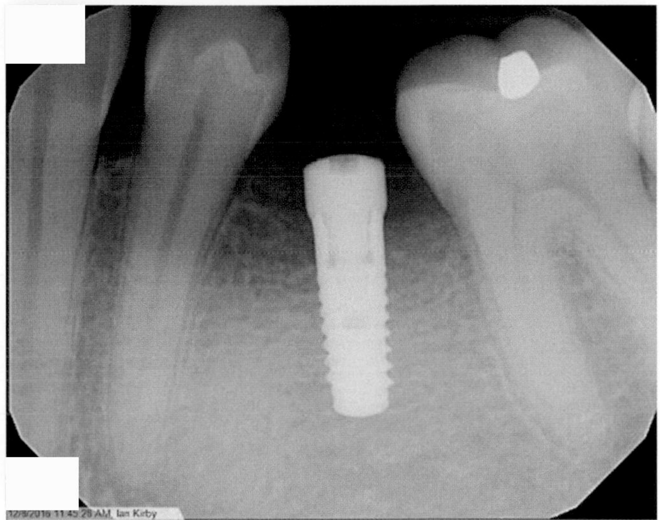

Figure 8.1.5: Implant with healing cap.

always entails some response from the body, varying as a function of the kind of application and the patient's characteristics (age, sex, etc.) (dos Santos et al. 2017).

Dental implants represent a reliable treatment option in oral rehabilitation of partially or fully edentulous patients in order to restore function and esthetics. Single tooth replacement with a dental implant has become the standard in esthetic treatment, providing advantages, but also challenges in some cases.

More than 45 years ago, Branemark et al. (2001) first described the process of osseointegration, which began an era of research on the shape and materials of dental implants. But more recently the focus of biomedical research shifted from shape and materials used to the oseoinductive potential of implant surfaces. Today there are over 1000 different implant systems with variations in shape, dimension, bulk, surface material, thread design, implant-abutment connection, surface topography and chemistry, wettability, and surface modification.

Although long-term survival rates of dental implants are excellent, failures do still occur in a small number of patients. Of these failures, 1–2% occur in the first few months due to insufficient osseointegration, and 5% of failures develop after several years due to peri-implantitis.

As with any disease process the presence of certain risk factors will increase the likelihood of disease development and progression, (Alani and Bishop 2014). Awareness of these risk factors when planning implant treatment is important in the prevention of peri-implantitis and failure of the implant. Among these factors both bone quality and poor oral hygiene may potentially play a role as a risk factor in peri-implantitis (Alani and Bishop 2014). Patients with advanced clinical conditions, such as those with diabetes mellitus, osteoporosis, bisphosphonate use, or those having undergone radiation therapy also continue to be a great challenge in terms of achieving successful osseointegration.

Patients need to be made aware that implants are susceptible to plaque related disease in much the same way as natural teeth. At the treatment planning stage it is critical that an objective assessment of oral hygiene is completed and that treatment should be postponed until adequate plaque control is achieved (Alani and Bishop 2014).

Among the other factors that may play a role in development of peri-implantitis is the quality of bone in the implant site. In the case of a congenitally missing tooth at the site of implant placement, several factors may lead to peri-implantitis and ultimately failure of the implant: inadequate consistency and quality of bone, a decreased collateral blood supply from remnant periodontal ligament, a missing tooth space larger than tooth to be replaced, and occlusal discrepancy.

Success in the case of a patient presenting with the above conditions will depend on several factors, among these, the skill of the clinician, the success of bone grafting, the stability and position of the implant and patient compliance, which should include regularly scheduled recare and maintenance visits as well as case specific oral hygiene instruction.

Research efforts have been focused on designing novel topographies of implant surfaces to increase osteoblastic migration, adhesion, proliferation, and differentiation.

Numerous studies have shown that use of particular surface modifications, such as laser ablation, and surface coatings with proteins, drugs, and growth factors may improve the success and survival rates of implants.

The goal of biomedical research on surface modifications is to promote early osseointegration and ensure a long-term bone-to-implant contact without substantial marginal bone loss.

Take-Home Hints

1. At the treatment planning stage it is critical that an objective assessment of oral hygiene is completed by the dental hygienist. If the patient has poor oral hygiene, implant placement should be postponed until the patient is compliant with home care, biofilm removal, and preventive procedures.
2. After implant placement, a case-specific oral hygiene regimen should be created for the patient based on individual needs.
3. Patients should be made aware that implant placement is a life-time commitment and implants require as much care, if not more, as natural teeth.
4. Regularly scheduled recare appointments are critical for maintenance and success of implants.

Self-Study Questions

1. Three major factors that are linked to the success of dental materials include all of the following except one. Which one is the exception?
- **A. Biocompatibility of the dental material**
- **B. Material properties**
- **C. Patients use of tobacco products**
- **D. Design of the dental device**

2. Current research has shown that peri-implantitis is of genetic origin:
- **A. True**
- **B. False**

3. Risk factors associated with peri-implantitis include all of the following except:
- **A. Poor oral hygiene**
- **B. Poor bone quality**
- **C. Decreased blood supply**
- **D. All of the above**

4. Periodontal pathogens will be UNABLE to colonize at implant site if implant placement is successful:
- **A. True**
- **B. False**

References

Alani, A. and Bishop, K. (2014). Peri-implantitis. Part 2: prevention and maintenance of peri-implant health. *British Dental Journal* 217 (6): 289–297. MEDLINE with Full Text, EBSCOhost, viewed 9 December 2016.

Anusavice, K.J., Shen, C., and Rawls, H.R. (2013). *Phillips' Science of Dental Materials*, Chapter 7, 111–147. St. Louis, MI: Elsevier.

Branemark, R., Branemark, P.I., Rydevik, B., and Myers, R.R. (2001). Osseointegration in skeletal reconstruction and rehabilitation: A review. *Journal of Rehabilitation Research and Development* 38 (2): 175–181.

dos Santos, V., Brandalise, R.M., and Savaris, M. (2017). *Engineering of Biomaterials*. Cham, Switzerland: Springer International.

Additional Resources

Canullo, L., Schlee, M., Wagner, W., and Covani, U. (2015). International brainstorming meeting on etiologic and risk factors of Peri-implantitis, Montegrotto (Padua, Italy), august 2014. *The International Journal of Oral & Maxillofacial Implants* 30 (5): 1093–1104. MEDLINE with Full Text, EBSCOhost, viewed 9 December 2016.

Hu, X., Li, J., Luo, J. et al. (2011). Multidisciplinary management of congenitally missing teeth with osseointegrated dental implants: a long-term report. *The Chinese Journal of Dental Research: The Official Journal of the Scientific Section of the Chinese Stomatological Association (CSA)* 14 (1): 29–36. MEDLINE with Full Text, EBSCOhost, viewed 9 December 2016.

Jepsen, S., Berglundh, T., Genco, R. et al. (2015). Primary prevention of peri-implantitis: managing peri-implant mucositis. *Journal of Clinical Periodontology* 42 (Suppl 16): S152–S157. MEDLINE with Full Text, EBSCOhost, viewed 9 December 2016.

Matsuda, S. (2015). The Patient with Dental Implants. In: Clinical Practice of the Dental Hygienist (ed. E.M. Wilkins), 533–546.

Monje, A., Aranda, L., Diaz, K. et al. (2016). Impact of maintenance therapy for the prevention of peri-implant diseases: a systematic review and meta-analysis. *Journal of Dental*

Research 95 (4): 372–379. MEDLINE with Full Text, EBSCOhost, viewed 9 December 2016.

Tonetti, M., Chapple, I., Jepsen, S., and Sanz, M. (2015). Primary and secondary prevention of periodontal and peri-implant diseases: introduction to, and objectives of the 11th European workshop on periodontology consensus conference. *Journal of Clinical Periodontology* 42 (Suppl 16): S1–S4. MEDLINE with Full Text, EBSCOhost, viewed 9 December 2016.

Warreth, A., Boggs, S., Ibieyou, N. et al. (2015). Peri-implant diseases: an overview. *Dental Update* 42 (2): 166. MEDLINE with Full Text, EBSCOhost, viewed 9 December 2016.

Wilson, V. (2013). An insight into peri-implantitis: a systematic literature review. *Primary Dental Journal* 2 (2): 69–73. MEDLINE with Full Text, EBSCOhost, viewed 9 December 2016.

Answers to Self-Study Questions

1. C

2. B

3. D

4. B

Case 2

Polishing Restored and Natural Teeth

CASE STORY
Mrs. X, a 52-year-old female, widow, will be getting married in two months "I am so excited about my wedding; I really want a make-over! But my teeth are another story; I don't know what I can do to improve my smile before my wedding. Is there anything I can do in the next month-and-a-half to improve the look of my front teeth?"

Review of Symptoms

- Vital signs
  - Blood pressure: 140/86 mmHg
  - Pulse: 74 beats/min
  - Respiration: 15 breaths/min

Medical History

The medical history reveals weight gain over the past two years and an increase in BP over the last six months. The patient is not on medication for high blood pressure. Currently the patient is seeing her physician to monitor blood pressure and has increased walking and began a low carbohydrate diet one month ago. She and her physician are hoping to lower blood pressure through a healthier lifestyle. The patient takes over-the-counter (OTC) medication for osteoarthritis in her right knee.

Social History

The patient has never smoked. She drinks two to three glasses of white wine, or a beer on weekends, and drinks two to three cups of tea daily

Extraoral Examination

No significant findings

Intraoral Examination

The intraoral exam reveals a slightly enlarged uvula and localized gingival recession of 2 mm on teeth #6, #22, and #27. Periodontal charting was completed and reveals two areas of probing depths 4 mm or greater, #1 with a distal-lingual reading of 5 mm and #16, mesial-lingual with a reading of 5 mm.

Dental examination reveals a Class III distal composite and Class IV mesial-incisal chip on tooth # 8 (see Figure 8.2.1), tooth #9 presents with a Class IV mesial-incisal composite with, mesial-incisal fracture, and irregular margins and a Class III distal composite with irregular margins and excess composite

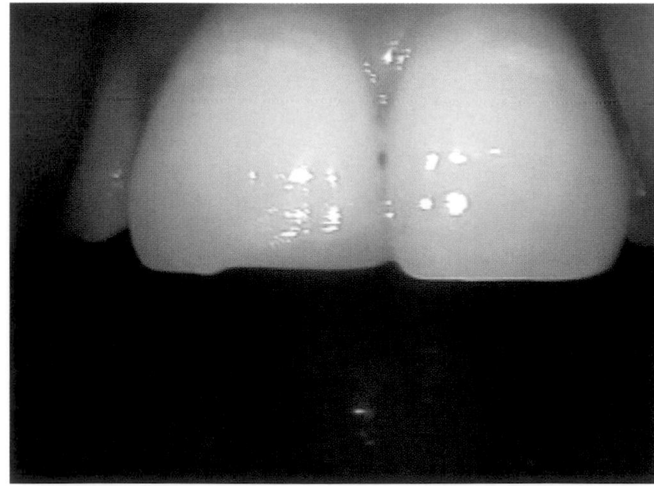

Figure 8.2.1: Intraoral photograph of Cl IV MI with mesial-incisal chip.

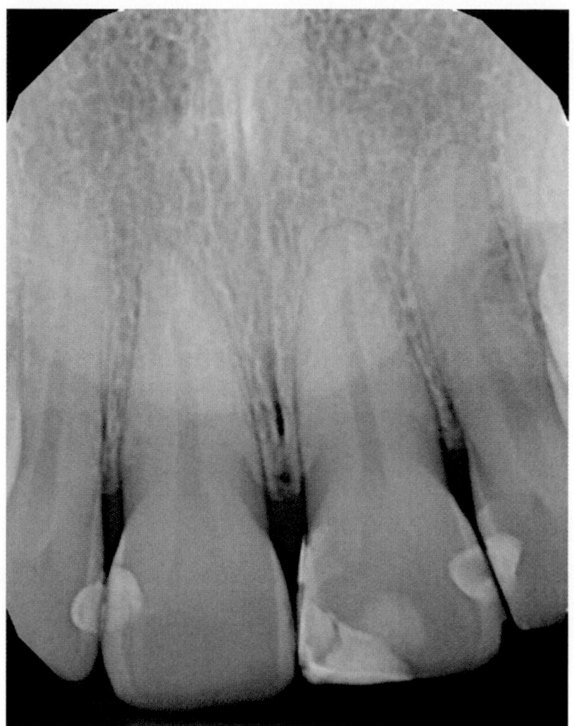

Figure 8.2.2: Periapical radiograph of #8, Class III, distal composite, Class IV MI composite with chip, #9 Class IV MI composite with fracture and irregular margins and CL III distal with excess composite.

The patient presents with generalized stain, most evident on lingual and facial surfaces of anterior teeth.

The patient's oral hygiene is good. She brushes twice daily, and flosses once daily.

Occlusion

Class I occlusion, with a slight overbite

Radiographic Examination

Four bitewings were prescribed and one periapical was prescribed of teeth #8 and #9. Tooth #8 reveals NSF in regards to caries, tooth 9 reveals a Class IV Mesial incisal with mesial incisal chip with no recurrent caries, the CL III distal presents with excess composite and rough margins (see Figures 8.2.2).

Diagnosis and Prognosis

The patient's general oral health is good. Localized inflammation is present in the areas of teeth #1 and #16.

Gingival recession present on teeth # 6, #11, and #22

Teeth present with moderate yellow extrinsic stain due to age, tea, and wine

Some localized brown extrinsic stain on mandibular lingual of anterior teeth and occlusal of posterior teeth due to tea drinking

Dental Hygiene Diagnosis

Problems	Related to Risks and Etiology
#8 Class IV mesial-incisal composite with mesial fracture	Sharp edge on incisal, further loss of tooth structure
# 9 Class IV mesial-incisal fractured composite with irregular margins	open margin, future recurrent caries, biofilm, excess material not removed, improper finishing, and polishing of restoration,
#9 Class III, distal composite with irregular margins and excess composite	open margin, future caries, loss of tooth structure, biofilm, excess material not removed, improper finishing and polishing of restoration,
Gingival recession on #6, #11, and #27	Use of medium toothbrush utilizing scrubbing technique
Bleeding on probing	Localized periodontal disease, difficulty removing biofilm in maxillary third molar areas
5 mm periodontal pockets on #1 and #16	Localized periodontal disease, difficulty removing biofilm in maxillary third molar areas
Generalized and localized staining	Tea and wine consumption

Planned interventions

Clinical	Educational/Counseling	Oral Hygiene Instructions
Evaluate soft and hard tissue Localized scaling and root planing with 4 to 6 week periodontal re-evaluation After localized SRP, prophy with polishing to remove extrinsic stain In-office whitening Refer to DDS for Tooth #8, placement of Cl IV mesial-incisal composite, #9, Cl IV mesial-incisal re-do of composite, possible future laminates Smooth and polish #8 Cl III distal to determine that margins are sealed, finish and polish restoration, removal of excess composite distal #9	Encourage brushing daily and flossing once daily, avoid further gingival recession through use of soft bristle toothbrush and proper technique Stress importance of maintaining recare visits, continued flossing daily and brushing twice daily Reduce tea consumption, increase brushing to three times daily Instruct patient that whitening should be done before redo of composite, since composite restorations will not whiten. Recommend use of dentifrice containing evidence based desensitizing agents (potassium nitrate, calcium sulfate) beginning 3 weeks before in–office whitening procedure and continued for 2 weeks after While resin and porcelain restorations are both durable and esthetic, care of esthetic restorations is still critical to enhance durability, function, and esthetics minimize attachment of bio-film and enhance esthetics of restoration	Soft bristle brush/ Modified Bass technique, Modified Stillman technique in areas of recession Emphasize importance of flossing and accessing third molar areas when brushing and flossing OTC whitening dentifrice with fluoride, after consuming tea and wine, rinse mouth with water Do not eat or drink for 1 hour after, avoid anything that can stain a white t-shirt for 1 week, reduce tea and wine intake, rinse mouth with water after consuming any foods with color Avoid biting into hard foods such as apples, instead, cut into smaller pieces to avoid fracture of resin/porcelain materials Emphasize use of soft bristle brush on teeth with restorations, utilizing Modified Bass technique

Discussion: Polishing Restored and Natural Teeth

Should we polish or not, and if yes, what should we use? These are the questions asked so often and discussed by many dental professionals. If you were to do a literature review you would find a variety of opinions and thoughts on the topic as related to the polishing of natural teeth, as a final step in dental prophylaxis, or as a necessary step in the finishing of a resin based restoration. Perhaps the following section will shed some light and address/answer your concerns and questions.

Polishing of Natural Teeth, Polishing vs Cleaning Agents

"Polishing" of natural teeth is performed in conjunction with dental prophylaxis to remove any remaining stain and/or dental biofilm. Every patient is unique, and products used for stain or biofilm removal are not "one size fits all."

The key point to keep in mind is that the least abrasive polishing agent or cleaning agent necessary to remove the remaining stains or biofilm is the product that should be used. If a very fine paste removes the stain, then that is all that is necessary.

Unlike traditional polishing paste, which contains irregularly shaped gritty particles, cleaning agents are made of nonabrasive particles, round, and flat in shape that do not scratch a surface and are able to produce a high luster. Because of their extremely low level of abrasion they can be used on natural teeth as well as restorations including implants. Cleaning agents are often made from a combination of feldspar, alkali, and aluminum silicates. The agent is mixed with water to create a slurry or flour consistency. For a patient who presents without stain, but feels that their prophy procedure has not been completed if a polishing procedure is not performed, a cleaning agent may be utilized (Barns 2013).

The use of cleaning and polishing agents for removal of stain and dental biofilm is a "selective procedure." Polishing is "selective" in that the teeth that need to be polished and the cleaning or polishing agent used must be selected based on the patient's individual needs (Barns 2013).

Polishing of Composite Restorations

As dental hygienists we are now caring for a population of patients who present with a scope of esthetic restorations, some which may be virtually undetectable. In fact, these restorations may look so natural; the only way to confirm that they are actually restorations will be by reviewing radiographs and the patient record (see Figures 8.2.1 and 8.2.2).

To be esthetically pleasing a composite restoration should be highly polished. This will make the restoration more lustrous and pleasing to the eye (those composites used today such as microfilled and nanofilled, are going to have the most esthetic appearance and will be most susceptible to polishing in achieving a highly lustrous finish).

A highly polished composite restoration however, has shown to provide other benefits besides enhanced esthetics; a decrease in accumulation of biofilm and reduction of staining of composite restorations has been noted (Mandikos 2007).

Some research also shows that roughness of a composite may be linked to the wear of the restoration, and by having a highly polished surface, wear incidence may be decreased (see Figure 8.2.1) (Mandikos 2007).

When a patient presents with composite restorations that exhibit stain, care should be taken to avoid roughening of the composite surface. Even a fine prophy paste can cause irregularities on the surface of a composite restoration. If necessary to remove surface stain, a cleaning agent such as a high-quality flour of pumice can be used. Luster of the restoration can be brought back by use of fine and ultrafine composite polishing disks, or use of a diamond luster paste.

Polishing Porcelain Veneers

Porcelain veneers routinely should not need polishing (see Figure 8.2.3).

Should a patient present with veneers that appear to be stained, it should first be determined that the discoloration is in fact stain and not a defect within the veneer.

Veneers may be polished with a rubber cup and use of a fine prophy paste for stain removal.

A urethane dimethacrylate-based point containing fine diamond powder or a ceramic finishing bur may also be utilized for polishing of the veneer (see Figure 8.2.4).

When polishing veneers, light pressure should always be used.

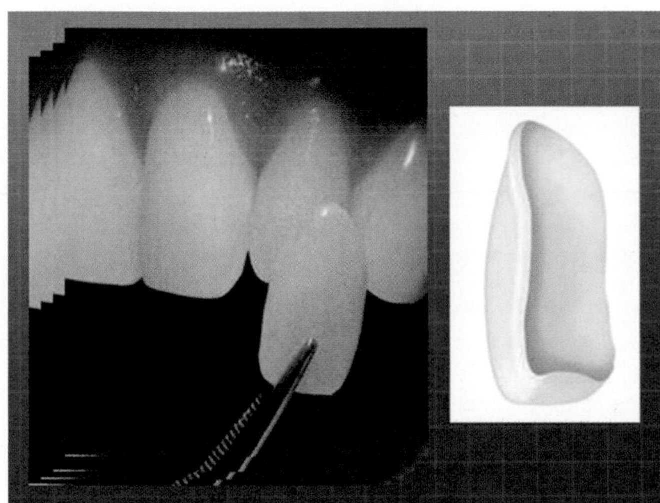

Figure 8.2.3: Veneers.

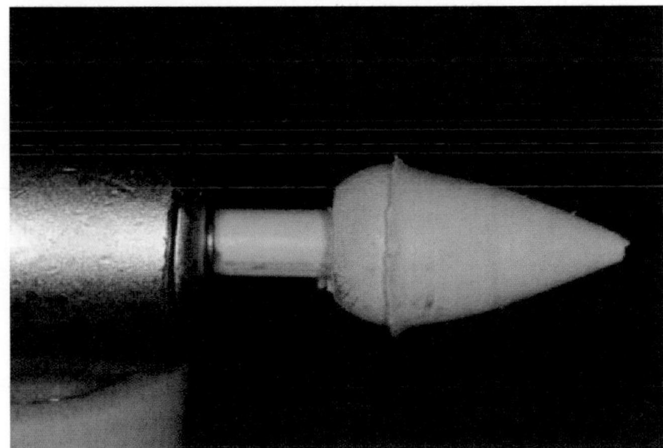

Figure 8.2.4: Veneer/composite polishing bur.

Take-Home Hints

1. For stain removal in pits and fissures of posterior teeth, prophy paste on a tapered polishing brush, instead of a rubber cup is very effective.
2. When determining the presence and location of composite restorations in a patient's mouth, light air should be utilized to dry teeth. In even the most esthetic restorations, it is easier to detect a margin on a dry tooth surface rather than wet.
3. Use air and a mirror utilizing transillumination technique to check for defects within a porcelain veneer.

Self-Study Questions

1. Cleaning agents are made of:
- **A. Round quartz particles**
- **B. Gritty irregular shaped particles**
- **C. Round flat particles**
- **D. Feldspar, alkali, and aluminum silicates**
- **E. Both C and D are true**

2. When removing stain from natural teeth, it is important to begin with the most abrasive polishing agent.
- **A. True**
- **B. False**

3. A highly polished composite restoration:
- **A. Exhibits enhanced esthetics**
- **B. Will be more resistant to stain**
- **C. Will have a decrease in biofilm attachment**
- **D. All of the above**

4. Luster of a composite restoration can be restored through:
- **A. Use of a coarse prophy paste**
- **B. Use of fine polishing discs**
- **C. Use of a coarse pumice paste mixed with water**
- **D. None of the above**

References

Barns, C.M. (2013). Extrinsic Stain Removal. In: Clinical Practice of the Dental Hygienist (ed. E.M. Wilkins), 689–708.

Mandikos, M.N. (2007). Polishing Composite Restorations. Australasian Dental Practice 122–124.

Additional Resources

Pelka, M., Altmaier, K., Petschelt, A., and Lohbauer, U. (2010). The effect of air-polishing abrasives on wear of direct restoration materials and sealants. *Journal of the American Dental Association (1939)* 141 (1): 63–70. MEDLINE with Full Text, EBSCOhost, viewed 9 October 2016.

Reis, A., Giannini, M., Lovadino, J., and dos Santos Dias, C. (2002). The effect of six polishing systems on the surface roughness of two packable resin-based composites. *American Journal of Dentistry* 15 (3): 193–197. MEDLINE with Full Text, EBSCOhost, viewed 9 October 2016.

Ryba, T., Dunn, W., and Murchison, D. (2002). Surface roughness of various packable composites. *Operative Dentistry* 27 (3): 243–247. MEDLINE with Full Text, EBSCOhost, viewed 9 October 2016.

Sen, D., Göller, G., and Işsever, H. (2002). The effect of two polishing pastes on the surface roughness of bis-acryl composite and methacrylate-based resins. *The Journal of Prosthetic Dentistry* 88 (5): 527–532. MEDLINE with Full Text, EBSCOhost, viewed 9 October 2016.

Turssi, C., Ferracane, J., and Serra, M. (2005). Abrasive wear of resin composites as related to finishing and polishing procedures. *Dental Materials: Official Publication of the Academy of Dental Materials* 21 (7): 641–648. MEDLINE with Full Text, EBSCOhost, viewed 9 October 2016.

Turssi, C., Rodrigues, A., and Serra, M. (2006). Textural characterization of finished and polished composites over time of intraoral exposure. *Journal of Biomedical Materials Research. Part B, Applied Biomaterials* 76 (2): 381–388. MEDLINE with Full Text, EBSCOhost, viewed 9 October 2016.

Watanabe, T., Miyazaki, M., Takamizawa, T. et al. (2005). Influence of polishing duration on surface roughness of resin composites. *Journal of Oral Science* 47 (1): 21–25. MEDLINE with Full Text, EBSCOhost, viewed 9 October 2016.

Answers to Self-Study Questions

1. E

2. B

3. D

4. B

Case 3

Alginate Impressions

CASE STORY

Ms. X, a single, 48-year-old female with a high-end career in finance presents with a chief complaint "As I get older my teeth are not the way they looked 20 years ago. I feel my teeth make me look older. I'm unhappy with my smile and want to know my options."

Review of Symptoms

- Vital signs
  - Blood pressure: 122/78 mmHg
  - Pulse: 72 beats/min
  - Respiration: 14 Breaths/min

Medical History

The medical history reveals no significant findings. The patient is not taking any medications.

Social History

The patient has a prior history of smoking. Patient quit smoking five years ago. She drinks two to three glasses of red wine on weekends, and drinks two cups of coffee daily.

Extraoral Examination

No significant findings.

Intraoral Examination

No abnormal findings with respect to intraoral structures, mucosa, and gingiva. Periodontal charting was completed and reveals five areas of probing depths 4 mm or greater, #2 distal with a reading of 5 mm, #14, distal with a reading of 5 mm, #15 distal with a reading of 5 mm, and #18 mesial and distal with a reading of 4 mm.

Patient completed orthodontic treatment 30 years ago and only wore retainer for first year after completion of treatment. She is not interested in retreatment.

Dental examination reveals a Class III distal composite on tooth #8 with a slight open margin and recurrent caries, tooth #9 reveals a large Class IV mesial-facial-incisal composite with open margins and recurrent caries, as well as a Class III distal composite with an open margin and recurrent caries. Tooth #9 also presents with a composite overhang on the mesial and distal surfaces.

The patient's oral hygiene is fair. She brushes twice daily, but flosses occasionally.

Occlusion

2 mm maxillary overjet Class (II) occlusion

Radiographic Examination

Anterior periapical was prescribed for tooth #8, #9. Posterior periapical of teeth #2, # 14, #15, and #18, molar and premolar bitewings were also prescribed but not shown (Figure 8.3.1).

Diagnosis and Prognosis

The patient's general oral health is fair.
Localized inflammation is present in the areas of teeth #2, #14, #15, and #18 with slight localized

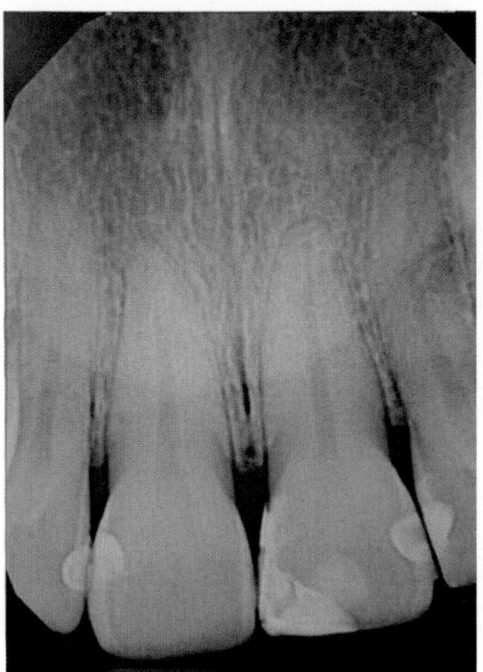

Figure 8.3.1: Radiographic image teeth #8 and #9.

bone loss on interproximal surfaces of teeth #2, #14, and #15.

Tooth #8 has caries, which has extended into dentin and can be seen on the radiograph.

Teeth present with yellow extrinsic stain due to age, coffee, and wine.

Dental Hygiene Diagnosis

Problems	Related to Risks and Etiology
2 mm overjet	Lack of orthodontic intervention and malocclusion
Bleeding on probing	Localized periodontal disease, poor oral hygiene management
4–5 mm periodontal pockets on teeth #2, #14, #15, #18	Localized periodontal disease, poor oral hygiene management
Generalized staining	Coffee and wine, biofilm accumulation, poor oral hygiene management

Planned Interventions

Clinical	Educational/counseling	Oral Hygiene Instructions
Evaluate soft and hard tissue for evidence of smoking	Encourage continued smoking cessation	Soft bristle brush/ Modified Bass technique
Localized scaling and root planing with 4 to 8 week periodontal re-evaluation	Stress importance of maintaining recare visits	Emphasize importance of flossing
Alginate impressions for fabrication of whitening trays	Discuss homecare technique for whitening trays	Wear whitening trays for 1 hour, once a day for 14 days
Refer to Doctor of Dental Surgery (DDS) for tooth #8, redo of existing Class III composite, tooth #9 redo of existing Class IV and Class III composites, possible future laminates	Instruct patient that whitening should be done before redo of composites, since composite restorations will not whiten. If sensitivity should occur, recommend dentifrice containing evidence based desensitizing agents (potassium nitrate, calcium sulfate)	Do not eat or drink for half an hour after, avoid anything that can stain a white t-shirt

Discussion: Alginate

Alginate is an elastic hydrocolloid impression material made from seaweed. It is also comprised of sodium alginate, calcium sulfate, and retarders. It is used to take primary or preliminary impressions. This colloidal material forms a gel when the powder is mixed with water. It solidifies into an elastic mass capable of producing a negative reproduction of the oral cavity (an impression) (Poling et al. 2008). Alginate is also referred to as an irreversible hydrocolloid because once it is mixed a chemical reaction occurs, known as gelation. Therefore, it can never return to its original state of powder and water. Alginate impressions are taken to obtain diagnostic study models, which are the positive reproductions of the teeth and surrounding structures. They are also used to fabricate bleaching trays and mouth guards. Alginate is the most universally utilized impression material in dentistry.

The following are characteristics of an ideal alginate impression material:

- cost effective,
- easy to mix,
- adequate flow properties,
- non-toxic or irritating,
- sufficient strength to avoid tearing material upon removal from the mouth, and
- acceptable working and setting times.

Taking Alginate Impressions

Positioning of Patient and Selection of Trays

Patient should be seated in an upright position.

Trays are selected, keeping in mind that proper fitting trays will allow the clinician to obtain all structures, including teeth and soft tissues. The tray should cover maxillary tuberosities and retromolar pads. The tray should also allow for room between the anterior teeth and anterior portion of tray approximately a space of 4 mm to allow for proper definition of anterior teeth.

Trays should be sprayed with a very light layer of alginate impression adhesive and allowed to dry for two to three minutes.

While waiting for adhesive to dry, have the patient rinse out well with a nonalcohol-based rinse to remove any debris.

Manipulation of Alginate Material

Alginate material comes in canisters and single-use packets. If using alginate in a canister, the canister should be turned gently upside down to fluff material before opening. If using premeasured single-use package, the bag may be lightly shaken before tearing open.

Alginate is mixed as a 1 : 1 ratio. Typically, three scoops of powder to three measures of water are used for a maxillary impression and two scoops of powder to two measures of water are used for a mandibular impression.

Proper mixing is critical: powder should be added to the bowl first and then cool water.

The first step is to incorporate the water and powder so powder particles are wet. This should be done quickly. Next, the mixture should be spatulated against one side of the bowl with the flat portion of the buffalo spatula, turning the spatula over at times to ensure a smooth bubble free mix (Poling et al. 2008) (see Figure 8.3.2).

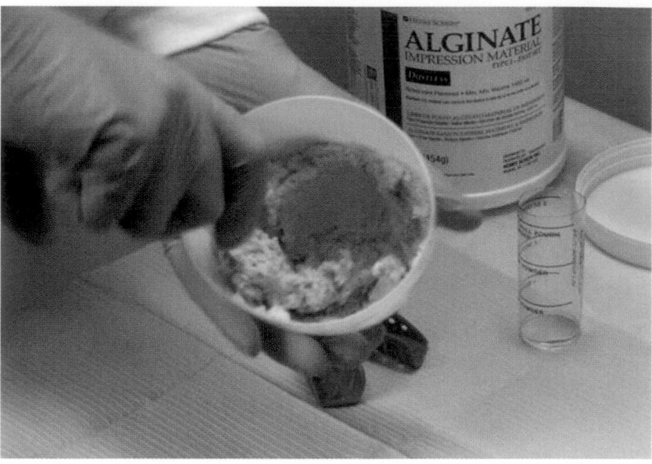

Figure 8.3.2: Proper spatulation technique.

Alginate setting time can be changed by altering the mixing time or water: powder ratio. However, due to nonconformities in mixing time or proportions of material utilized, certain properties of the gel can be effected and diminish. The best way to alter gelation time is to change the temperature of the water in the mix. The higher the temperature of the water the shorter the gelation time of the alginate.

Taking the Impression

The mandibular impression is always taken first to introduce the patient to the procedure as it is easier and less likely to cause gagging (Poling et al. 2008) (see Figure 8.3.3).

The material is scooped up and loaded into the tray from the lingual portion of the tray (it should only take two-three portions of material to fill tray).

The clinician stands at about 8.00 o'clock, in front of the patient and retracts the patient's cheek with index and middle finger, the tray is inserted into the patient's mouth sideways, and seated in posterior area first and then anterior. Soft tissues, lips and cheeks, should then be maneuvered over tray gently.

The maxillary impression is taken with the clinician standing at about 10.00–11.00 o'clock, beside and slightly behind the patient. The procedure for taking the impression is repeated (see Figure 8.3.4).

Patient should rinse and all alginate should be removed from the patient's face.

Alginates should be rinsed immediately, disinfected with a broad spectrum disinfectant, and then wrapped in damp paper towels and preferably stored in a sealed plastic bag for no longer than 30 minutes (Demajo et al. 2016; Hiraguchi and Hirose 2016; Iwasaki and Iwasaki 2016; Walker et al. 2010).

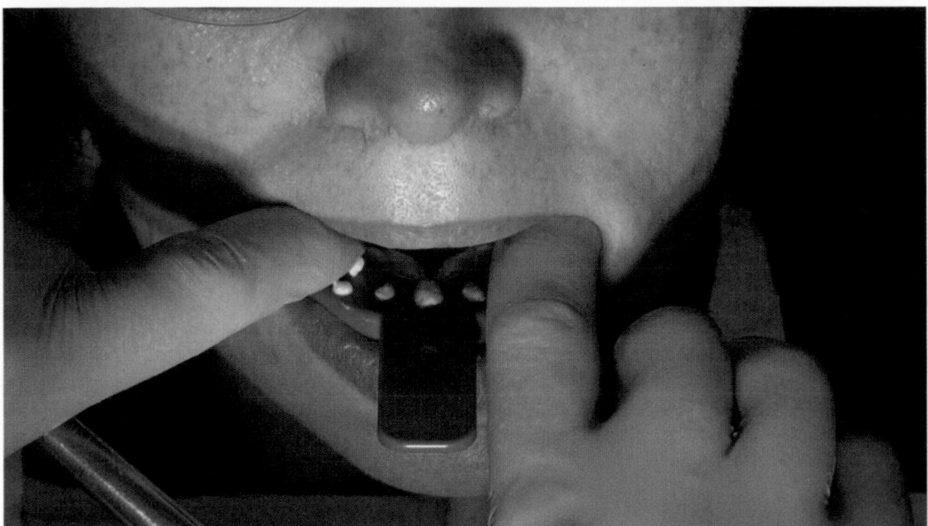

Figure 8.3.3: Placement of mandibular tray.

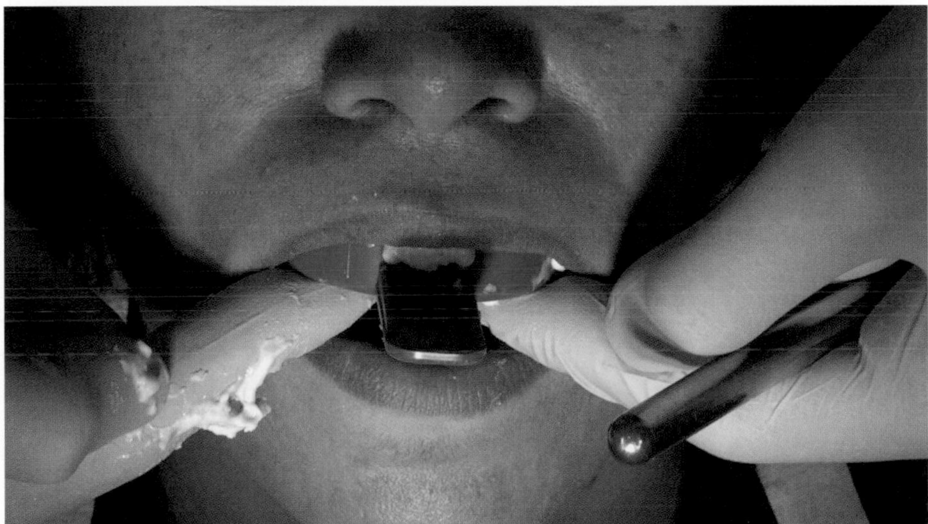

Figure 8.3.4: Placement of maxillary tray.

Alginate should be poured immediately as it is subject to deformation, which can include imbibition, an uptake of water that results in swelling, or syneresis, a loss of water that results in shrinkage (Rohanian et al. 2014).

Criteria of an Ideal Alginate Impression

Surface texture; moist, elastic, strong (proper thickness of material), and without voids.

The maxillary impression is aligned with the maxillary facial upper midline, the mandible, with the mandibular dental midline, most often between central incisors the borders of the impression should be rolled, round and thick, one-quarter thickness of alginate material covering the borders of the tray and extending into all vestibular spaces and including soft tissue attachments, such as frenula, maxillary tuberosity, hard palate, and retromolar pads, and detail of the gingival margin, no distortion, and no tray visible, including the borders of the tray (Figure 8.3.5).

The Future of Impressions

Technology is advancing in our greater world, as we move into a more digital arena in all aspects of our lives. The same holds true in dentistry; digital impressions are taking the place of conventional alginate impressions.

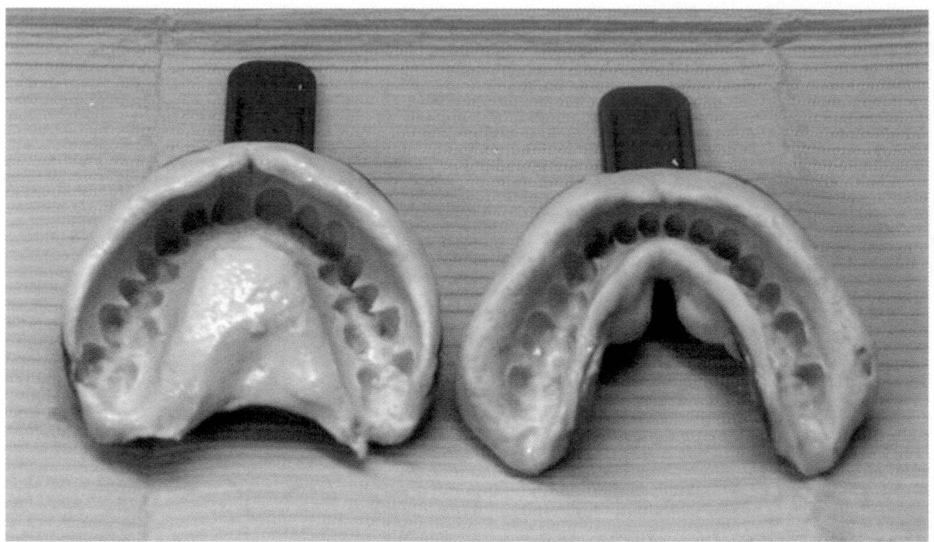

Figure 8.3.5: Acceptable maxillary and mandibular impressions.

Two types of systems are available today: Computer aided design/computer aided manufacture (CAD/CAM) and dedicated three-dimensional digital impressions (3D). These systems are used for restorative dentistry, implant dentistry, and orthodontics. While there are many systems available, the one thing is common is that they all provide potential for greater accuracy, precision, speed, and patient comfort when compared to traditional impressions. CAD/CAM dental systems are able to supply data obtained from digital scanning of teeth directly into milling systems which carve restorations out of ceramic or composite blocks, for example, CEREC. There are also dedicated 3D digital dental impression scanners, for example, iTero, that utilize lasers and imaging technology to capture tooth and gingival structure. Conventional impression success depends on many factors; material, tray selection, and technique. Each step involves potential risk of human and material error. Using digital scanners eliminates these problems; however, digital scanners have their own types of errors that can occur. A few systems use powders to coat the abutment teeth prior to scanning. This helps to eliminate reflection and allow for accurate measurements. The powder also adds thickness of 13–85 μm to the surfaces. Other scanners do not use the powder because their software is able to interpret the shiny surfaces of the abutment teeth. Either system can be affected by saliva, blood, poor soft-tissue isolation, humidity, and patient movement (Renne et al. 2017).

Take-Home Hints

1. Utility wax may be placed around the border of the impression tray. This enhances patient comfort and promotes proper fit of tray so that all oral structures are obtained in the impression
2. Before placing your impression tray, take a small scoop of alginate with your fingers and place on anterior facial surfaces, and posterior occlusal surfaces. This will help you achieve good detail of these areas and help to prevent voids
3. For patients with overactive gag reflex do the following: instruct patient to breathe deeply through the nose and focus on an object about 2–3 ft away or raise one leg and lower up and down as if exercising. These simple procedures help to take the patient's focus off the tray in their mouth and can help to minimize gagging.

Self-Study Questions

1. Alignate impression material is a:
- **A. Silicone material**
- **B. Hydrocolloid material**
- **C. Rigid Impression material**
- **D. None of the above**

2. Alginate impressions should obtain all of the following structures except
- **A. Frenula**
- **B. Hard palate**
- **C. Uvula**
- **D. Maxillary tuberosity**

3. The maxillary impression is always taken first
- **A. True**
- **B. False**

4. An uptake of water associated with a hydrocolloid impression is
- **A. Calcination**
- **B. Syneresis**
- **C. Imbibition**
- **D. Hydration**

References

Demajo, J.K., Cassar, V., Farrugia, C. et al. (2016). Effectiveness of disinfectants on antimicrobial and physical properties of dental impression materials. *International Journal of Prosthodontics* 29 (1): 63–67. doi: 10.11607/ijp.4358.

Hiraguchi, K. and Hirose, Y. (2016). Effect of immersion disinfection of alginate impressions in sodium hypochlorite solution on the dimensional changes of stone models. *Dental Materials Journal* 31 (2): 280–286.

Iwasaki, H. and Iwasaki, Y. (2016). Effects of immersion disinfection of agar-alginate combined impressions on the surface properties of stone casts. *Dental Materials Journal* 35 (1): 45–50.

Poling, R., Zimmerman, C., and Stauffer, D. (2008). *Alginate Impressions.* The International Training Institute.

Renne, W., Ludlow, M., Fryml, J. et al. (2017). Evaluation of the accuracy of 7 digital scanners: an *in vitro* analysis based on 3-dimensional comparisons. *The Journal of Prosthetic Dentistry* 118 (1): 36–42. doi: 10.1016/j.prosdent.2016.09.024 [Early Epub 2016 Dec 23].

Rohanian, A., Ommati Shabestari, G., Zeighami, S. et al. (2014). Effect of storage time of extended-pour and conventional alginate impressions on dimensional accuracy of casts. *Journal of Dentistry* 11 (6): 655–664.

Walker, M.P., Burckhard, J., Mitts, D.A., and Williams, K.B. (2010 Nov). Dimensional change over time of extended-storage alginate impression materials. *The Angle Orthodontist* 80 (6): 1110–1115. doi: 10.2319/031510-150.1.

Additional Resources

Anusavice, K.J., Shen, C., Rawls, H.R. (2013) Phillips' *Science of Dental Materials*, Chapter 7, pp 111–147. St. Louis, MI: Elsevier.

Birnbaum, N., Aaronson, H.B., Stevens, C., and Cohen, B. (2009). 3D digital scanners: a high-tech approach to more accurate dental impressions. *Inside Dentistry* 5 (4): Available from: www.insidedentistry.net.

Guiraldo, R.D., Moreti, A.F., Martinelli, J. et al. (2015). Influence of alginate impression materials and storage time on surface detail reproduction and dimensional accuracy of stone models. *Acta Odontológica Latinoamericana* 28 (2): 156–161. doi: 10.1590/S1852-48342015000200010.

Hansen, P., Franco, R., and Beatty, M. (2016). Wax lining in an impression tray and accuracy in gypsum cast fabrication. *Journal of Prosthodontics* 25 (1): 44–48. doi: 10.1111/jopr.12347 Epub 2015 Oct 23.

Kulkarne, M.M. and Thombare, R.U. (2015). Dimensional changes of alginate dental impression materials-an in-vitro study. *Journal of Clinical and Diagnostic Research* 9 (8): Zc88–ZC102. doi: 10.7860/JCDR/2015/13627.6407.

Polido, W.D. (2010). Digital impressions and handling of digital models: the future of dentistry. *Dental Press Journal of Orthodontics* 15 (5): 18–22.

Yuzbasioglu, E., Kurt, H., Turunc, R., and Bilir, H. (2014). Comparison of digital and conventional impression techniques: evaluation of patients' perception, treatment comfort, effectiveness and clinical outcomes. *BMC Oral Health* 14: 10. doi: 10.1186/1472-6831-14-10.

Answers to Self-Study Questions

1. B

2. C

3. B

4. C

Case 4

Dentinal Hypersensitivity

CASE STORY

A 42-year-old female patient presents to the office with the chief concern of "I've forgotten to wear my nightguard for the last two weeks, I was on vacation. Sighs. For the last few days, I've had a sensitivity to cold on this tooth." Patient points to the lower the left molar, tooth #19.

PROBLEM-BASED LEARNING GOALS AND OBJECTIVES

- Describe the oral hygiene instructions necessary for a patient with symptoms of dentinal hypersensitivity
- Describe the best practices for treatment planning and scheduling of patients with dentinal hypersensitivity
- Understand the etiology of dentinal hypersensitivity
- Explain best practices for choosing effective dental materials for desensitizing teeth that are experiencing dentinal hypersensitivity

Medical History

Patient is in good health. Not currently taking any medications. No known medication allergies. Has seasonal allergies. Takes over-the-counter antihistamines when necessary.

Review of Systems

- Vital signs:
  - Blood pressure: 117/78 mmHg
  - Pulse: 62 beats/min
  - Respiration: 15 breaths/min
  - Height: 5′ 6″
  - Weight: 135 lbs

Social History

Patient reports a history of clenching and grinding. Patient has had a preventive night guard appliance for two years that she wears to sleep. Patient reports of headaches when she forgets to wear her night guard appliance. She also develops swelling in the muscle on the lower left jaw. Patient reports that she tries to wear it regularly. Patient says that she drinks socially on the weekend, two to four drinks. She also occasionally socially smokes a few cigarettes, one to three. Her diet consists of low carbohydrate and high protein intake. She reports she eats a Paleo diet and chooses to buy only organic foods. Her daily snack consists of a handful of almonds and prefers to juice her vegetables. Patient says she prefers and only purchases 76% dark chocolate. Patient reports two to three cups of coffee and day, with two packets of "sweet and low." Otherwise, she drinks water throughout the day. Patients reports she brushes twice daily and occasionally flosses.

Patient lives with her boyfriend of seven years and has four children. Her children's ages range from 11 to 21 years. She solely owns her home. She has a full-time job as a childcare worker in a local daycare center.

The patient's current dental home care regimen consists of brushing in the morning with an electric toothbrush. Patient reports she is unaware when to replace the toothbrush heads. She believes her current brush head is over six months old. She occasionally flosses, no other dental aids used. She only uses a rinse to freshen her breath.

Extraoral Examination

Patient presents with normal findings upon palpation of her lymph nodes and glands. Patient presents with slight swelling in masseter muscle on the mandibular left side. There is no clicking or deviation in the temporomandibular joint. However, patient reports slight tenderness. Normal findings upon the assessment of other facial features.

Intraoral Examination

Three intraoral pictures were taken. Please see intraoral images in Figure 8.4.1. This includes a maxillary palatal view, mandibular occlusal view (tori present), and an occlusal view of the left side.

- Soft and hard tissues of the oral cavity:
  - Bilateral linea alba buccal mucosa
  - Tongue is slightly coated otherwise no significant findings
  - Hard palate, soft palate, tonsils, and oropharynx appear normal
  - Salivary glands appear normal
  - Bilateral mandibular tori
- Occlusal examination:
  - Class I occlusion with attrition noted on all posterior teeth especially #19. #10 is labioverted with 2 mm diastema
- Gingival examination:
  - Maxillary arch presents with pink stippled tissue, papilla knife shaped, erythematous and edematous gingiva on the buccal of #2, #3, #14, and #15
  - Mandibular arch presents with pink stippled tissue, with erythematous and edematous gingiva on the mandibular anterior lingual of teeth #s 22–27
  - Patient has light to moderate generalized staining, with stain highly visible on lingual of maxillary and mandibular anterior.

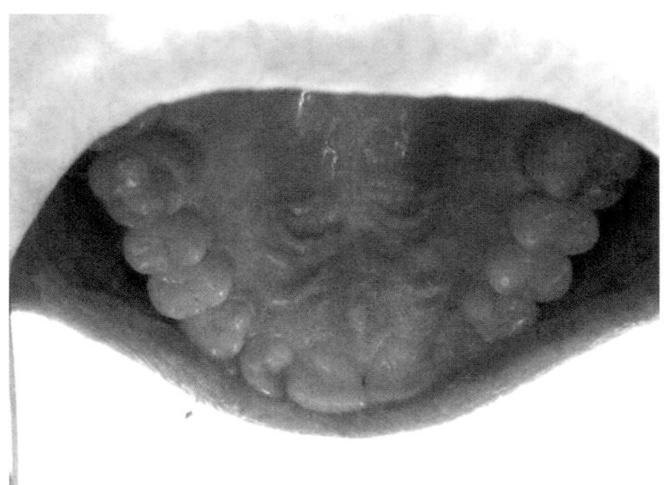

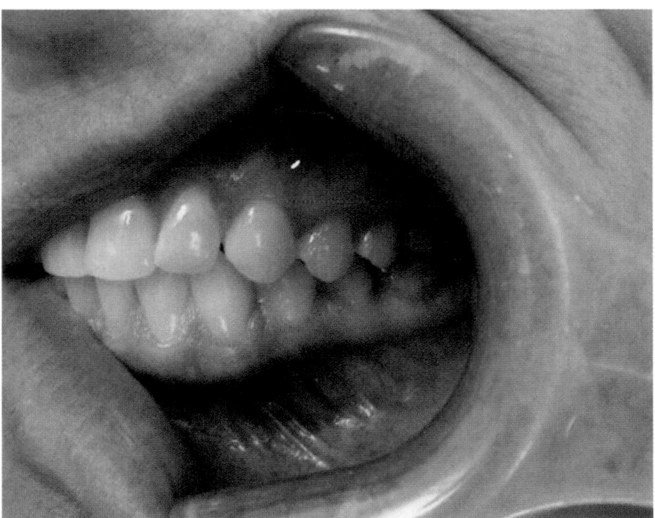

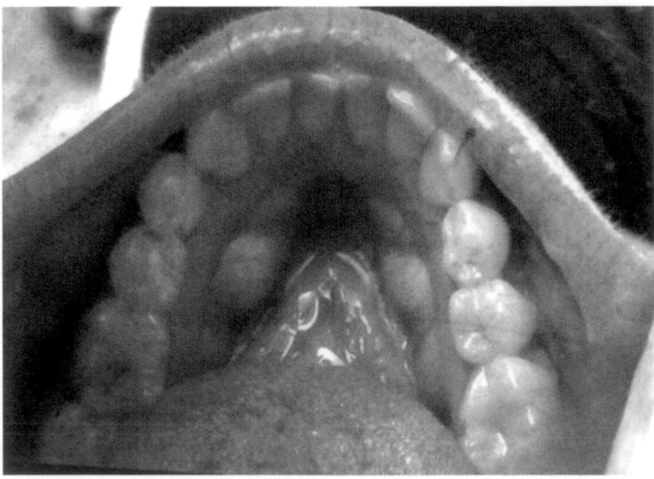

Figure 8.4.1: Intraoral pictures (left to right) show maxillary and mandibular arches, and occlusion on the lower left side, noting the significant recession on #19.

- Light localized calculus deposits noted on the mandibular anterior teeth lingual and the buccal of maxillary molars.
- Periodontal evaluation reveals generalized 1–3mm pocketing with 4mm on #2, #3, #14, and #15. Patient has generalized 1mm recession, with the exception of tooth #19, which has 3mm recession. A notable change since her last visit six months ago.

- Dental examination:
  - Patient is missing teeth #1, #16, #17, and #32
  - Minimal number of Class I and II composite restorations
  - No current caries are seen
  - Patient has visible signs of occlusal wear facets on all posterior teeth

Radiographic Evaluation

Three digital photographs (Figure 8.4.1), one horizontal bitewing of the left side (Figure 8.4.2).

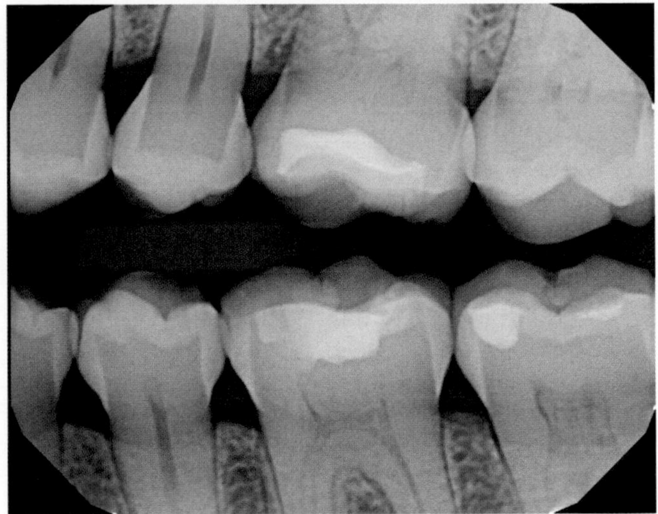

Figure 8.4.2: Horizontal bitewing of the left side.

Dental Hygiene Diagnosis

Problems	Related to Risks and Etiology
Dentinal hypersensitivity on tooth #19	Clenching and grinding at night (bruxism), not wearing night guard regularly
Occlusal wear facets	Clenching and grinding, bruxism
Swollen masseter muscle on left side	Clenching and grinding, bruxism
Bleeding on probing #2, #3, #14, and #15	Lack of interproximal cleansing
Social smoking Increased stain	Potential health risks, including periodontal disease
Coated tongue	Biofilm accumulation

Planned Interventions

Clinical	Education/Counseling	Oral Hygiene Instructions
Take blood pressure once yearly Adult prophylaxis with a 4-month re-evaluation of tissue #2, #3, #14, and #15 Place a desensitizing agent on tooth #19 Refer to DDS for planned examination	Encourage smoking cessation Emphasize importance of routinely scheduled dental care visits Encourage evening use of night guard appliance to prevent continued recession and flare-up of hypersensitivity Recommend increase of fluoridated water and toothpaste that contains potassium, stannous fluoride, calcium sodium phosphosilicate, and arginine to block/occlude dentin tubules to prevent hypersensitivity	Continued use of electric toothbrush Use of a tongue scraper Recommend toothpaste that contains fluoride as well as potassium, stannous fluoride, calcium sodium phosphosilicate, and arginine Once daily flossing or the use of another form of interdental cleaners Instruction of proper use, cleaning, and care of night guard

Discussion

Dentinal hypersensitivity is a prevalent clinical condition that is experienced by 10–20% of the population (Argawahl et al. 2016; Zhong et al. 2015; Kunam et al. 2016; Pathan et al. 2016). Kachalia (2016) suggests that 50% of the population suffers from dentinal hypersensitivity. Dentinal hypersensitivity is characterized by short, often sharp pain originating from exposed dentin in response to stimuli (Argawahl et al. 2016; Zhong et al. 2015; Kunam et al. 2016; Pathan et al. 2016). These stimuli can present as thermal, evaporative, tactile, osmotic, or chemical and cannot be attributed to any other form of dental defect or pathology (Argawahl et al. 2016; Zhong et al. 2015; Kunam et al. 2016; Pathan et al. 2016). Correct diagnosis of dentinal hypersensitivity is crucial for dental professionals. Assessment begins with a differential investigation to exclude some dental defects such as a fractured tooth, dental caries, and periodontal diseases in order to administer the correct form of treatment (Argawahl et al. 2016; Zhong et al. 2015; Kunam et al. 2016; Pathan et al. 2016). Dentinal hypersensitivity is related to exposed dentinal tubules, and the most common clinical cause of exposed dentinal tubules is gingival recession (Argawahl et al. 2016; Zhong et al. 2015; Kunam et al. 2016; Pathan et al. 2016). See intraoral images (Figure 8.4.1) for gingival recession on tooth #19. Aggressive brushing habits, high acidic or sugar intake in the diet, all types of tobacco use, and some other illnesses including gastroesophageal reflux may also cause dentin hypersensitivity (Argawahl et al. 2016; Zhong et al. 2015; Kunam et al. 2016; Pathan et al. 2016). It also results from abfraction, abrasion, or erosion and denudation of the root surface. See Figure 8.4.2 for excessive wear facets on mesial cusp. It has also been indicated as a result of nonsurgical and surgical periodontal treatment (Argawahl et al. 2016; Zhong et al. 2015; Kunam et al. 2016; Pathan et al. 2016).

The treatment for dentinal hypersensitivity has been classified by mode of delivery as at-home (patient-applied) therapy and in-office (professional) therapy (Argawahl et al. 2016; Zhong et al. 2015; Kunam et al. 2016; Pathan et al. 2016). There are many products available on the market that claim to reduce dental hypersensitivity effectively. It is a dental hygienist's responsibility to use evidence-based literature as a guide to making clinical decisions regarding what to recommend to patients. Numerous researchers have provided a concise overview of various approaches to occlude the dentinal tubules (Argawahl et al. 2016; Zhong et al. 2015; Kunam et al. 2016; Pathan et al. 2016). Researchers have determined that there are two ways of reducing hypersensitivity: one is that the occlusion of dentinal tubules occurs by natural mineralization *in situ* and two by the blockage of tubules by fine particle layers (Argawahl et al. 2016). In other words, products either reduce the fluid flow within the dentin tubules by occluding the tubules, while others interrupt the neural response to stimuli (Jena and Shashirekha 2015). Most products are intended to control the hydrodynamic mechanisms of pain (Jena and Shashirekha 2015).

According to Bae et al. (2016) meta-analysis indicated that there is sufficient evidence to support the use of potassium, stannous fluoride, calcium sodium phosphosilicate, and arginine-containing desensitizing toothpaste for dentin hypersensitivity, but not the use of strontium-containing desensitizing toothpaste (Bae et al. 2016). The clinical relevance of meta-analysis provides support for dental professionals and best-practice decision making for recommending a desensitizing toothpaste to patients (Bae et al. 2016). Many of these potassium, stannous fluoride, calcium sodium phosphosilicate, and arginine products in toothpaste offer only short-term relief to patients by means of dentinal hypersensitivity reduction (Kachalia 2016). In fact, other at-home products such as oxylates, in strips, have been determined to have no effect on dentine hypersensitivity in a single treatment when compared to placebos (Arnold et al. 2015). However, dental professionals have products available that can be applied to the teeth that resolve sensitivity for a longer period. These products are considered in-office varnishes. Pathan et al. (2016) suggests reduced dentinal hypersensitivity can last one month after one treatment with in-office products, as opposed to brushing with a sensitive toothpaste whereby reduction of dentinal hypersensitivity begins after two weeks of twice daily use. In-office desensitizing agents provide immediate, provisional relief from symptoms of dentinal hypersensitivity (Pathan et al. 2016). Currently, there is no "gold standard" for dentinal hypersensitivity treatment (Jena and Shashirekha 2015). A consultation with a dental professional regarding best treatment options along with a recommended home-care regimen and regularly scheduled dental recare appointments are highly recommended.

Take-Home Hints

1. Dental hygienists can recommend desensitizing toothpaste for dentin hypersensitivity in patients, and give other knowledgeable information regarding the effects of desensitizing toothpaste on dentin hypersensitivity with evidence-based research. This recommendation consists of toothpaste that contain potassium, stannous fluoride, and calcium sodium phosphosilicate, as well as arginine-containing desensitizing toothpastes, reduce the symptoms of dentin hypersensitivity.
2. Patients presenting with dentinal hypersensitivity should have a comprehensive examination and assessment to determine if a possible fracture or recurrent caries is related to pain.
3. A patient's progress with dentinal sensitivity should be monitored during regularly scheduled recare visits.

Self-Study Questions

1. A dental hygienist should always look for evidence-based research when recommending home care products for their patients.
- **A. True**
- **B. False**

2. Which active ingredients are proven to help reduce dentinal hypersensitivity in patients?
- **A. Potassium nitrate**
- **B. Calcium sodium phosphosilicate**
- **C. Arginine**
- **D. All of the above**

3. If a patient complains of cold sensitivity a dental hygienist should immediately recommend:
- **A. An in-office desensitizer (varnish)**
- **B. An at-home sensitive toothpaste containing either potassium nitrate, calcium sodium phosphosilicate, or arginie**
- **C. A clinical examination**
- **D. A radiographic examination**
- **E. All of the above**

4. Dentinal hypersensitivity is related to:
- **A. Gingival recession**
- **B. Abfraction**
- **C. Brushing habits**
- **D. All of the above**

References

Agarwal, J.H., Gupta, A., Garg, A. et al. (2016). Assessment and comparison of two different desensitizing agents for treating dentin hypersensitivity: a randomized clinical study. *Journal of International Oral Health* 8 (5): 615–618.

Arnold, W.H., Prange, M., and Naumova, E.A. (2015). Effectiveness of various toothpastes on dentine tubule occlusion. *Journal of Dentistry* 43 (4): 440–449.

Bae, J.H., Kim, Y.K., and Myung, S.K. (2016). Desensitizing toothpaste versus placebo for dentin hypersensitivity: a systematic review and meta-analysis. *Journal of Clinical Periodontology* 42: 131–141. doi: 10.1111/jcpe.12347.

Jena, A. and Shashirekha, G. (2015). Comparison of efficacy of three different desensitizing agents for in-office relief of dentin hypersensitivity: a 4 weeks clinical study. *Journal of Conservative Dentistry* 18: 389–393.

Kachalia PR (2016) Sensitive approaches: Treatment options can make our patients more comfortable by combating sensitivity [Online]. Available at: http://www.rdhmag.com/articles/print/volume-36/issue-7/contents/sensitive-approaches.html (May 22, 2018).

Kunam, D., Manimaran, S., Sampath, V., and Sekar, M. (2016). Evaluation of dentinal tubule occlusion and depth of penetration of nano-hydroxyapatite derived from chicken eggshell powder with and without addition of sodium fluoride: an *in vitro* study. *Journal of Conservative Dentistry* 19: 239–244.

Pathan, A.B., Bolla, N., Kavuri, S.R. et al. (2016). Ability of three desensitizing agents in dentinal tubule obliteration and durability: an *in vitro* study. *Journal of Conservative Dentistry* 19: 31–36.

Zhong, Y., Lui, J., Li, X. et al. (2015). Effect of a novel bioactive glass–ceramic on dentinal tubule occlusion: an *in vitro* study. *Australian Dental Journal* 60: 96–103. doi: 10.1111/adj.12241.

Answers to Self-Study Questions

1. A

2. D

3. E

4. D

9

Management of Special Needs Patients

Clinical Cases in Dental Hygiene, First Edition. Edited by Cheryl M. Westphal Theile, Mea A. Weinberg and Stuart L. Segelnick.

Case 1

Older Adult

CASE STORY

A 73-year-old Hispanic female patient presents to the clinic with the chief concern of "I had a partial denture made back home in my own country and it does not fit well, because it rocks from side to side when I am trying to eat. I also have cold sensitivity when I am drinking cold beverages. My teeth are shorter and wearing down in the front of my mouth so I am self-conscious when I talk to people."

PROBLEM-BASED LEARNING GOALS AND OBJECTIVES

- Describe the oral hygiene instructions necessary for a patient with removable prosthesis
- Describe best practices for treatment planning and scheduling of the older adult patient
- Demonstrate effective time schedule management of patients with osteoarthritis
- Explain best practices for effective biofilm removal for the older adult patient

Medical History

Patient was diagnosed with high blood pressure 10 years ago and is taking 50 mg of metoprolol succinate (Toprol) once a day. She also takes atorvastatin (Lipitor) 10 mg once a day. She was also diagnosed with osteoarthritis 10 years ago that affects dexterity of her hands and has limited mobility when walking. Patient is also taking over-the-counter 325 mg of aspirin as needed for the osteoarthritis. She has no known medication allergies.

Social History

Patient reports quitting smoking cigarettes about five years ago, and prior to quitting, was smoking one-pack a day for approximately 50 years. She drinks three cups of coffee throughout the day. Patient also drinks alcohol socially. Patient also reports that she has a dry mouth, and tries to drink some type of liquid drink of water or juice during the day. Her daily diet consists of soft foods such as noncruciferous vegetables, fish, and dairy products, due to difficulty chewing while using her removable partial prosthesis. Patient snacks regularly on sugary candies and desserts, and does not brush during the day.

Patient currently lives alone in an apartment building, located within an older adult community. Patient is able to take care of her own dental needs and is able to travel independently to scheduled dental appointments by public transportation.

The patient's current dental home care regimen involves brushing her own teeth once a day in the morning using a medium-bristled manual toothbrush. Patient replaces her toothbrush infrequently, approximately once a year. Patient rinses her partial prosthesis under tap water on a daily basis. She does not brush the prosthesis daily or take out at night and soak. She does not use floss, interdental aids, or mouthrinses.

The patient reports that her last dental visit was five years ago back in her own country to make the removable partial prosthesis. She was not given any specific home care instructions or follow-up care for the removal partial prosthesis.

Review of Systems

- Height: 5′ 4″
- Weight: 120 lbs

- Vital Signs
  - Blood pressure: 148/90 mmHg
  - Pulse: 64 beats/min
  - Respiration: 18 breaths/min

Extraoral Examination

Patient presents with bilateral clicking of the temporomandibular joint but does not express any discomfort. Her lips are dry and cracked. Patient presents with normal findings upon palpation of her lymph nodes, as well as the assessment of other facial features.

Intraoral Examination

Five intraoral pictures were taken.

- Soft tissues of the oral cavity:
  - Maxillary posterior ridges appear erythematous and tender upon palpation.
  - Tongue is enlarged and slightly coated on its dorsal surface.
  - Salivary output examination reveals hyposalivation of her major salivary glands.
- Occlusion Examination:
  - Edge-to-edge bite with attrition noted on all anterior teeth (Figure 9.1.1)
- Gingival examination:
  - Maxillary arch presents with localized recession with rolled margins, with erythematous and edematous gingiva on #6–7
  - Patient has generalized 3–4 mm probing depths, and localized areas of recession:
    - 4 mm recession on #6 facial
    - 2 mm recession on #8 facial
    - 3 mm recession on #9 facial
    - 3 mm recession on #11 distofacial
    - 3 mm on #23–26 lingual surfaces (Figure 9.1.2)

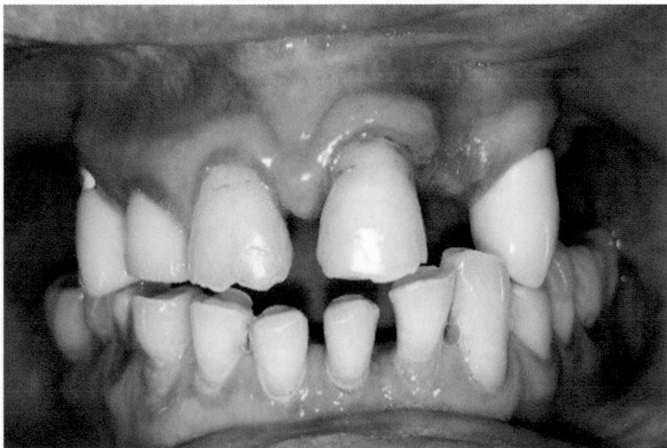

Figure 9.1.1: Front view.

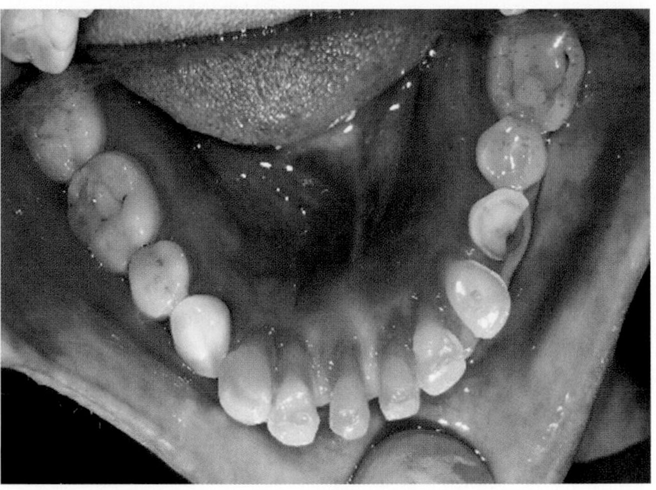

Figure 9.1.2: Mandibular occlusal view.

  - Generalized bleeding upon probing.
  - Patient has a diastema between #8 and #9, as well as open contacts on mandibular anterior teeth.
  - Gingival festooning on labial gingiva of #8 and #9.
- Dental examination:
  - Patient has crowns on #s 6, 7, 11, and 21
  - Patient has missing teeth #s 1–5, 10, 12–17, 31–32.
  - Patient presents with buccal surface abrasions on mandibular posterior teeth (Figures 9.1.3, 9.1.4, 9.1.5).

Radiographic Examination

A panoramic radiograph was taken and, upon examination, a retained root tip was found in the area of tooth #31 (Figure 9.1.6).

Dental Hygiene Diagnosis

Table 9.1.1 provides details of the problems and related risks

Planned Interventions

Table 9.1.2 provides details of the planned interventions

Discussion

The number of adults over the age 65 in the United States continues to increase, as people are living longer – 13% of the United States population is aged at least 65 with 7% of the population between 65 and 74 years, 4% between 75 and 84 years of age, and 2% older or equal to 85 years of age (Oong and An 2014; "Quick facts, United States" n.d.). Older adults are retaining more of their natural dentition because of increased access to dental care during their younger years (CDC 2010; LaSpina and Towle 2016). However,

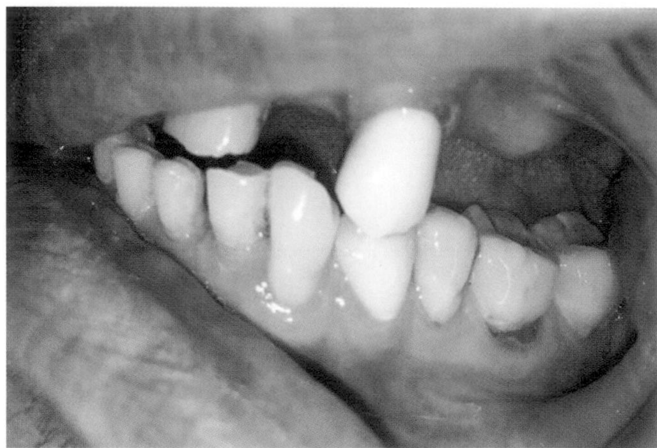

Figure 9.1.3: Right side.

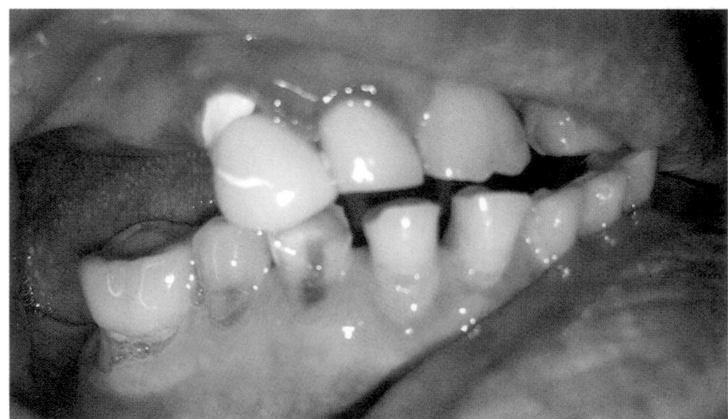

Figure 9.1.4: Left side.

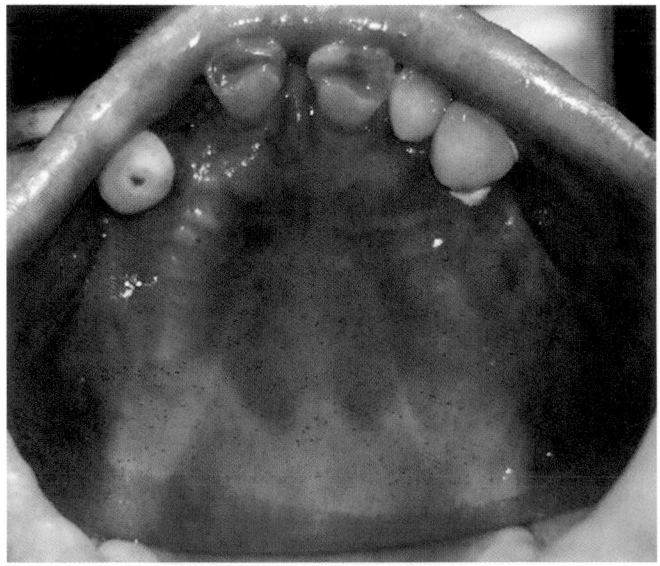

Figure 9.1.5: Maxillary occlusal view.

Table 9.1.1: Dental hygiene diagnosis.

Problems	Related to risks and etiology
Ill-fitting removable partial prosthesis	Nutritional deficiency, traumatic lesions
Osteoarthritis	Limited dexterity, poor oral hygiene management
Bleeding upon probing	Periodontal disease, poor oral hygiene management
Localized abrasions	Aggressive toothbrushing with medium-bristled toothbrush
Localized attrition	Bruxism
Coated tongue	Biofilm accumulation
Past history of smoking	Periodontal disease
Medication for hypertension	Xerostomia, biofilm accumulation

this population continues to need proper home care regimens, including preventative measures to maintain their dental health. Medicare, which provides healthcare insurance for adults 65 and older, provides no basic dental coverage. This population of adults who do not have supplemental insurance are at the greatest risk of having unmet health-care needs (Cohen et al. 1997). The lack of access to care is compounded by many other factors, such as: a shortage of skilled health-care providers for the older adult, limited transportation options to appointments, and lack of financial resources (Dolan et al. 2005).

Due to the complex needs of this aging population, older adult patients can often present with multiple medical and periodontal conditions. A thorough review of the patient's medical and dental history, including periodontal examination, must be completed to facilitate proper diagnosis. As a person ages, metabolic changes occur, and the adverse effects of long-term pharmaceutical usage will have an impact on the oral cavity (Yellowitz and Schneiderman 2014).

The dental hygienist needs to be prepared and be competent in treating this aging population – they must remain current in their knowledge of pharmaceutical products, while providing preventive and therapeutic services in all types of dental practices. For example, xerostomia is a very common side effect of many medications and is one of the factors of an increased caries risk in older adults (Moore 2016). Interprofessional communication needs to be improved among all health-care providers in order to manage and maintain the older adult patients' quality of care and medications – especially among dental and medical health-care providers.

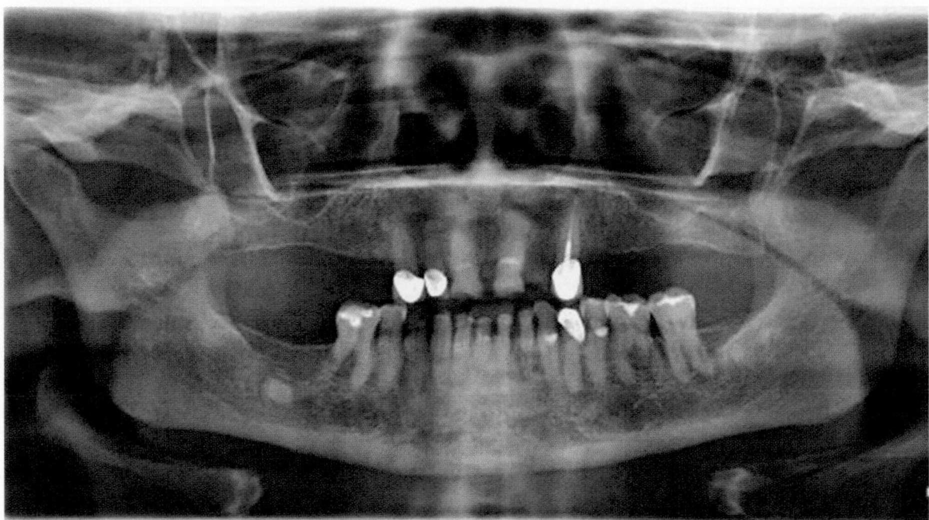

Figure 9.1.6: Panoramic radiograph.

Table 9.1.2: Planned interventions.

Clinical	Education/Counseling	Oral Hygiene Instructions
Take blood pressure at every visit Scaling and root planing with 4 to 8 week periodontal reevaluation of initial therapy. Refer to Doctor of Dental Surgery (DDS) or Doctor of Dental Medicine (DMD) for planned extractions, fabrication of crowns, and removable partial prosthesis	Encourage continued smoking cessation Stress importance of routine primary care visits and scheduled dental recare visits Recommend increased intake of fluoridated water for hydration, relief of xerostomia, remineralization of hard tooth surfaces Nutritional counseling for increasing calcium and/or Vitamin D intake	Soft-bristled toothbrush usage with modified Stillman technique Toothbrush with tongue scraper Recommend use of fluoride toothpastes Recommend use of lubricating mouthrinse for xerostomia Design of adaptive aids for effective brushing and functional control Instruction of proper removable partial prosthesis cleaning and care

Patients in this aging population frequently present with degenerative joint disease (DJD), or osteoarthritis, and this can affect their motor function. Manual dexterity and the timing of the appointment are important to consider when treating these patients. Considerations of limited manual dexterity from DJD or osteoarthritis should include: the design of adaptive aids that are easier to grip and are of enlarged and wider size to promote grip strength and functional control (Muzzin 2014). It is recommended that these patients have shorter appointments, and be scheduled during the late mornings or in the afternoons (LaSpina and Towle 2016).

In many cases, the older adult patient may require a fabrication of a removable prosthesis. This can be the result of periodontal disease, trauma, and/or decay. Removable prosthesis can restore the aesthetic appearance of the older adult, as well as their quality of life and dental function (Yellowitz and Schneiderman 2014). In order to maintain the integrity of the removable prosthesis, it is recommended that it be cleaned daily using a dedicated removal prosthesis toothbrush with soft end-rounded filaments. Proper cleaning, along with daily removal of the prosthesis overnight will prevent denture stomatitis and other related oral infections (Donnelly 2014; Swecker 2016).

Take-Home Hints

1. Daily care of removable prosthesis should include: nightly removal of the prosthesis with rinsing, immersing, and brushing with a designated partial denture toothbrush for proper biofilm removal.
2. Degenerative joint disease or osteoarthritis can influence the patient's dexterity required for effective biofilm removal. Adjunct aids should be introduced and custom-designed for the patient's individual needs.
3. Scheduling/dental appointment times for older adult patients with degenerative joint disease or osteoarthritis

4. Patients presenting with periodontal disease should be regularly scheduled for recare appointments at three-month intervals to ensure periodontal maintenance.
5. Considerations for improved access to dental care for the older adult patient; transportation, finances, scheduling of appointments, and interprofessional teamwork.

Self-Study Questions

1. Which of the following effects do degenerative joint diseases or osteoarthritis have on the patient's ability to perform daily brushing and interdental care?
- **A. Limited dexterity and strength**
- **B. Xerostomia**
- **C. Periodontal disease**
- **D. Excessive motor activity**

2. What is the best time to schedule a dental appointment for an older adult patient who has degenerative joint disease, or osteoarthritis?
- **A. Early morning appointments**
- **B. Late morning or afternoon appointments**
- **C. Evening appointments**
- **D. A and C**
- **E. B and C**

3. What barriers to care can impact recare appointments of the older adult patient?
- **A. Financial constraints**
- **B. Insurance coverage**
- **C. Transportation options**
- **D. A and B**
- **E. All of the above**

4. What are proper daily home care instructions for care of full and partial removable prosthesis for the older adult patient?
- **A. Daily removal of prosthesis overnight**
- **B. Soak in alcoholic mouthrinse**
- **C. Brush daily with dedicated toothbrush**
- **D. A and C**
- **E. B and C**

References

CDC. (2010, January 26). *New series of reports to monitor health of older Americans* [Online]. Available at: http://www.cdc.gov/nchs/pressroom/01facts/olderame.htm (May 16, 2016).

Cohen, R.A., Bloom, B., Simpson, G., and Parsons, P.E. (1997). Access to health care. Part 3: older adults. *Vital and Health Statistics. Series 10, Data from the National Health Survey* 198: 1–32.

Dolan, T.A., Atchison, K., and Huynh, T.N. (2005). Access to dental care among older adults in the United States. *Journal of Dental Education* 69 (9): 961–974.

Donnelly, L.R. (2014). Persons with fixed and removable dental prosthesis. In: *Dental Hygiene: Theory and Practice* (ed. M.L. Darby and M.M. Walsh), 1006–1021. United States: Elsevier Health Sciences.

LaSpina, L.M. and Towle, J.H. (2016). The older adult patient. In: *Clinical Practice of the Dental Hygienist* (ed. E.M. Wilkins), 899–916. United States: Wolters Kluwer.

Moore, J.C. (2016). Sealants. In: *Clinical Practice of the Dental Hygienist* (ed. E.M. Wilkins), 619–632. United States: Wolters Kluwer.

Muzzin, K.B. (2014). Persons with disabilities. In: *Dental Hygiene: Theory and Practice* (ed. M.L. Darby and M.M. Walsh), 786–804. United States: Elsevier Health Sciences.

Oong, E.M. and An, G.K. (2014). Treatment planning considerations in older adults. *Dental Clinics of North America* 58 (4): 739–755.

Quick facts, United States n.d. [Online] Available at: https://www.census.gov/quickfacts/table/PST045215/00. (October 2, 2016).

Swecker, T.K. (2016). Care of dental prosthesis. In: *Clinical Practice of the Dental Hygienist* (ed. E.M. Wilkins), 511–531. United States: Wolters Kluwer.

Yellowitz, J.A. and Schneiderman, M.T. (2014). Elder's oral health crisis. *The Journal of Evidence-Based Dental Practice* 14: 191–200.

Answers to Self-Study Questions

1. A

2. B

3. E

4. D

Case 2

Psychiatric Disability

CASE STORY

A 19-year-old female college student presents to the clinic with the chief concern of "my upper front teeth seem thin and are really sensitive to cold drinks, and my tongue feels like its burning." She reports that she is very self-conscious of her front teeth and hasn't seen a dental provider in the last few years because of her insecurities.

PROBLEM-BASED LEARNING GOALS AND OBJECTIVES

- Define and identify concepts and key terms related to patients exhibiting symptoms of a feeding and eating disorder, bulimia nervosa
- Identify intra and extraoral signs and symptoms related to patients with bulimia nervosa
- Demonstrate effective dental hygiene treatment for patients exhibiting symptoms of bulimia nervosa
- Understand the key role of the dental hygienist in the treatment and recare of patients with bulimia nervosa

Medical History

Patient was diagnosed with anxiety disorder in high school, and is taking 20 mg of duloxetine hydrochloride (Cymbalta) twice daily. The patient is currently under the care of a physician for her medications. She does not have any other significant medical history findings.

Social History

Patient reports that she has a habit of biting her nails. Patient also reports drinking socially with her college friends, as well as frequently eating at fast-food restaurants. She has a membership to the college fitness facility, and frequents it often because she feels that she is overweight. She states that she goes through phases of uncontrollable binge eating and reports vomiting on occasion or uses laxatives after the binges. Patient reports only drinking bottled water and carbonated soft drinks.

Since she has been away in college, the patient reports that she hasn't visited her dentist in over a year. Her daily home care consists of brushing once a day in the morning. She reports flossing occasionally and uses a generic-brand mouth rinse on a daily basis, but cannot recall the name of the mouth rinse and what it contains.

Review of Systems

- Blood pressure: 110/65 mmHg
- Pulse rate: 60 beats/min
- Respiration: 17 breaths/min

Extraoral Examination

Nail biting is evident. There is evidence of ecchymosis and calluses on the back and knuckle area of the patient's right hand. Patient also presents with dry, cracked lips. There is bilateral swelling of the zygomatic facial regions.

Intraoral Examination

- Lingual surface erosion of #s 7–10, appearing translucent and glasslike, especially on the incisal edges of the teeth with slight chipping.
- Generalized interproximal caries
- Bilateral swollen parotid glands
- Hyposalivation
- Inflamed and erythematous pharyngeal tonsillar area

Intraoral Pictures

Figure 9.2.1 and Figure 9.2.2 provide images in palatal view.

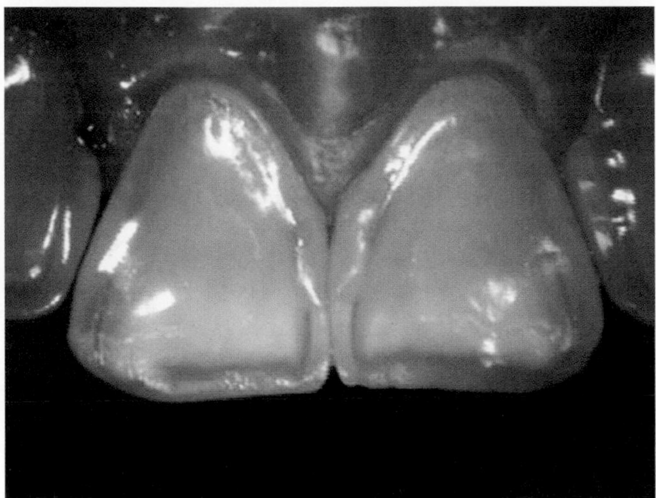

Figure 9.2.1: Maxillary incisors palatal view 01.

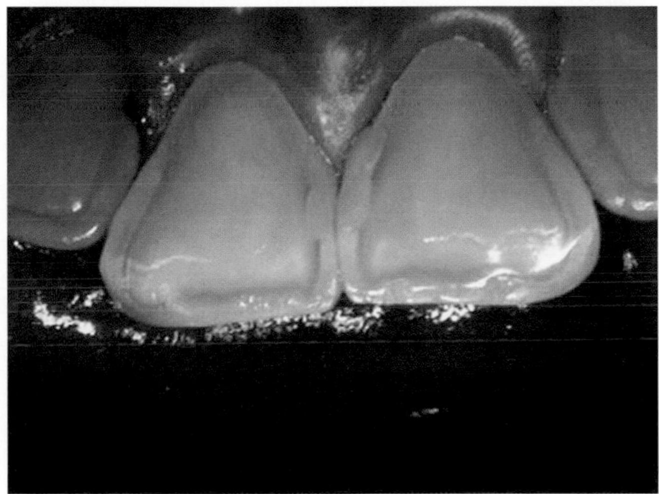

Figure 9.2.2: Maxillary incisors palatal view 02.

Table 9.2.1: Dental hygiene diagnosis.

Problems	Related to risks and etiology
Increased caries risk	Xerostomia and hyposalivation Dehydration Poor oral hygiene: brushing once a day and occasional flossing Infrequent dental visits High carbohydrate diet
Lingual erosion of maxillary incisors	Perimylolysis
Chipping of maxillary incisors, #s 7 and 8	Nail biting and perimylolysis
Increased hypersensitivity	Chemical erosion

Dental Hygiene Diagnosis

Table 9.2.1 gives details of the diagnosis.

Planned Interventions

Table 9.2.2 gives details of the interventions planned for this patient.

Discussion

In the psychiatric literature, bulimia nervosa, and anorexia nervosa are interconnected by the term eating disorder (Pantzari et al. 2015). Of the patients suffering from bulimia nervosa 80% are female, and in that 80%, 1–2% are adolescents and young adult women (National Eating Disorders Association 2016). Bulimia nervosa presents as a psychiatric compulsive disorder, and is frequently linked to depression and changes in social adjustment (National Eating Disorders Association 2016). Risk of death from suicide or medical complications is significantly increased for eating disorders (National Eating Disorders Association 2016).

Table 9.2.2: Planned interventions.

Clinical	Education/counseling	Oral hygiene instructions
Radiographic examination Adult prophylaxis In-office fluoride treatment using fluoride varnish containing 5% neutral sodium fluoride Refer to DDS for planned caries restorations and aesthetic maxillary anterior teeth fixed prosthodontic restorations Three to four month recare schedule to monitor new incidence of caries and erosion	Avoidance of brushing immediately after vomiting Sugar-free mints or xylitol gum to promote salivary flow Increase intake of fluoridated water Encourage increased compliance to specialist visits for psychiatric counseling Nutritional counseling	Nonalcoholic fluoridated mouth rinse Lubricating mouth rinse for xerostomia Brushing twice daily with extra-soft toothbrush using fluoridated toothpaste Daily interdental care

Bulimia nervosa has two defined types: nonpurging and purging. In the nonpurging type, the patient can engage in inappropriate behaviors, such as excessive exercise and fasting but does not involve the usage of laxatives and vomiting behaviors. In the purging type, the patient frequently engages in self-induced vomiting, usage of diuretics, enemas, or overuse of laxatives (Boyd and Wilkins 2016). The profile of the bulimic patient can include: normal body weight and/or slightly overweight, severe dehydration, and electrolyte imbalance from excessive purging, swollen salivary glands especially in the parotid region, with a commonly swollen and inflamed throat. Teeth can also show signs of chemical erosion, sensitivity, and increased caries (Lasater and Mehler 2001). These eating disorder characteristics/profiles can lead to a pathological control of body weight, and can cause systemic and oral alterations (Schlueter et al. 2012).

Patients with eating disorders are typically treated with antidepressant medications that can result in xerostomia or hyposalivation (Hunter and Wilson 1995; Sreebny and Schwartz 1997). It should be noted that a dry oral cavity, coupled with poor home care, may enhance dental plaque accumulation on teeth surfaces facilitating cariogenic bacterial growth on fermentable carbohydrates (Romanos et al. 2012).

Developing erosive lesions on teeth and dental wear is a notable finding of eating disorder patients, especially with bulimia nervosa, and early diagnosis is essential. In literature, the erosive lesion typically seen in these patients is called perimylolysis (Boyd and Wilkins, 2016). Perimylolysis is defined as a chemical erosion by acid to the tooth surface, typically from regurgitation of stomach contents (Boyd and Wilkins 2016). It most frequently affects the lingual surfaces of the maxillary anterior teeth. The tongue protects the mandibular teeth from the erosive effects of vomiting (Spear 2008). The maxillary anterior teeth lingual surfaces appear glasslike and translucent, and can become sensitive to thermal changes (Boyd and Wilkins 2016).

For patients, it is difficult to detect early enamel erosion due to its smooth and shiny appearance, and lack of symptoms. It is the responsibility of the dental professional to identify early stages of enamel erosion and implement preventive treatment measures (Baheti and Toshniwal 2015). Treatment should begin with identifying the underlying medical disorder and level of disease progression (Baheti and Toshniwal 2015). Supportive referrals to appropriate specialists are necessary to address the medical well-being of the patient (Romanos et al. 2012).

Dental hygienists are often the first health-care professionals to recognize signs of chemical erosion of the teeth. Dental hygienists are able to provide preventive measures to minimize the effects of chemical erosion, and make necessary referrals for caries restoration. Preventive measures can include: caries risk assessment, application of fluoride varnish, and nutritional counseling with dietary analysis. Preventive measures that can be employed by the patient should include: avoidance of toothbrushing after regurgitation, use of a low-abrasive fluoridated toothpaste, and salivary stimulation by using sugarless candies or gum (Baheti and Toshniwal 2015).

Depending on the degree of tooth wear, restorative options can range from localized composite restorations to prosthodontic reconstruction of the affected teeth (Baheti and Toshniwal 2015). A three to four month recare schedule is recommended to maintain patient compliance, and to monitor/assess new incidence of caries and erosion.

Take-Home Hints

1. Females are at higher risk of developing bulimia nervosa than males.
2. Early detection of dental erosion can be indicators of an underlying feeding/eating disorder.
3. Vomiting associated with a feeding/eating disorder can be related to dehydration, xerostomia, and perimylolysis.
4. Teeth surfaces most affected by vomiting are maxillary anterior lingual surfaces.
5. Identification of early dental erosion by the dental professional is important in identifying an underlying medical condition that can be detrimental to the patient's health.

Self-Study Questions

1. Identify the chemical erosion of the tooth surfaces by increased exposure to acid from vomiting?
A. Attrition
B. Lanugo
C. Perimylolysis
D. Prodromal

2. Which surfaces are most vulnerable to chemical erosion after vomiting?
A. Mandibular anterior lingual surfaces
B. Mandibular posterior lingual surfaces
C. Maxillary anterior lingual surfaces
D. Maxillary posterior lingual surfaces

3. What is the best advice in regards to her chief concern of "thin, chipping, and really sensitive to cold drinks"?
A. Have more frequent dental prophylaxis
B. Avoid mouthrinses with fluoride
C. Brush teeth as much as possible
D. Do not brush teeth immediately after vomiting

4. What is the eating disorder that this patient has?
A. Bulimia nervosa purging type
B. Bulimia nervosa nonpurging type
C. Anorexia nervosa Restrictive type
D. Bipolar disorder

References

Baheti, M.J. and Toshniwal, N.G. (2015). Acidity and dentistry: problems and solutions. *International Dental Journal of Students Research* 3 (3): 113–119.

Boyd, L.D. and Wilkins, E.M. (2016). The patient with a mental health disorder. In: *Clinical Practice of the Dental Hygienist* (ed. E.M. Wilkins), 1069–1083. United States: Wolters Kluwer.

Hunter, K. and Wilson, W. (1995). The effects of antidepressant drugs on salivary flow and content of sodium and potassium ions in human parotid saliva. *Archives of Oral Biology* 40 (11): 983–989.

Lasater, L. and Mehler, P. (2001). Medical complications of bulimia nervosa. *Eating Behaviors* 2 (3): 279–292.

National Eating Disorders Association. (2016). *Bulimia Nervosa* [Online]. Available at: http://www.nationaleatingdisorders.org/bulima-nervosa (August 4, 2016).

Pantzari, F., Kamposiora, P., and Papavasiliou, G. (2015). A multidisciplinary approach to the functional and esthetic rehabilitation of a patient with bulimia nervosa: a clinical report. *International Journal of Dentistry and Oral Science* 53–58.

Romanos, G., Javed, F., Romanos, E., and Williams, R. (2012). Oro-facial manifestations in patients with eating disorders. *Appetite* 59 (2): 499–504.

Schlueter, N., Ganss, C., Pötschke, S. et al. (2012). Enzyme activities in the oral fluids of patients suffering from bulimia: a controlled clinical trial. *Caries Research* 46 (2): 130–139.

Spear, F. (2008). A patient with severe wear on the anterior teeth and minimal wear on the posterior teeth. *The Journal of the American Dental Association* 139 (10): 1399–1403.

Sreebny, L. and Schwartz, S. (1997). A reference guide to drugs and dry mouth – 2nd edition. *Gerodontology* 14 (1): 33–47.

Answers to Self-Study Questions

1. C

2. C

3. D

4. A

Case 3

Abuse

CASE STORY

A seven-year-old male Caucasian child presents to the dental office for emergency care. The child is accompanied by his 26-year-old mother. While the child is waiting his turn for treatment, the dental professional takes note that the child is wearing a long sleeve shirt on a warm summer day, is withdrawn, and is discreetly watching other children's behavior in the waiting room while covering his mouth. Upon examination the dental hygienist notes lip and labial trauma to the labial frenum, as well as caries on the posterior teeth.

PROBLEM-BASED LEARNING GOALS AND OBJECTIVES

- Identify what constitutes child abuse, maltreatment, and neglect
- Describe the facial and oral injuries consistent with physical and sexual child abuse
- Describe the behavioral characteristics of child abuse and maltreatment
- Assess the scope and incidence of the child abuse in the United States
- Identify the perpetrators of child abuse/ maltreatment and neglect
- Identify the role of the dental professional and mandated state reporting procedures of child abuse and neglect
- List the physical/ psychological, behavioral, and social consequences of child abuse

Medical History

The seven-year-old child presents with a negative medical history reported by his mother.

Social History

This child has two siblings, a five-year-old brother and a four-year-old sister and lives with his parents. The mother is unemployed and the father works as a landscaper.

The mother describes the child as a thumb sucker, and tends to breathe through his mouth. She also mentions that he just started second grade, but misses many classes due to frequent colds.

Review of Systems

- Blood pressure: 106/66 mmHg
- Pulse rate: 80 beats/min
- Respiration: 25 breaths/min

Extraoral Examination

Edematous and erythematous upper lip.

Intraoral Examination

Patient presents with:

- Dental caries
- Caries on teeth #19 and #30, as well as primary teeth A, J, K, and T.
- Severed maxillary labial frenum.
- Short maxillary labial frenum resulting in anterior diastema between #8 and #9.
- Tissue trauma around tooth #9.
- Class II Division I occlusion with anterior open bite.

Radiographic Examination

None available, as the child's mother refused to give permission to take intraoral radiographs at this appointment. Furthermore, she stated that she brought her son to "take care of the swollen and cut lip and not for the cavities" (see Figure 9.3.1).

Dental Hygiene Diagnosis

Table 9.3.1 details the diagnosis

Planned Interventions

Table 9.3.2 details the interventions planned for the case.

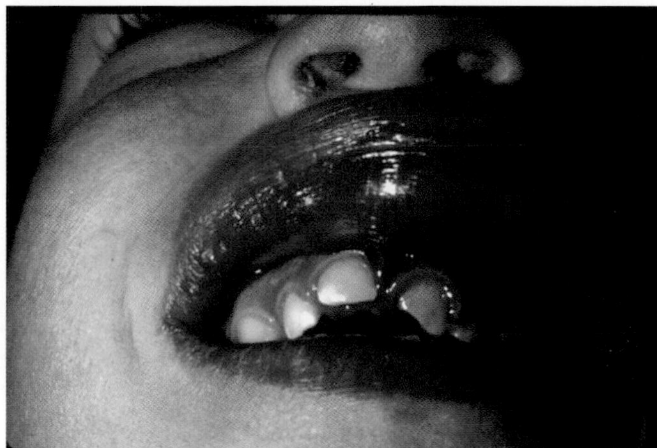

Figure 9.3.1: Upper lip.

Table 9.3.1: Dental hygiene diagnosis.

Problems	Related to risks and etiology
Difficulty in eating	Malnutrition, underweight, caries
Diminished social interaction with peers, neglect	Low self-esteem, unwillingness to talk or complain
Caries, pain	Poor diet, lack of daily oral hygiene, absence of dental care
Gingival bleeding	Lack of daily home care
Mouth breathing	Malocclusion
Lacerated frenum	Possible trauma to the upper lip

Discussion

In the United States the reporting of child abuse and neglect are mandated in all 50 states, including the District of Columbia and the Commonwealth of Puerto Rico (Child Welfare Information Gateway 2016c). This responsibility mandates professionals, including dentists and dental hygienists, to report suspected child maltreatment of children younger than 18 years of age to Child Protective Services, or law enforcement (Katner and Brown 2012).

Each state has its own definition of child abuse and neglect that is based on the federal law standards. The Child Abuse Prevention and Treatment Act (CAPTA), provides a foundation by identifying a set of acts or behaviors that define child abuse and neglect. The CAPTA Reauthorization Act of 2010 retained the existing definition of child abuse and neglect at minimum as "any recent act or failure to act on the part of a parent or caretaker which results in death, serious physical or emotional harm, sexual abuse or exploitation; or an act or failure to act, which presents an imminent risk of serious harm" (Child Welfare Information Gateway 2016a).

In the United States in 2014, there were an estimated 1580 children who died of abuse and neglect; 75% of these were three years of age or younger. The number of fatalities account for 2.13 per 100,000 children. Among these fatalities, cases involving at least one parent accounted for 79.3%. Children in their first year of life have the highest rate of victimization at 24.4 per 1000 children of the same age. Boys have a higher rate of fatality than girls at 2.48 boys versus 1.82 girls per 100,000 in the population. Of all child abuse victims that resulted in fatalities, 43% were Caucasian, 30.3% African American, and 15.1% were Hispanic (Child Maltreatment 2014).

Table 9.3.2: Planned interventions.

Clinical	Education/Counseling	Oral Hygiene Instructions
Identifying suspected child abuse and report	Deliver home care instructions to the parent and the patient	Soft-bristled toothbrush
Determine cause of neglect and maltreatment	Reduce consumption of cariogenic and sugary foods	Fluoridated toothpaste
Report the potential child abuse incidence to the State child protective services, or law enforcement authorities	Nutritional counseling	Daily fluoridated mouthrinses
Refer to DDS to address torn labial frenum		Increase consumption of fluoridated water
Refer to DDS for restoration of caries		
Refer to DDS for orthodontic consultation		
Fluoride varnish treatment		
Periodic dental visits		
Proper documentation of patient behavior, and extraoral and intraoral examination findings		

From 2010 to 2014, there was a 7.4% increase in the number of reported cases of child abuse. Of the reported cases in 2014, 75% of child victims were neglected, 17% were physically abused, and 8.3% were sexually abused (Child Maltreatment 2014).

The ethnicities of the majority of the child abuse victims were white (44.0%), Hispanic (22.7%), and African American (21.4%). The perpetrator is defined as the person who is responsible for the abuse or neglect of the child. Of the reported perpetrators 83.2% are between the ages of 18 and 44 years of age, 54.1% are women, 44.8% men, 48.8% are Caucasian, 20% African American, and 19.8% Hispanic (Child Maltreatment 2014).

Dental health-care providers have the unique opportunity to identify and report child abuse since approximately 65% of all physical manifestations of abuse are found around the neck and head areas. In addition, abused children are more likely to continue to visit the same dentist, while the parents frequently change physicians in order to prevent detection of child abuse (Thomas et al. 2006). Medical professionals receive minimal training in oral health, oral diseases, identifying injury or trauma of the oral cavity, and may not as readily be able to recognize dental aspects of abuse or neglect. Therefore, medical professionals and dental professionals are encouraged to collaborate interprofessionally in identifying child abuse and increase the prevention, detection, and treatment of these child abuse cases (American Academy of Pediatrics Committee on Child Abuse and Neglect and American Academy of Pediatric Dentistry Council on Clinical Affairs 2010).

Most states recognize four major types of child maltreatment: neglect, physical abuse, psychological (emotional), and sexual abuse. Any of these forms of maltreatment may be committed separately or in combination (Child Maltreatment 2014).

Neglect

The most frequent maltreatment is child neglect. It is defined as the "failure to provide for a child's basic physical, emotional, medical/dental or educational needs or combination thereof, by the parent or legal guardian, and neglect to protect the child from harm or potential harm, ensure a child's safety within and outside the home given the child's emotional and developmental needs" (Child Welfare Information Gateway 2016a). It is also be defined as the omission and deprivation of providing shelter, clothing, adequate food, appropriate supervision, and medical and dental care (Merrick and Latzman 2014).

Dental neglect, as defined by the American Academy of Pediatric Dentistry, is "the willful failure of parents or guardian to seek and follow through with treatment necessary to ensure a level of oral health essential for adequate function and freedom from pain and infection" (American Academy of Pediatric Dentistry 2005).

Physical Abuse

Physical abuse is defined as the "intentional use of physical force against a child that results, or has the potential to result in, physical injury" (Nagelberg 2015). Craniofacial, head, face, and neck injuries occur in more than half of the cases (American Academy of Pediatric Dentistry 2004).

Psychological (Emotional) Abuse

Psychological (emotional) abuse is defined as "intentional caregiver behavior that conveys to a child that he/she is worthless, flawed, unloved, unwanted, endangered, or valued only in meeting another's needs" (Nagelberg 2015). It involves overt verbal abuse or covert acts of extreme punishment such as confinement of child in a closet or dark room or being tied to a chair for long periods of time. Psychological (emotional) abuse includes patterns of scapegoating, threatening, scaring, discriminating, ridiculing, or other nonphysical forms of hostile or rejecting treatment (Mathur and Chopra 2013).

Sexual Abuse

Sexual abuse is defined as "any completed or attempted (non-completed) sexual act, sexual contact with, or exploitation (i.e. non-contact sexual interaction) of a child by a caregiver" (Nagelberg 2015).

General Indicators Seen in Victims of Child Maltreatment Cases

Table 9.3.3 gives details of indicators seen in victims for the four types of abuse discussed.

General Caregiver Indicators Seen in Maltreatment Cases

Table 9.3.4 gives details of indicators seen in caregivers for the four types of abuse discussed.

Child abuse and neglect impact on child's physical and psychosocial development (Child Welfare Information Gateway 2016b) and there can be significant consequences to their long-term health.

Table 9.3.3: General indicators seen in victims of child maltreatment cases.

Neglect	Physical	Behavioral	Sexual Abuse
• Lack of dental care, untreated caries present • Lack of medical care • Malnourishment, listlessness, or fatigue • Stealing or begging for food • Lack of personal care, poor hygiene, torn or soiled cloths • Inappropriately dressed for the season • Untreated need for dental care, glasses or other medical attention • Frequent absence or tardiness to school • Child inappropriately left unattended or without supervision (Child Welfare information Gateway 2016a)	• Unexplained injuries that are inconsistent with the explanation • Delays in seeking care • Child blames someone else for injury • Contusions and lacerations of the tongue • Trauma to the hard and soft palate, buccal mucosa • Laceration to the labial frenum • Cuts and lacerations to the lips • Frequently appearing injuries such as cuts, bruises, burns, especially if child is unable to provide an adequate explanation. (The injuries may appear in distinctive patterns such as, cigarette burns, grab marks, or other instruments.) • Human bite marks – human bites cause compression of flesh and can cause abrasions, contusions and lacerations but rarely avulsions of tissue caused by dog bites. • Chipped or discolored teeth • Missing teeth • Injuries to eyes or both sides of the head or body (accidental injuries usually only seen on one side of the body) • Traumatic alopecia (bald spots) • Lichenification (thickening of the skin and scarring at the corners of the mouth from repeated use of gags) • Multiple injuries, injuries in different stages of healing • History of fractures (American Academy of Pediatric Dentistry 2004; Mathur and Chopra 2013)	• Wears clothing to conceal injury, that is, long sleeves • Does not make eye contact • Avoids physical contact with others • Apprehensive when other children cry • Refuses to undress for gym • Gives inconsistent explanation about the injury or burn • Appears frightened by parents • Comes early to school stays late • Frequently late or absent from school • Dramatic mood changes • Has difficulty getting along with other children • Overly compliant, withdrawn, gives in readily, and allows others to do for him/her without protest • Plays aggressively, frequently hurting others • Complains of pain on movement or contact • Has history of running away from home	• Although the oral cavity is a frequent site of sexual abuse in children, visible damage or infections are rare (Mathur and Chopra 2013) • Symptoms of sexually transmitted diseases • Injury to genital area • Difficulty when walking and/or sitting • Sexually suggestive, inappropriate or promiscuous behavior or verbalization • Expressing age-inappropriate knowledge of sexual relations • Sexual victimization of other children

Table 9.3.4: General caregiver indicators seen in maltreatment cases.

Parental/Caregiver	Nonspecific Caregiver
• Explanation of injury not believable and inconsistent • Child has been previously abused • Understates the seriousness of the condition • Delays in seeking attention • Cannot be located • History of drug or alcohol abuse • Parents were abused as children • Economic stress or unemployed • Personal or marital problems • Social isolation, no family or friend supportive network • Does not respond appropriately to child's pain • Antagonistic, suspicious, and fearful of other people • Constantly criticizes and has inappropriate expectations of child • Views child as bad or evil • Blames child for maltreatment • Takes child to different physicians and hospitals for each injury	• Hostile and aggressive attitude • Compulsive • Inflexible • Unreasonable and cold • Passive and dependent • Unrealistic expectations of child • Overreaction to child's behavior

Source: Mathur and Chopra (2013).

There is a causal relationship between abuses that were nonsexual abuse as risk factors for depressive disorders, anxiety disorders, suicide behavior, lifestyle risk factors such as alcohol and drug abuse, higher risk of sexually transmitted diseases, and/or risky sexual behavior. It had been determined that those who were physically abused had a higher risk of type II diabetes, hypertension, cardiovascular disease, neurological disorders, cancer, malnutrition, and chronic pain. For those who were sexually abused, there was an increased risk for diabetes, oral health problems, vision problems and poor lung function, and risky sexual behavior (Norman et al. 2012; Widom et al. 2012). In addition, it is estimated approximately one-third of abused and neglected children will eventually victimize their own children (Child Welfare Information Gateway 2016a).

Awareness and Identification

Dental health-care professionals should be aware of what constitute child abuse and neglect. Dental practitioners should develop a clinical protocol including behavioral assessment of the child and parent/guardian, patient history, general physical assessment, oral examination, and injury documentation. It is critical that practitioners be aware of the child's behavioral indicators when assessing a potential case of child abuse and neglect.

Filing a Report

Dentists and dental hygienists are mandated to report when they suspect a child is abused or neglected. In case of a suspected case, the parent or caregiver and patient should be questioned separately as to what happened and their responses should be recorded. In all cases of suspected child abuse there should be a complete documentation noted in client's records, including examination, radiographs, photographs, date of examination, description, size, and location of the injury. The documentation should be cosigned by another witness of the examination. "The law provides protection for mandated reporters who make their report in good faith; there are also harsh penalties for not reporting abuse, including fines and prison time. Failure by a mandated reporter to report suspected abuse is a misdemeanor in most states" (Rayman et al. 2012). All health-care professionals should visit their state's Child Protective Services website for a complete list of state-specific definitions of child maltreatment, as well as the websites for the Children's Bureau, Administration for Children and Families, US Department of Health and Human Services for a complete list of definitions and individual state requirements on the topic of child maltreatment (Rayman et al. 2012).

Self-Study Questions

1. Mandated reporters are required to make an oral report of suspected child abuse, maltreatment, or neglect by telephone:
- **A. Within 24 hours**
- **B. Within seven days**
- **C. Immediately**
- **D. After completing a child abuse reporting form**

2. Perhaps the most serious consequence of a mandated reporter's failure to report a case of suspected child abuse is:
- **A. Being charged with a Class A misdemeanor**
- **B. Facing criminal penalties**
- **C. Leaving oneself open to a civil suit for monetary damages**
- **D. Leaving a child vulnerable to further harm**

3. "Reasonable cause" to suspect child abuse or maltreatment requires:
- **A. Certainty that the injury is non-accidental**
- **B. Doubting what is personally observed or stated about an injury**
- **C. Believing what a parent says happened to an injured child**
- **D. Thinking it possible that an injury occurred because of abuse or neglect**

4. The general definition of neglect is:
- **A. Failure to provide for child's basic physical needs**
- **B. Failure to provide for a child's emotional needs**
- **C. Failure to provide for a child's educational needs**
- **D. All of the above**

5. The likelihood of child abuse increase when:
- **A. There are inconsistent descriptions of how an injury occurred**
- **B. There is inconsistency between the history of the trauma and the type of injury observed**
- **C. There have been multiple medical and dental evaluations for trauma**
- **D. All of the above**

References

American Academy of Pediatric Dentistry (2004). Clinical guideline on oral and dental aspects of child abuse and neglect. *Pediatric Dentistry* 26 (7 Suppl): 63–66.

American Academy of Pediatric Dentistry (2005). *Pediatric Dental Reference Manual*. New York: American Academy of Pediatric Dentistry.

American Academy of Pediatrics Committee on Child Abuse and Neglect and American Academy of Pediatric Dentistry Council on Clinical Affairs (2010). Guideline on oral and dental aspects of child abuse and neglect. *Clinical Guidelines: Reference Manual* 33: 147–150.

Child Maltreatment. (2014) *Child Maltreatment | Children's Bureau | Administration for Children and Families* [Online]. Available at: http://www.acf.hhs.gov/cb/research-data-technology/statistics-research/child-maltreatment (October 2, 2016).

Child Welfare Information Gateway, (2016a). *Definitions of Child Abuse and Neglect in Federal Law - Child Welfare Information Gateway* [Online]. Available at: https://www.childwelfare.gov/topics/can/defining/federal (October 2, 2016).

Child Welfare Information Gateway, (2016b). *Impact of Child Abuse and Neglect* [Online]. Available at: https://www.childwelfare.gov/topics/can/impact (October 2, 2016).

Child Welfare Information Gateway, (2016c). *Mandatory Reporters of Child Abuse and Neglect* [Online]. Available at: https://www.childwelfare.gov/pubPDFs/manda.pdf (June 3, 2018).

Katner, D. and Brown, C. (2012). Mandatory reporting of oral injuries indicating possible child abuse. *The Journal of the American Dental Association* 143 (10): 1087–1092.

Mathur, S. and Chopra, R. (2013). Combating child abuse: the role of a dentist. *Oral Health & Preventive Dentistry* 11 (3): 243–250.

Merrick, M.T. and Latzman, N.E. (2014). Child maltreatment: a public health overview and prevention considerations. *Online Journal of Issues in Nursing* 19 (1): 2.

Nagelberg, R.H. (2015). Child abuse awareness in the dental profession. *Dental Economics* 105 (11): ZC28–ZC30.

Norman, R.E., Byambaa, M., De, R. et al. (2012). The long-term health consequences of child physical abuse, emotional abuse, and neglect: a systematic review and meta-analysis. *PLoS Medicine* 9 (11): e1001349.

Rayman, S., Dincer, E., and Almas, K. (2012). Child abuse: concerns for oral health practitioners. *The New York State Dental Journal* 79 (4): 30–34.

Thomas, J.E., Straffon, L., and Inglehart, M.R. (2006). Knowledge and professional experiences concerning child abuse: an analysis of provider and student responses. *Pediatric Dentistry* 28 (5): 438–444.

Widom, C.S., Czaja, S.J., Bentley, T., and Johnson, M.S. (2012). A prospective investigation of physical health outcomes in abused and neglected children: new findings from a 30-year follow-up. *American Journal of Public Health* 102 (6): 1135–1144.

Answers to Self-Study Questions

1. A

2. D

3. D

4. D

5. D

Case 4

Substance-Related Disorder

CASE STORY

A 32-year-old male presents with a white lesion in the mandibular vestibule area of the left molar region. Patient states that he has chewed smokeless tobacco for over 10 years, since college ... He works in finance and has very stressful and long work days.

PROBLEM-BASED LEARNING GOALS AND OBJECTIVES

- Understand health risks associated with usage of smokeless tobacco
- Identify possible oral lesions associated with long-term smokeless tobacco
- Discuss the incidence and global health impact of smokeless tobacco
- Describe the role of the dental professional in identifying the risks related to smokeless tobacco usage

Medical History

Patient has a negative medical history and does not take any medication

Social History

Patient reports being a social drinker consuming three to four beers a week. He was recently married and has no children. He uses smokeless tobacco three to four times a week and sometimes chews up to two times a day depending on his work day.

Patient reports that he tries to go to the gym two or three times a week.

He brushes with a soft-bristled toothbrush twice a day and flosses three to four times a week. He has occlusal composites on the posterior teeth and has completed with professional whitening treatments. He also had orthodontic treatment as a teenager.

Review of the Systems

- Vital signs
  - Blood pressure: 130/87 mmHg
  - Pulse: 61 beats/min
  - Respiration: 16 breaths/min

Extraoral Exam

Within Normal Limits

Intraoral Exam

- Mandibular buccal to #18 and #19, vestibular area: evidence of tobacco pouch keratosis, dimensions 12 × 6 mm. Clinical appearance of lesion is wrinkled, white, nonfriable.

Intraoral Images

See Figure 9.4.1 and Figure 9.4.2 for lower left vestibule views.

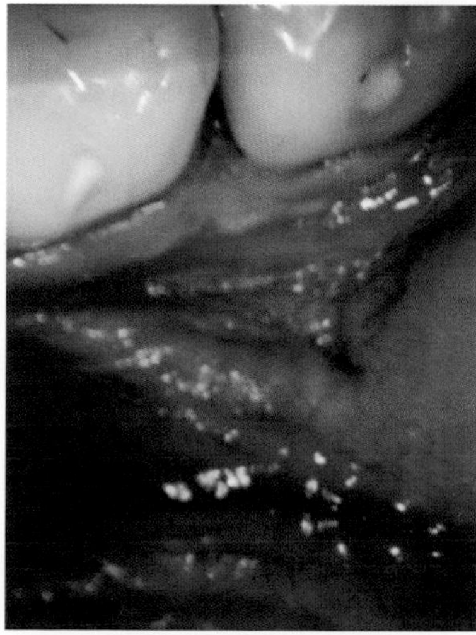

Figure 9.4.1: Lower left vestibule view 01.

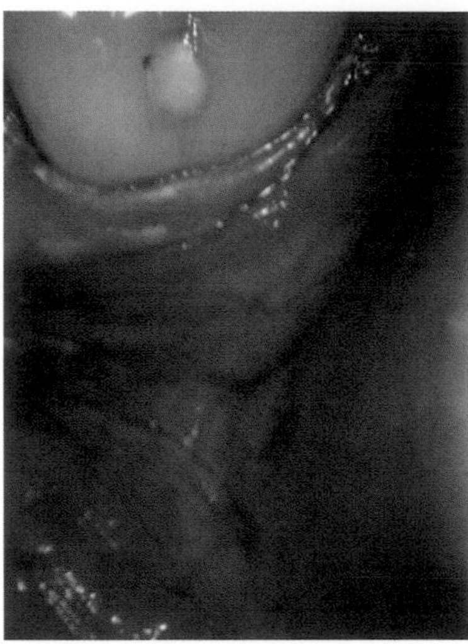

Figure 9.4.2: Lower left vestibule view 02.

Gingival Examination

- Generalized 1–3 mm probing depths and localized areas of recession
- 4 mm pocket on #4 distal-lingual
- 4 mm pocket on #31 mesial-facial
- See Figure 9.4.3 Periodontal Chart

Radiographic Examination

- A full mouth series of radiographs were taken (see Figure 9.4.4)
- Four existing composite restorations on occlusal surfaces of posterior molars
- No recurrent or active caries

Odontogram

Full record is shown in Figure 9.4.5.

Dental Hygiene Diagnosis

Problems	Related to Risks and Etiology
Usage of smokeless tobacco	Dysplasia of the oral cavity Increased risk for oral cancer
Lack of knowledge regarding risks associated with smokeless tobacco use	Increased risk of periodontal disease Increased risk of caries

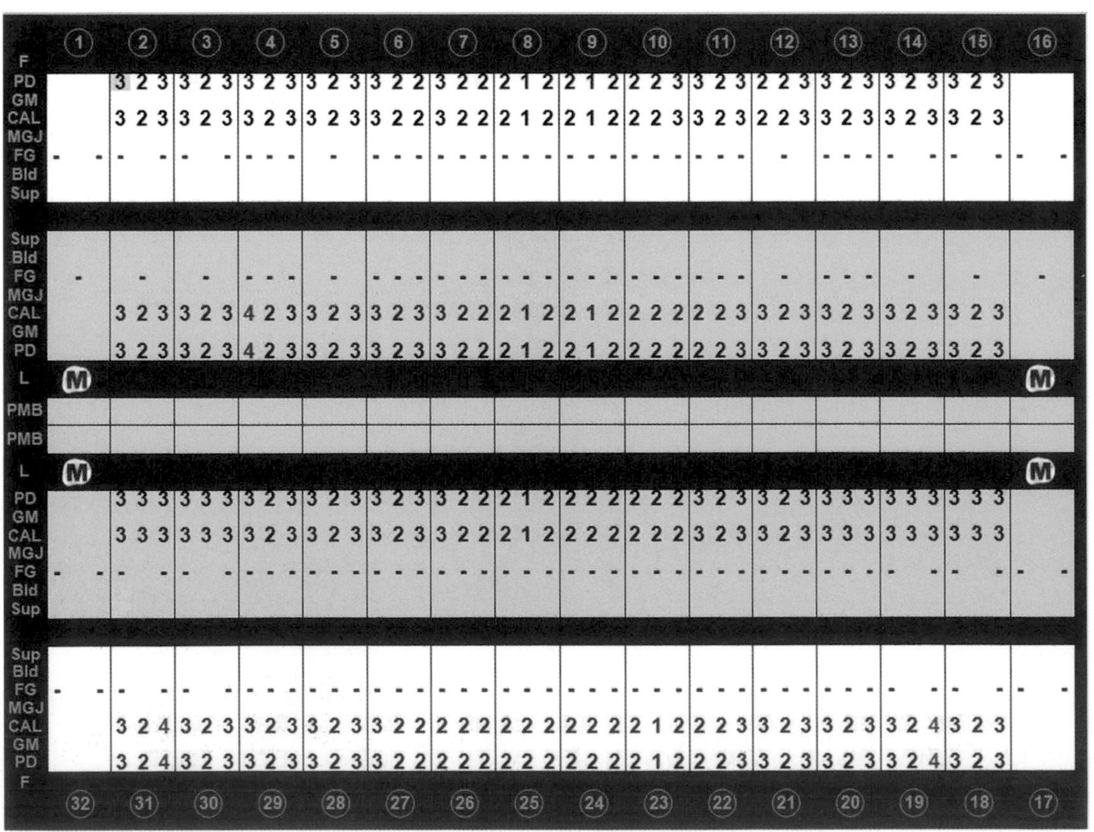

Figure 9.4.3: Periodontal Chart.

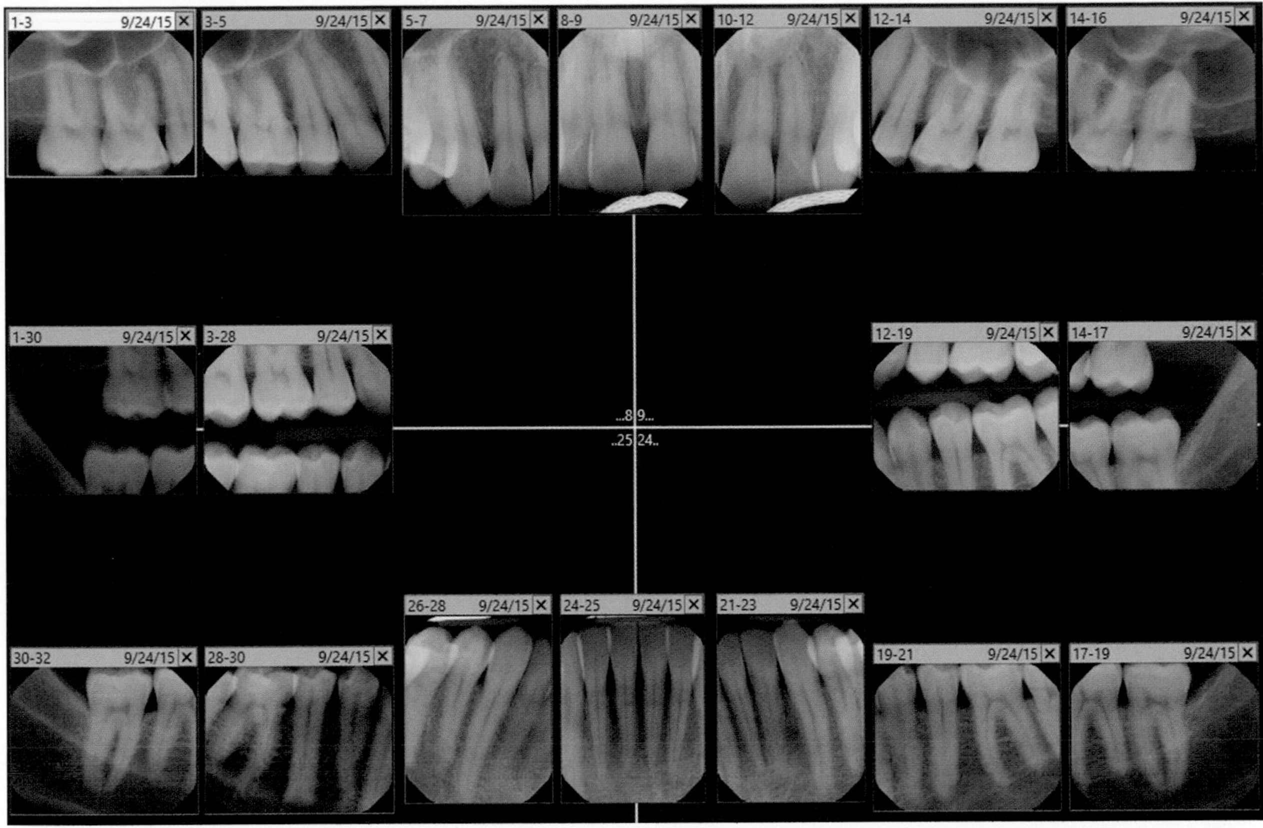

Figure 9.4.4: Full mouth series.

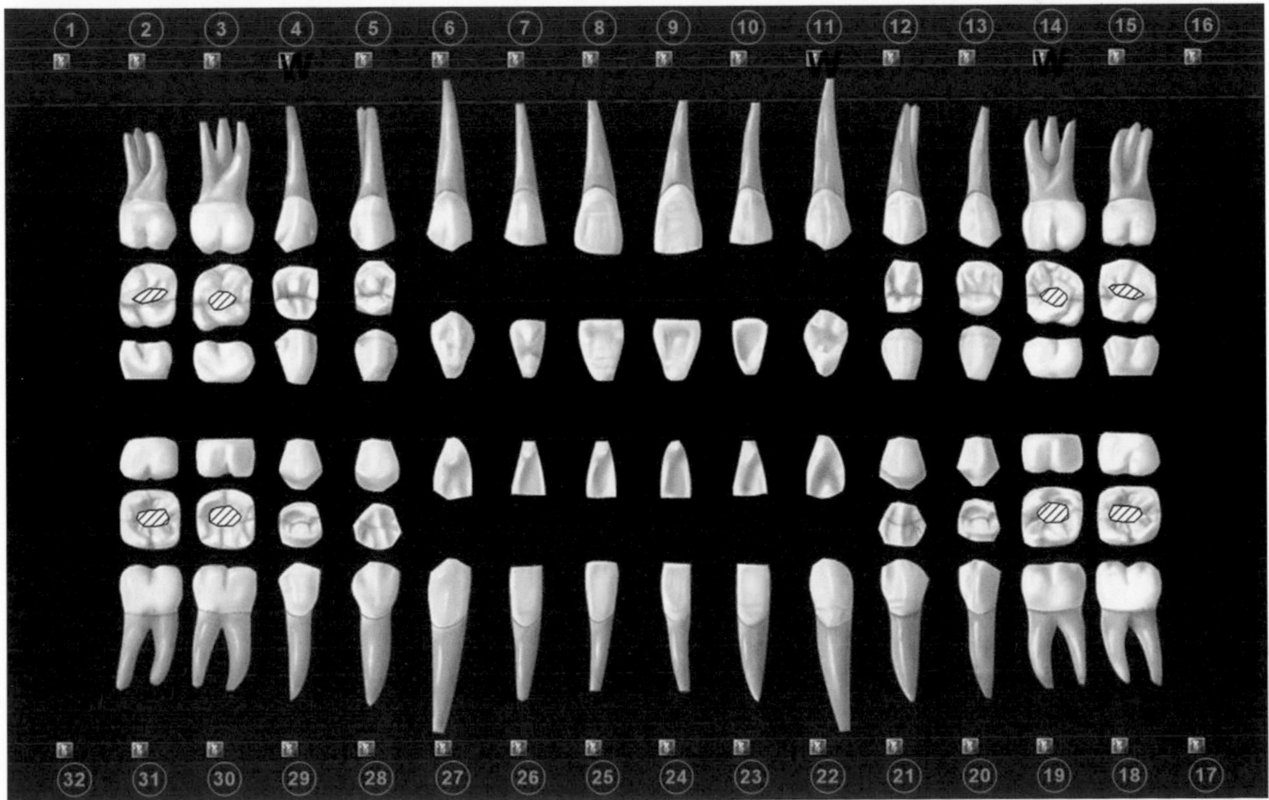

Figure 9.4.5: Odontogram.

Planned Interventions

Clinical	Education/Counseling	Oral Hygiene Instructions
Refer to DDS for pathology diagnosis of affected area Six-week re-evaluation of affected area Adult prophylaxis Six-month periodontal recare visits	Cessation of smokeless tobacco Explain increased risks of oral dysplasia, caries, and periodontal disease with usage of smokeless tobacco Monitoring of affected area caused by usage of smokeless tobacco Importance of fluoride usage in daily home care	Continue usage of soft-bristled toothbrush using Modified Bass brushing technique Increase frequency of interdental care

- A brush biopsy was performed
- Brush biopsy results:
  - Findings revealed nonhyperplastic cells with negative findings.
  - Evidence showed keratinized tissue
- Patient was advised to immediately discontinue use of smokeless tobacco and referred to specialist for counseling and cessation.

Treatment Plan

- Oral hygiene instructions
- Routine adult prophylaxis
- Six-week evaluation of mandibular left vestibular area

Discussion

There are two forms of smokeless tobacco: snuff, also known as "dip," and chewing tobacco (Bhattacharyya 2012). All smokeless tobacco products contain the carcinogen N-nitrosonornicotine (NNN), and it is an accepted cause of oral cancer (Greer 2011; Lee and Hamling 2009). Oral cancer is defined as a term affecting the tissues of the oral cavity or those of the oropharynx, which includes part of the throat and the back of the mouth ("Head and neck cancer" 2011).

The use of smokeless tobacco is associated with dysplasia of the oral cavity and oral squamous cell carcinoma (Greer 2011; Lee and Hamling 2009). Smokeless tobacco can also be associated with periodontal inflammation, gingivitis, and dental caries. There an estimated one-quarter million new cases of oral cancer worldwide each year attributed to the use of smokeless tobacco, with an estimated increase of 275,000 new cases each year (Balbo et al. 2013; Warnakulasuriya 2009).

In the United States, one in five white adolescent males between the ages of 18 and 25years old, and 7% of all men, use smokeless tobacco. Smokeless tobacco comes in the form of teabag-like sachets of moist snuff and is usually placed in the vestibular areas between gingiva and buccal mucosa (CDC 2014; International Agency for Research on Cancer 2007; US Department of Health and Human Services 2012). With long-term usage, the area that the smokeless tobacco is placed can exhibit a white plaque-like lesion that cannot be wiped off, sometimes referred to as leukoplakia (Jones et al. 2014). Most leukoplakia lesions are the result of hyperkeratosis, which is the thickening of the keratin layer or a combination of epithelial hyperplasia (thickening of the prickle cell or the spinous layer) and hyperkeratosis (Jones et al. 2014). Epithelial dysplasia and even squamous cell carcinoma may even be seen in a microscopic investigation of leukoplakia (Jones et al. 2014). However, the cytopathology of lesions associated with smokeless tobacco are unique (Carroll 2012). Long-term use of smokeless tobacco may result in white lesions called "smokeless-tobacco associated keratosis, rather than leukoplakia because the direct cause of the lesion is known" (Jones et al. 2014). A differential diagnosis, including a biopsy of the area, needs to be established in order to determine the etiology of the lesion.

The global health impact of tobacco use, in smokeless and smoked forms, is significant – it constitutes about 90% of all drug-caused deaths and is most conspicuous reason of health inequalities (Jarvis and Wardle 2006). Tobacco use also has an impact on economic development, resulting in families spending less money on basic items, such as health care, food, and education (Agbor et al. 2013).

The role of the dental professional is essential in identifying possible patient risks for developing precancerous/cancerous lesions in the oral cavity. Each patient must be provided with a thorough extra/intraoral examination and review of medical and social histories. Recommendations for intervention include: continued monitoring of lesion for any significant changes, possible brush biopsies, or specialist referrals. The patients who present with significant lesions should be put on a frequent recare schedule.

The dental professional has an essential role in eliminating the use of tobacco products. Education of the patient on the risks of tobacco usage is recommended, with an emphasis on the potential detrimental effects on the oral tissues and the oropharynx. Sometimes smokeless tobacco may even be used as a safe alternative to cigarette smoking, which poses a public health threat in many ways (Bhattacharyya 2012). Dental professionals can assist tobacco users to quit by establishing partnerships with patients to promote healthier habits (Rainchuso et al. 2016). When indicated, tobacco cessation programs should also be recommended (Rainchuso et al. 2016).

Smokeless tobacco is often used by professional sports figures at major sporting events (Greer, 2011; Lee and Hamling 2009). The media exposure creates a false impression that tobacco usage is popular and is acceptable, without any detrimental health effects.

In response to the health hazards of smoking tobacco products and as an aid to smoking cessation, advertisement and usage of electronic cigarettes also called e-cigarettes or electronic nicotine delivery systems are increasing in popularity. These battery-operated devices often contain nicotine, different flavorings, and other chemicals that can expose the lungs to a variety of chemicals with unknown health effects (NIH 2017). Exposure to electronic cigarettes with nicotine is becoming increasingly common in adolescents and can lead to nicotine addiction and risk to other drugs (Leventhal et al. 2015). E-cigarettes are now the most commonly used form of tobacco in adolescents in the United States and may serve as an introductory product for adolescents before the use of other tobacco products (NIH 2017).

More research is needed as e-cigarettes have not been thoroughly evaluated in scientific studies and also to find out whether they may be as effective, as advertised, smoking cessation aids (NIH 2017).

Take-Home Hints

1. Smokeless tobacco use is most prevalent in white males, ages 18–25.
2. Long-term use of smokeless tobacco is often associated with oral cavity dysplasia and can lead to oral squamous cell carcinoma.
3. The use of smokeless tobacco can be most associated with erythroplakia.
4. Smokeless tobacco is most commonly placed on the mandibular buccal vestibular area.
5. All dental professionals should perform a thorough intraoral examination to identify early signs of oral dysplasia caused by possible use of smokeless tobacco.

Self-Study Questions

1. The use of smokeless tobacco can be associated with the following except:
- **A. Leukoplakia**
- **B. Erythroplakia**
- **C. Dysplasia of the oral cavity**
- **D. Oral squamous cell carcinoma**

2. What is the role of the dental professional in treating a patient who is using smokeless tobacco?
- **A. Oral hygiene instructions/education**
- **B. Administration of brush biopsy/specialist referral**
- **C. Frequent recare appointments**
- **D. All of the above**

3. Smokeless tobacco is more predominantly used among which population?
- **A. White males ages 18–25**
- **B. White males ages 45–60**
- **C. Hispanic males ages 18–25**
- **D. Hispanic males ages 45–60**

4. Leukoplakia can be defined as:
- **A. A result of hyperkeratosis**
- **B. White-plaque lesion that cannot be rubbed off**
- **C. Idiopathic leukoplakia**
- **D. All of the above**
- **E. A and C**

References

Agbor, M., Azodo, C., and Tefouet, T. (2013). Smokeless tobacco use, tooth loss and oral health issues among adults in Cameroon. *African Health Sciences* 13 (3): 785–790.

Balbo, S., James-Yi, S., Johnson, C.S. et al. (2013). (S)-N'-Nitrosonornicotine, a constituent of smokeless tobacco, is a powerful oral cavity carcinogen in rats. *Carcinogenesis* 34 (9): 2178–2183.

Bhattacharyya, N. (2012). Trends in the use of smokeless tobacco in United States, 2000–2010. *The Laryngoscope* 122 (10): 2175–2178.

Carroll, D.J. (2012). Cytological diagnosis of benign lesions of the oral cavity. *Oral Cytology* 49–71.

CDC. (2014, November 4). Types of smokeless tobacco [Online]. Available at: http://www.cdc.gov/tobacco/data_statistics/fact_sheets/smokeless/products_marketing/index.htm (June 3, 2018).

Greer, R.O. (2011). Oral manifestations of smokeless tobacco use. *Otolaryngologic Clinics of North America* 44 (1): 31–56.

Head and neck cancer. (2011). [Online]. Available: http://www.cancer.gov/types/head-and-neck (October 2, 2016).

International Agency for Research on Cancer (ed.) (2007). *Smokeless Tobacco and Some Tobacco-Specific N-Nitrosamines*, vol. 89. World Health Organization.

Jarvis, M.J. and Wardle, J. (2006). Social patterning of health behaviors: the case of cigarette smoking. In: *Social Determinants of Health* (ed. M. Marmot and R.G. Wilkinson), 224–237. Oxford: Oxford University Press.

Jones, A.C., Freedman, P.D., Phelan, J.A., and Kacher, J.E. (2014). Neoplasia. In: *Oral Pathology for the Dental Hygienist* (ed. O.A.C. Ibsen and J.A. Phelan), 222–261. United States: Elsevier Saunders.

Lee, P.N. and Hamling, J. (2009). Systematic review of the relation between smokeless tobacco and cancer in Europe and North America. *BMC Medicine* 7 (1): 36.

Leventhal, A., Strong, D., Kirkpatrick, M. et al. (2015). Association of electronic cigarette use with initiation of combustible tobacco product smoking in early adolescence. *JAMA* 314 (7): 700.

NIH. (2017, June). Electronic cigarettes (E-cigarettes) [Online]. https://www.drugabuse.gov/publications/drugfacts/electronic-cigarettes-e-cigarettes (August 4, 2018).

Rainchuso, L., Benton, E., and Cotter, J. (2016). The patient who uses tobacco. In: *Clinical Practice of the Dental Hygienist* (ed. E.M. Wilkins), 547–570. United States: Wolters Kluwer.

US Department of Health and Human Services (2012). *Preventing Tobacco Use among Youth and Young Adults: A Report of the Surgeon General.* Atlanta, GA: US Department of Health and Human Services, Centers for Disease Control and Prevention National Center for Chronic Disease Prevention and Health Promotion, Office on Smoking and Health, 3.

Warnakulasuriya, S. (2009). Global epidemiology of oral and oropharyngeal cancer. *Oral Oncology* 45 (4–5): 309–316.

Answers to Self-Study Questions

1. B

2. D

3. A

4. D

10

Management of Medically Complex Patients

Clinical Cases in Dental Hygiene, First Edition. Edited by Cheryl M. Westphal Theile, Mea A. Weinberg and Stuart L. Segelnick.

Case 1

Patient with Diabetes

CASE STORY

A 43-year-old Hispanic male presented with the dental concern of "my gums are bleeding and one of my teeth is moving." He explained that his last dental visit was five years ago when he was recommended to have "deep cleanings to fix the problem with his gums." He had the scaling and root planing and then was recommended to have surgery to "lower pockets" in the bottom right side "one of the molars." Patient went back for cleaning every three months for first year and then did not continue.

PROBLEM-BASED LEARNING GOALS AND OBJECTIVES

- How to determine level of control in the diabetic patient – well controlled, moderately controlled, or poorly controlled
- To understand the clinical symptoms of diabetes
- To identify the side effects of drugs used to treat diabetics
- Learn how to be prepared for hypoglycemic events
- Medical management of the poorly controlled diabetic

Medical History

This patient gives a history of a diagnosis of diabetes and hypertension five years ago. He states that his blood pressure is well controlled, but his diabetes "goes up and down." He checks his blood sugar at home three times/week and sees the numbers >225 on a regular basis. His last visit to his physician was two months ago for examination and blood work.

- Vital signs:
  - Blood pressure: 130/79 mmHg
  - Pulse: 83 beats/min
  - Height: 5′ 10″
  - Weight: 250 lbs
  - BMI: 35.9
- Medications: Glucophage® (metformin), Victoza® (luraglutide), Coreg® (carvedilol), Diovan® (valsartan), and fish oil.

Dental History

Patient has not had a dental exam or prophylaxis in five years. He brushes once daily with a soft toothbrush. He tells you that his last dental office had recommended scaling and root planing but he did not follow through with treatment. He tells you he has a feeling of "bad breath" and a "bad taste" in his mouth.

Social History

He currently smokes half a pack of cigarettes/day but used to smoke two packs per day. He rarely drinks alcohol and used marijuana in his teens and 20s.

Dental Examination

The intra and extraoral soft tissue exam was unremarkable. The patient is missing teeth #s 2,3,14, 18, 19, and 30. No caries visible radiographically or clinically. Probing depths vary from 3 to 5 mm with localized pocketing of 4–6 mm and attachment loss in the lower anterior teeth. In addition, there is 50% bleeding on probing and calculus is visible radiographically as well as clinically.

Radiographic examination revealed the presence of generalized moderate horizontal bone loss, with localized severe vertical bone loss on tooth #22 (Figure 10.1.1).

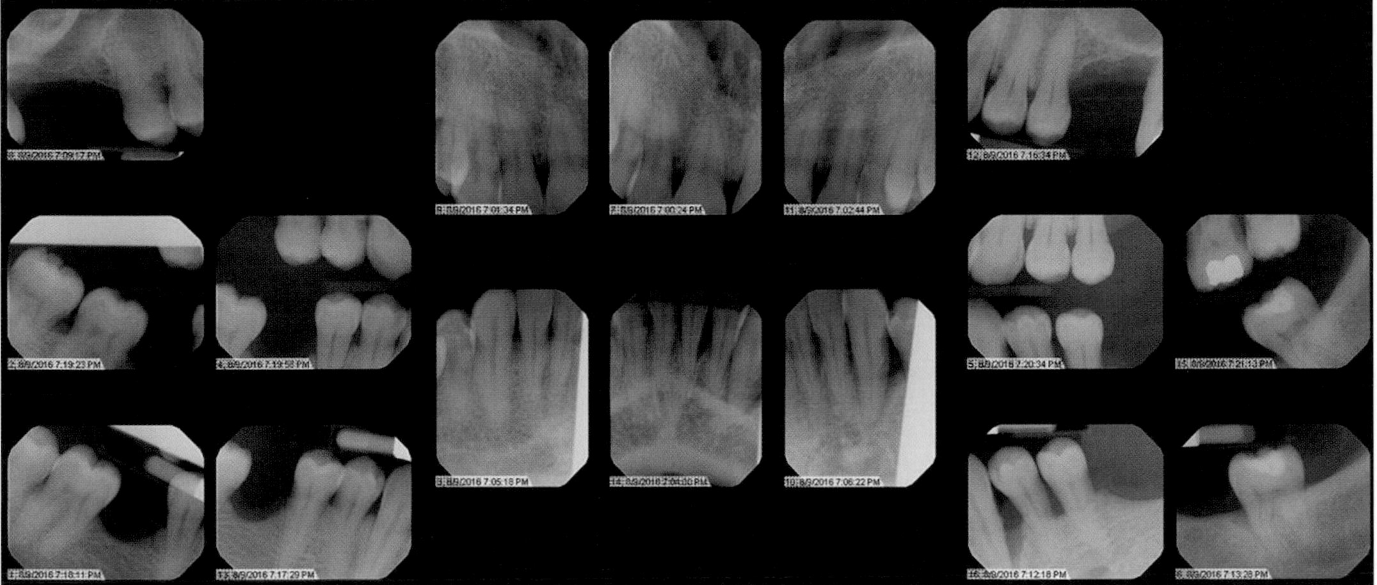

Figure 10.1.1: Periapical radiographic series showing generalized moderate horizontal bone loss, with localized severe vertical bone loss on tooth #22.

Treatment Plan

- Oral hygiene instructions to reduce plaque, bleeding on probing, and sensitivity.
- Initial scaling and root planing to eliminate calculus and reduce periodontal pockets.
- Further assessment after six weeks as to the results of scaling and root planing and assessment as to overall prognosis of teeth – extraction(s), periodontal surgery, assessment for prosthetics.

Discussion

Medical Considerations: Diabetes

Diabetes is caused by the lack of insulin production or decrease or inability of tissue to respond to insulin. It is divided into three categories: Type 1 (body doesn't make enough insulin) and can develop at any age; Type 2 (body doesn't use insulin properly); and gestational diabetes (diabetes that develops during pregnancy). According to the Center for Disease Control and Prevention (CDC), as of 2012, 29.1 million people in the United States have been diagnosed with diabetes and one-quarter are unaware they have the disease. Periodontal disease is more common in diabetics with about one-third having severe periodontal disease with loss of attachment >5mm. These patients are also at risk of other systemic issues such as heart disease, stroke, hypo/hyperglycemia, renal disease, and blindness. An increased risk of postoperative infection and poor wound healing are also concerns. Undiagnosed or poorly controlled diabetics may have complaint of polydipsia (excessive thirst), polyuria (excessive urination), and polyphagia (excessive hunger). Keep in mind that not all diabetics have periodontal disease, despite how controlled or uncontrolled they are.

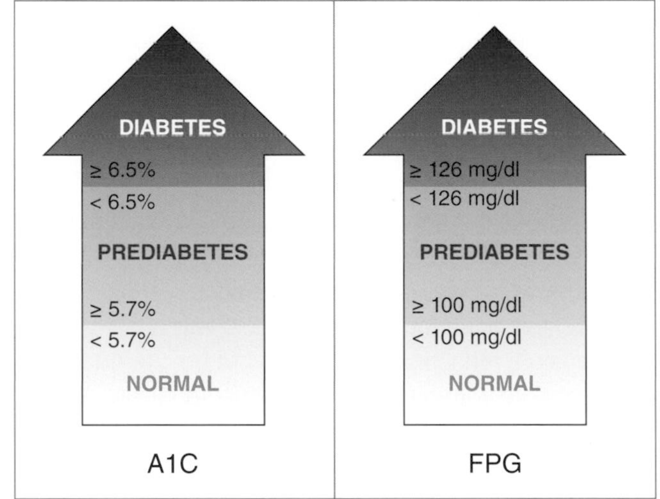

Figure 10.1.2: A1C and fasting plasma glucose normal values.

How do we as oral health professionals assess the control of our patients who are diagnosed with diabetes, as well as the undiagnosed diabetic? The "Gold Standard" is the hemoglobin A1c (HbA1c) blood test. This test assesses the average blood glucose for the past three months. Patients are diagnosed as normal, prediabetic, and diabetic (Figure 10.1.2). Diabetics with A1c results of seven or less are considered well controlled. As the A1c increases, the patient is considered less controlled.

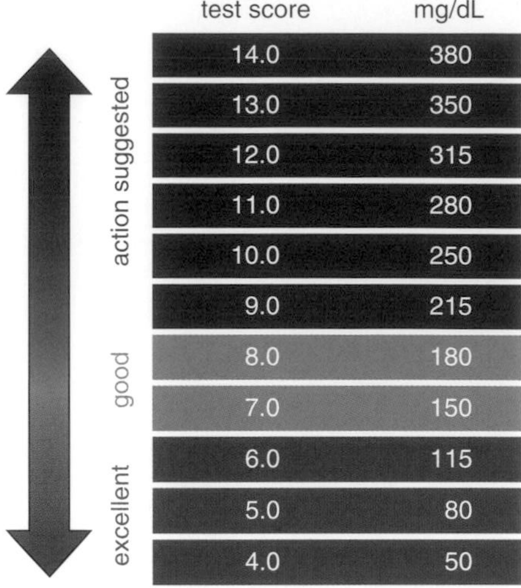

Figure 10.1.3: The A1c test score (%) on left as compared to the fasting blood sugar (mg/dl).

A1c results >9 (Figure 10.1.3) are indicative of a patient who is poorly controlled. In the dental setting, oral complications may include poor wound healing, post-operative bacterial infections and fungal infections.

Fasting plasma glucose (FPG) or fasting blood sugar (FBS) is another means of assessment although not as accurate for assessing overall control as the hemoglobin A1c (Figure 10.1.2). Patients can perform this test at home. Normal FBS should be less than 100. As these numbers climb, so does the hemoglobin A1c. FBS levels that are consistently >200–250 result in a hemoglobin A1c>9.

Treatment for well-controlled diabetics without comorbidities or serious complications (e.g., hypertension, renal disease) should not be altered. For those patients with diabetes who have serious complications, treatment may need to be altered after consultation with a physician. The decision regarding nonemergency surgical procedures for patients whose diabetes is poorly controlled should be assessed on a case-by-case basis. Recommendations may include scaling and root planing and extractions. Consideration should also be given to patient's ability to eat following surgery and as to whether their medication dose needs altering, especially insulin. It is the responsibility of the oral health-care provider to collect a thorough medical history, carry out appropriate bloodwork and, if warranted, have a conversation with the primary care provider to assess the patient's health status. (Little et al. 2013)

The dental health professional must consider precautions for this patient as they are on two medications (Table 10.1.1 and Table 10.1.2) that have the potential of causing orthostatic hypotension as a side effect. During procedures where the patient is reclined for a long period of time, even for a simple prophylaxis visit, the chair should be raised slowly to minimize the risk of syncope (fainting). It is important to keep in mind that all antidiabetic medications do not cause hypoglycemia and those that do cause it to differing degrees (Table 10.1.3). The dental professional should always be prepared to treat a hypoglycemic event (Table 10.1.4) by maintaining a glucose source handy. Some examples of these sources are glucose tablets and icing.

Table 10.1.1: Oral health concerns as they relate to risks and etiology.

Problems	Related to Risks and Etiology
Periodontal disease	Poor oral hygiene, poorly controlled diabetes
Taste disorder	Side effects of metformin
Orthostatic hypotension	Side effects of antihypertensive medication
Increased risk of postoperative infection and poor wound healing	Poorly controlled diabetes
Hypoglycemic Event	Side effect of antidiabetic medications
Increased risk of periodontal disease	Generalized heavy biofilm, slight supra, and subgingival calculus with bleeding upon probing in select anterior and posterior sites

Table 10.1.2: Medical management considerations: antihypertensive medications.

Antihypertensive Medication	Class	Side Effect
Coreg	Beta blocker	Orthostatic hypotension
Diovan	Angiotensin II Receptor Blocker (ARB)	Orthostatic hypotension

Specific Considerations

1. Proper assessment of the diabetic patient includes the following questions:
   - Did you take your medication today?
   - When did you last eat?
   - Do you check your blood sugar at home? If so, how often and do you ever see numbers >200.
   - When was your last visit to the doctor and your last A1c? Do you know the results of that test?
2. The risk of poor wound healing and increased risk of infection is assessed with hemoglobin A1C
3. The risk of hypoglycemia – be alert for signs and symptoms and be ready to treat hypoglycemia if it occurs.

Table 10.1.3: Common antidiabetic medications.

Short-acting insulin
- regular insulin (Humulin and Novolin)

Rapid-acting insulins
- insulin aspart (NovoLog, FlexPen)
- insulin glulisine (Apidra)
- insulin lispro (Humalog)

Intermediate-acting insulin
- insulin isophane (Humulin N, Novolin N)

Long-acting insulins
- insulin degludec (Tresiba)
- insulin detemir (Levemir)
- insulin glargine (Lantus)
- insulin glargine (Toujeo)

Combination insulins
- NovoLog Mix 70/30 (insulin aspart protamine-insulin aspart)
- Humalog Mix 75/25 (insulin lispro protamine-insulin lispro)
- Humalog Mix 50/50 (insulin lispro protamine-insulin lispro)
- Humulin 70/30 (human insulin NPH-human insulin regular)
- Novolin 70/30 (human insulin NPH-human insulin regular)
- Ryzodeg (insulin degludec-insulin aspart)

Medications for type 2 diabetes

Alpha-glucosidase inhibitors

These medications help your body break down starchy foods and glucose in the diet resulting in lower blood glucose levels.
- acarbose (Precose)
- miglitol (Glyset)

Biguanides

Biguanides decreases glucose production by the liver. They decrease how much sugar your intestines absorb, make your body more sensitive to insulin, and help your muscles absorb glucose. The most common biguanide is metformin (Glucophage, Metformin Hydrochloride ER, Glumetza, Riomet, Fortamet). Metformin can also be combined with other drugs for type 2 diabetes. Hypoglycemia risk is decreased unless combined with other antidiabetic medications.
- metformin-alogliptin (Kazano)
- metformin-canagliflozin (Invokamet)
- metformin-dapagliflozin (Xigduo XR)
- metformin-empagliflozin (Synjardy)
- metformin-glipizide
- metformin-glyburide (Glucovance)
- metformin-linagliptin (Jentadueto)
- metformin-pioglitazone (Actoplus)
- metformin-repaglinide (PrandiMet)
- metformin-rosiglitazone (Avandamet)
- metformin-saxagliptin (Kombiglyze XR)
- metformin-sitagliptin (Janumet)

DPP-4 inhibitors

DPP-4 inhibitors help the body continue to make insulin. They work by reducing blood sugar without causing hypoglycemia.
- alogliptin (Nesina)
- alogliptin-metformin (Kazano)
- alogliptin-pioglitazone (Oseni)
- linagliptin (Tradjenta)
- linagliptin-empagliflozin (Glyxambi)
- linagliptin-metformin (Jentadueto)
- saxagliptin (Onglyza)
- saxagliptin-metformin (Kombiglyze XR)
- sitagliptin (Januvia)
- sitagliptin-metformin (Janumet and Janumet XR)
- sitagliptin and simvastatin (Juvisync)

Glucagon-like peptides (incretin mimetics)

These drugs are similar to the natural hormone called incretin. They increase B-cell growth and how much insulin your body uses. They decrease your appetite and how much glucagon your body uses.
- albiglutide (Tanzeum)
- dulaglutide (Trulicity)
- exenatide (Byetta)
- exenatide extended-release (Bydureon)
- liraglutide (Victoza)

Table 10.1.4: Signs and symptoms of hypoglycemia.

SIGNS AND SYMPTOMS OF HYPOGLYCEMIA (BLOOD SUGAR < 70 mg dl^{-1})
• Sweating/chills/diaphoresis • shakiness • Nervousness/anxiety • Irritability/impatience • Rapid heart beat • Nausea • Headache • Weakness • Seizure • Unconsciousness

Take-Home Hints

1. It is important to assess the current status of patients diagnosed with diabetes prior to any treatment.
2. Be well versed in drug side effects and how they impact your patient and how you develop your management plan.

Self-Study Questions

1. The "Gold Standard" blood test for assessing diabetic control is:
- **A. Fasting blood sugar (FBS)**
- **B. CBC with differential**
- **C. A1c (glycosylated hemoglobin)**
- **D. International normalized ration (INR)**

2. Signs and symptoms of hypoglycemia include all but one of the following EXCEPT one. Which one is the exception?
- **A. Sweating/chills/diaphoresis**
- **B. Rapid heart beat**
- **C. Nausea**
- **D. Shortness of breath**

3. Diabetics who are poorly controlled are at increased risk of:
- **A. Poor wound healing and infection**
- **B. Nausea and vomiting**
- **C. Hypothyroidism**
- **D. Caries**

4. All of the following HbA1c results reflect reasonably good control except one. Which one is the exception?
- **A. 6.3**
- **B. 5.4**
- **C. 7.8**
- **D. 9.2**

5. Diabetes develops as a result of all of the following except one. Which one is the exception?
- **A. Decreased insulin production**
- **B. Increased insulin production**
- **C. Decreased tissue response to insulin**
- **D. Excessive sweets in the diet**

References

Little, J., Falace, D., Miller, C., and Rhodus, N. (2013). *Dental Management of the Medically Compromised Patient*, 8e, 219–239. London: Elsevier Health Sciences.

Additional Resources

American Diabetes Association. 2016. Diabetes Basic [Online]. Accessed at: http://www.diabetes.org/diabetes-basics/diagnosis/?loc=symptoms (June 4, 2018).

Archives of Medicine and Health Science (2015) Oral health management considerations in patients with diabetes mellitus [Online]. Available at: http://www.amhsjournal.org/article.asp?issn=2321-4848;year=2015;volume=3;issue=1;spage=72;epage=79;aulast=Kaur (May 31, 2018).

Lamster, I. (2014) Diabetes mellitus and oral health: an interprofessional approach [Online]. Accessed by subscription at: https://ebookcentral-proquest-com.ezproxy.med.nyu.edu/lib/nyulibrary-ebooks/reader.action?docID=1652942&query= (May 31, 2018).

Rhodus, N., Vibeto, B., and Hamamoto, D. (2005). Glycemic control in patients with diabetes mellitus upon admission to a dental clinic: Considerations for dental management. *Quintessence International* 36 (6): 474–482.

The Dental Clinics in North America (2006) Dental management of patients with diabetes [Online]. Available at: https://www.dental.theclinics.com/article/S0011-8532(06)00050-4/pdf (May 31, 2018)

Answers to Self-Study Questions

1. C. Glycosylated hemoglobin test, a1c, is the Gold Standard because it measures the use of glucose in red blood cells over 90-120 days (the life of the RBCs). This is a better assessment of how the patient's body is processing glucose.

2. D. All of the above choices except for shortness of breath are signs and symptoms of hypoglycemia.

3. A. Wounds tend to heal more slowly and get worse faster in diabetics. Factors that affect the rate of healing in a diabetic include blood glucose levels, poor circulation, diabetic neuropathy, immune system deficiency, and infection.

4. D. The normal HbA1c range in patients without diabetes is between 4 and 5.6%. HbA1c levels between 5.7 and 6.4% indicate there is a higher change of developing diabetes. Levels of 6.5% or higher indicates the patient has diabetes.

5. B. Diabetes develops due to decreased insulin production or absolutely no insulin production, insulin resistance (decreased tissue response to insulin), and increased sweets in the diet.

Case 2

Patient with Asthma

CASE STORY

A 27-year-old female presents for an in-office dental whitening appointment. Her last recare appointment was three months ago and, at that time, her oral hygiene was noted to be good with moderate calculus present on the lingual of her lower incisors and bleeding on probing on her anterior gingiva with pocket depths <3 mm. She inquired about whitening her teeth and after discussing the options, has selected chairside bleaching to be followed by home bleaching using custom trays and gel once a week for maintenance. She is excited about having "brighter teeth."

PROBLEM-BASED LEARNING GOALS AND OBJECTIVES

- Recognize factors that may precipitate an episode of asthma
- List the oral complications associated with the use of common asthma medications
- Understand implications of dental management for asthma
- Describe strategies to prevent an acute attack in the dental setting

Medical History

Her medical history is pertinent for mild persistent extrinsic asthma (precipitated by dust, strong odors, tree pollen, and aspirin) that was diagnosed when she was a teenager. She is currently taking Flovent® (flucticasone) steroid inhaler, Singulair® (montelukast) leukotriene inhibitor, and Serevent® (salmeterol) long-acting ®-2 agonist inhaler twice a day. She uses Proventil HFA® (albuterol) inhaler (short acting ®-2 agonist) as needed (two or three times a week most of the year but daily in the springtime when her allergies are most severe). Her last emergency room visit for asthma was 18 months ago, precipitated by an upper-respiratory infection. She also takes birth control pills and a multivitamin.

- Allergies:
  - No known drug allergies (NKDA)
- Vital signs:
  - Blood pressure: 135/85 mmHg
  - Pulse: 72 beats/min
  - Respiration: 12 breaths/min
  - Height: 5′5″
  - Weight: 135 lbs
  - BMI: 22.5

Social History

Never used tobacco, uses alcohol socially two to three times a month.

Dental History

She uses an electric toothbrush twice a day and flosses occasionally. She had orthodontics as a teenager with four third-molar extractions to correct "buck teeth." She has routine periodic exams and cleanings. She has intact occlusal restorations on all molars, as well as buccal restorations on her mandibular molars. Periodontal probing depths <3 mm.

Dental Examination

Extraoral examination is unremarkable. Oral hygiene appears good with no visible plaque. Intraoral soft tissue exam reveals marginal inflammation present on maxillary anterior gingiva. Patchy erythema is noted on posterior palate and oropharynx as well as patchy depapillation of the posterior dorsum of the tongue. Her saliva appears frothy. Upon questioning, the patient states that she often feels that her mouth is dry, especially when she wakes up, and that she frequently "mouth breathes" at night.

Medical Considerations

Asthma is a chronic inflammatory disorder of the airways that affects 17.7 million (7.4%) adults and 6.3 million (8.6%) children living in the United States (Centers for Disease Control and Prevention 2013.) It is characterized by a hyperactive response to stimuli that results in periodic episodes of contractions of bronchial smooth muscle that causes reversible narrowing of airways leading to wheezing, coughing, chest tightness, and difficulty in breathing. Exposure to a variety of triggers (allergens such as dust, pet dander, mold and pollen; respiratory irritants such as tobacco smoke or pollution; upper-respiratory infections, exercise, cold air) result in the release of histamine and cytokines that cause bronchospasm, hypersecretion of mucus, and impaired mucociliary clearance in the bronchi and bronchioles. Most patients have mild to moderate disease and have normal function with minimal symptoms between acute exacerbations. Classification of severity of disease is based on presence of symptoms (particularly nocturnal symptoms), interference with normal activity, decrease in lung function, and need for short-acting (or rescue) medications. There are four levels of asthma severity: intermittent, mild persistent, moderate persistent, and severe persistent based on the frequency of symptoms, presence of nocturnal symptoms, and the effect on pulmonary function before treatment (National Asthma Education Program 2007).

Medical management of asthma includes reduction in risk factors by minimization of exposure to triggers and management of inflammation and acute symptoms. The goals of treatment are to:

- prevent chronic symptoms and progressive loss of lung function,
- maintain normal activity levels,
- decrease the need for rescue medications, and
- prevent exacerbation of acute attacks and minimize hospital visits (National Asthma Education Program 2007).

Pharmacologic management of asthma is divided into controller or maintenance drugs that are taken chronically to control and prevent asthma symptoms and reliever or rescue drugs that are used to relieve acute symptoms. Medications with different pharmacologic actions are added in a controlled manner depending on the severity of the symptoms. Common medications include:

Reliever/Rescue Drugs

- Rapid-onset/short-acting drugs that are used to treat acute symptoms and have immediate effect
- Short-acting β2 agonists
  - Albuterol (Proventil®, Ventolin®, ProAir®) levalbuterol (Xopenex®), metaproterenol, pirbuterol, terbutaline

Controller/Maintenance Drugs

- Slow-onset/long-acting drugs that are used to treat the underlying inflammatory component but have no immediate effect
  - Long acting β2 agonists
    - Arformoterol, (Brovana®), formoterol (Fordil®), salmeterol (Serevent®)
  - Anti-cholinergics
    - Ipratropium bromide (Atrovent®), tiotropium (Spiriva®), methylxanthines, theophylline
  - Mast cell stabilizers
    - Cromolyn, nedocromil
  - Corticosteroids (inhaled)
    - Beclomethasone (Qvar®), budesonide (Pulimcort®), fluticasone (Flovent), mometasone
  - Corticosteroids (systemic)
    - Dexamethasone, fludrocortisone, methylprednisolone, prednisone
  - Leukotriene receptor antagonists
    - Montelukast (Singulair®), zafirlukast, zileuton (Zyflo®)
  - Combination inhalers
    - Fluticasone/salmeterol (Advair Diskus®), ipratropium/albuterol (Combivent®), budesonide/formoterol (Symbicort®)

Oral side effects of asthma drugs include xerostomia and potential increased caries risk (short- and long-acting β2 agonists and anticholinergics) and oropharyngeal candida (inhaled steroids).

Dental Considerations

Elective care should only be done on asymptomatic, well-controlled patients. Patients exhibiting symptoms (wheezing, coughing or history of an acute attack within the last 24 hours) should be rescheduled. Patients should be asked about:

- Triggers of acute attacks
- Frequency and severity of symptoms and acute attacks
  - Emergency room visit and hospitalizations
  - Attack management
- Treatment
  - Controller drugs
  - Rescue drugs and frequency of use
- Presence of symptoms currently
- If patient uses a short-acting bronchodilator, is the inhaler present?

Reduction or elimination of agents known to be triggers for the patient should be attempted. These include

- Minimizing exposure to materials with strong or irritating odors (disinfectants, methylacrylate).
- Be careful when using particulate irritants like prophy paste.
- Avoid having the patient sit with mouth open for prolonged periods of time to avoid drying out the oropharynx and precipitating coughing.
- Carefully position cotton rolls and suction tips to avoid stimulating the cough reflex.
- Temperature in the operatory should be kept moderate.
- Positioning patients who have difficulty breathing when fully reclined in a semisupine position.

Patients with drug-related xerostomia should be educated about the potential of increased caries risk and an aggressive prevention plan should be initiated including regular dental appointments and daily fluoride supplements. Strategies such as sipping water frequently, using sugarless gum and mints, avoiding alcohol containing oral products and using over the counter salivary substitutes can be initiated (Table 10.2.1) to increase patient comfort but do not decrease the risk of caries. Patients who use inhaled steroids should be monitored for candidiasis and treated with antifungal medications as needed. Use of a spacer and instructing patients to rinse their mouths out with water immediately after use can help decrease the incidence of fungal infections.

Take-Home Hints

1. Update medical history at every visit in terms of asthma activity, increased frequency of use of rescue medications and any changes in or presence of symptoms.
2. Elective dentistry should only be performed on asymptomatic patients. The presence of coughing, wheezing or an upper-respiratory infection necessitates reappointment.

Table 10.2.1: Specific Considerations for this Case.

Issue	Potential problem	Management
Asthma	• Acute Attack	• Make sure patient is asymptomatic and has taken all her daily medications • Have patient take puff of rescue medication before procedure • Have patient's rescue inhaler on bracket table
Bleaching procedure	Potential triggers • Pumice/prophy paste • Bleaching chemicals • Prolonged time in chair with mouth open	• Make sure that smell is not potential trigger • Keep patient in semi-supine position • Careful positioning of suction tip • Use rubber dam • Apply oral lubricant to prevent oral and airway drying
Acute attack	• Airway compromise • Desaturation • Hypoxia	• Wipe off bleach, remove lip retractors, dental dam and saliva evacuator. • Make note of time attack started • Sit patient up and allow them to assume position that makes them comfortable (usually will be sitting slightly forward) • Administer the short-acting β_2 agonist (repeat as needed) and administer low-flow oxygen (3–4 L/min) via a nasal cannula or hood • Activate emergency response if no response after several minutes or condition deteriorates

Medication induced xerostomia	• Increase caries risk and gingival disease
	• Patient comfort
		• Regular dental maintenance appointments
		• Excellent oral hygiene
		• Daily fluoride supplements
		  ○ Toothpaste
		  ○ Gel
		  ○ Rinse
		• Daily application of CPP-ACP
		• Avoid alcohol containing mouthrinses
		• Salivary replacements

Inhaled steroid use	• Oropharyngeal candidiasis	• Treat with topical antifungals • Use a spacer • Instruct patient to rinse mouth out immediately after use
Mouth breathing	Anterior gingival inflammation	Nightly application of dry mouth treatment gel to affected area

3. Make sure patient has taken most recent scheduled dose of antiasthma medications.
4. Be aware of potential triggers present in the office and reduce or eliminate exposure.
5. The patient's own short-acting β2 agonist should be readily available.
6. Have the patient take a prophylactic dose of short-acting β2 agonist immediately prior to procedure.

Self-Study Questions

1. A patient presents for a cleaning. You notice that he appears to have a cold and has a slight expiratory wheeze. How should you proceed?

A. Proceed with the cleaning as long as the patient has taken all his asthma medications.
B. Have the patient take a few puffs of Flovent (inhaled corticosteroid) prior to beginning the treatment
C. Use cotton rolls and high-speed suction to reduce airway stimulation from aerosolized particles
D. Reschedule the appointment

2. A 33-year-old man with a history of asthma presents for a periodic cleaning. As you are polishing his teeth with prophy paste, he starts coughing and wheezing. He leans forward in the chair and you notice that he is lifting his shoulders up with each breath. You should do all of the following EXCEPT one. Which one is the exception?

A. Have the patient use a short-acting β-2 agonist inhaler
B. Place the patient supine in the rescue position
C. Establish and maintain a patent airway if necessary
D. Provide low flow oxygen via nasal cannula

3. A patient with a history of asthma is noted to have multiple carious lesions. Which of the following is/are TRUE concerning the caries?

A. Side effects from inhaled β2 agonists may be a contributing factor
B. Using a spacer and rinsing her mouth after using inhaled steroids should help decrease the development of caries
C. Topical fluoride should be prescribed for daily use
D. A and C
E. All of the above

References

Centers for Disease Control and Prevention (2013). *Asthma Facts—CDC's National Asthma Control Program Grantees*. Atlanta, GA: US Department of Health and Human Services, Centers for Disease Control and Prevention.

National Asthma Education Program. Expert Panel on the Management of Asthma. Expert Panel report 3: guidelines for the diagnosis and management of asthma. Bethesda, MD. NIH Publication No. 08–5846. 2007:9. Available at: https://www.nhlbi.nih.gov/files/docs/guidelines/asthsumm.pdf (May 31, 2018).

Answers to Self-Study Questions

1. D. The appointment should be rescheduled. Elective care should only be done on asymptomatic patients.

2. B. Sit patient up and allow them to assume position that makes them comfortable, usually sitting slightly forward. Placing the patient supine can make breathing more difficult and increase patient anxiety.

3. D. Xerostomia is a common adverse side effect of inhaled short and long acting β2 agonists and anticholinergics and can contribute to an increased caries rate. Daily application of topical fluoride and/or casein phosphopeptide/amorphous calcium phosphate (CPP-ACP) can help to prevent the development of caries. Using a spacer and rinsing after use can help minimize the development of a candidal infection.

Case 3

Patient with Hypertension

CASE STORY

A 67-year-old male came with a chief concern of: "my gums started bleeding and I'm concern about bad breath." He reports his last dental visit was two years ago. A deep cleaning was done and he complains that since then he has generalized sensitivity. He further explains that sensitivity made him avoid seeking further treatment.

PROBLEM-BASED LEARNING GOALS AND OBJECTIVES

- To review the effect of high blood pressure during dental treatment
- To identify the potential interactions of high blood pressure medications during dental treatment
- To plan adequate management

Medical History

His medical history is positive for hypertension diagnosed three years ago. He blames it on gaining weight after quitting smoking five years before. He sees his doctor four times a year. The physician prescribed medications that he confessed taking sometimes and forgetting sometimes. He denies any other medical issue. His blood pressure today was 165/95 and 170/93. He claims he rushed to the appointment that he did not take his medications. His medications are amlodipine (Norvasc) and hydrochlorothiazide and a daily multivitamin.

Dental History

He manually brushes at least once a day, in the morning, does not use any interdental cleaning device, but uses an alcohol containing mouthwash twice a day. He is concerned that brushing aggravates the bleeding.

Social History

He smoked more than a pack a day for 40 years. He drinks alcohol socially.

Dental Examination

The intra- and extraoral soft tissue exam were unremarkable.

Little saliva is observed present but the patient does not report dry mouth.

All teeth were present besides #17. All posterior buccal surfaces had some degree of loss of attachment. Teeth #16 and #31 have visible caries. Plaque is present in 40% of posterior surfaces. There is 75% bleeding and probing, calculus is present on the lingual surfaces of lower anterior teeth and probing depths range 3–6 mm. Radiographic examination shows the presence of generalized mild to moderate bone loss, especially in the lower incisors (Figure 10.3.1).

Dental Considerations

The patient will require:

- Oral hygiene instructions to reduce plaque, bleeding on probing, and sensitivity
- Extraction of #16 and possibly #31 because of a poor prognosis
- Periodontal treatment to reduce plaque and calculus and reduce periodontal pockets.

Medical Considerations: Hypertension

Hypertension (HTN) is a very prevalent medical condition affecting one every three adults overall, although that prevalence increases drastically with age. Among the adults with HTN only about half are under control. Up to 95% of patients have what is known as

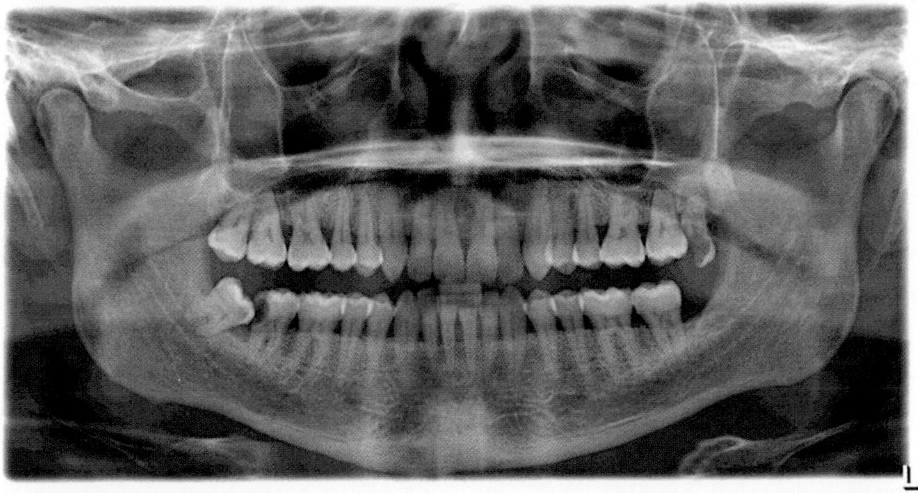

Figure 10.3.1: Panoramic image of the patient.

Table 10.3.1: Blood pressure categories defined by the American Heart Association.

What is the AHA recommendation for healthy blood pressure?
This blood pressure chart reflects categories defined by the American Heart Association.

Blood Pressure Category	Systolic mmHg (upper#)		Diastolic mmHg (lower #)
Normal	less than 120	and	less than 80
Prehypertenslon	120–139	or	80–89
High Blood Pressure (Hypertension) Stage 1	140–159	or	90–99
High Blood Pressure (Hypertension) Stage 2	160 or higher	or	100 or higher
Hypertensive Crisis (Emergency cere needed)	Higher than 180	or	Higher than 110

Source: http://www.heart.org/HEARTORG/Conditions/HighBloodPressure/AboutHighBloodPressure/About-High-Blood-Pressure_UCM_002050_Article.jsp#.V5V0RldVK0h.

primary or essential hypertension where there is no single identifiable cause.

The American Heart Association establishes the categories of blood pressure ranging from normal all the way to hypertensive crisis (Table 10.3.1). Uncontrolled HTN can lead to myocardial infarction, stroke, renal failure, and death. It is also known as "the silent killer" because for most patients it has no symptoms.

Accurate measurement of the blood pressure is vital during dental evaluation and during follow up. Blood pressure should be taken following recommendations from the American Heart Association as follows:

- Patients should be seated with back supported and arm bared and supported
- Patients should refrain from smoking or ingesting caffeine for 30 minutes before measurement
- Measurement should be done after at least five minutes of rest
- Appropriate cuff size and calibrated equipment should be used
- Systolic and diastolic values should be recorded
- Additional readings are recommended if >140/90

There are special considerations that need to be taken during dental treatment depending on blood pressure values (Table 10.3.2).

Medical Considerations: Medications

Multiple pharmacological options are available for the treatment of hypertension with different mechanism of action. Patients can be treated with single agents but, in many cases, they require more than one drug (polypharmacy).

Providers need to become familiar with each medication including learning about side effects and potential interactions that may affect treatment or require modifications to the dental treatment.

Table 10.3.2: Special considerations during dental treatment regarding blood pressure values.

BP values	Treatment Recommendations
<120 or <80	All dental treatment
>120/80 but <140/90	All dental treatment.
>140/90 but <165/95 without target organ disease (e.g. kidney)	Monitor BP. May include some modifications (e.g., limit vasoconstrictor) Recommend following up with primary care provider. Most dental treatment is safe.
>160/100 but <180/110	Monitor BP and limit epinephrine Medical Consultation before elective treatment. Palliative care of pain and infections

For values above 180/110 they require immediate referral to the primary care provider or the ER.

Table 10.3.3: Side effects and interactions of high blood pressure medications.

Classes of Blood Pressure Medications	Examples of Relevant Side Effects and Interactions
Diuretics	Orthostatic hypotension NSAIDs may diminish the therapeutic effect of these drugs
Beta-blockers	Limit vasoconstrictor use with noncardioselective beta-blockers (e.g., propranolol, naldolol, pindolol, penbutolol, sotalol, timolol) NSAIDs may diminish the therapeutic effect of these drugs
ACE inhibitors	Orthostatic hypotension Dry cough
Angiotensin II receptor blockers	Orthostatic hypotension NSAIDs may diminish the therapeutic effect of these drugs and affect kidney function Systemic antifungals may decrease drug metabolism
Calcium channel blockers	May cause gingival overgrowth Systemic antifungals may decrease drug metabolism Macrolide antibiotics may decrease drug metabolism
Alpha blockers	Orthostatic hypotension Dry mouth
Alpha-2 receptor agonist	Orthostatic hypotension Dry mouth Sore tongue
Combined alpha and beta-blockers	Orthostatic hypotension NSAIDs may diminish the therapeutic effect of these drugs
Central agonists	Orthostatic hypotension Dry mouth
Peripheral adrenergic inhibitors	Orthostatic hypotension Dry mouth Caution w/vasoconstrictor
Vasodilators	Orthostatic hypotension NSAIDs may diminish the therapeutic effect of these drugs

A summary of relevant adverse effects and interactions from high blood pressure medications related to dental treatment are present in Table 10.3.3.

Specific Considerations

It is important before treatment plan to first identify all the medical issues and conditions that may require management and plan appropriately.

Self-Study Questions

1. All of the following statements pertain to the appropriate monitoring of blood pressure EXCEPT one. Which one is the exception?
- **A. Measuring BP should be done on all patients during the first dental visit**
- **B. Monitoring of BP during dental procedures is necessary on all patients during local anesthetic administration.**
- **C. It is important to establish a baseline BP**
- **D. It is not necessary take BP on a patient that does not report hypertension on the initial visit**

2. Dental treatment modifications should be planned based on:
- **A. Current blood pressure values**
- **B. Medication/s the patient may be taking**
- **C. Age of the patient**
- **D. All of the above**

3. High blood pressure medications potentially interact with all the following medications EXCEPT one. Which one is the exception?
- **A. Nonsteroidal anti-inflammatory drugs (NSAIDs)**
- **B. Epinephrine**
- **C. Systemic antifungals**
- **D. Penicillin**

4. If a patient comes to a regular dental visit with a blood pressure of 165/95 you should:
- **A. Refer immediately to the primary care provider**
- **B. Delay all nonemergency treatment**
- **C. Retake the blood pressure first**
- **D. Immediate referral to the ER**

Answers to Self-Study Questions

1. D. Monitor BP should be done on ALL patients during first visit. This is very important not only to establish a baseline but also because hypertension is highly prevalent (one-third of adults) and only half of the patients diagnosed as hypertensive are under control.

2. D. All of the above.

3. D. Patients treated for HTN may be taking single or multiple drugs that require the use of a reputable drug reference resource to verify side effects and potential interactions. Penicillin seems to be a safe drug, regardless of what HTN medication the patient is on.

4. C. Blood pressure should be obtained following the AHA recommendations and multiple readings are recommended if the initial value is above 140/90.

Case 4

Patient Taking Antithrombotic Drugs – Valve Replacement

CASE STORY

A 52-year-old female presents with a dental chief complaint "I need a checkup and a cleaning. My gums bleed when I'm flossing." She was going regularly for dental check-ups but after moving to a different state, she needs a new dentist. Most of her past dental visits were for dental cleanings. She brushes and flosses regularly. Her last caries was many years ago.

PROBLEM-BASED LEARNING GOALS AND OBJECTIVES

- Understand the current guidelines for antibiotic prophylaxis for patients at risk of developing infective endocarditis and the evidence supporting them
- Recognize which medical conditions the American Heart Association (AHA) requires antibiotic prophylaxis before some dental procedures
- Identify which dental procedures warrant antibiotic prophylaxis
- Know the impact of antithrombotic agents on hemostasis and their management in dental patients taking them
- Identify necessary laboratory data to make clinical management decisions within the context of planned dental therapy

Medical History and Review of Systems

The patient has a history of a congenital heart defect that caused an abnormality in the mitral valve. Due the severity of the condition and the associated symptoms (patient was suffering with severe shortness of breath, fatigue, palpitations, and swollen feet), the valve was replaced one year ago.

A summary of her medical history:

- Mitral valve replaced with a mechanical valve due to a previously damaged valve due to a congenital heart defect
- Seasonal allergies

Medications

Warfarin (Coumadin) 5 mg once a day for thromboembolic events prevention.

Low-dose aspirin (acetylsalicylic acid, 81 mg) once a day for thromboembolic events prevention.

Occasional over-the-counter antihistaminic: cetirizine (Zyrtec) which is a histamine H_1 antagonist for seasonal allergies.

Allergies

Penicillin (since childhood, she reported a history of severe rash)

- **Vital signs:**
  - Blood pressure: 126/85 mmHg
  - Pulse: 62 beats/min
  - Respiration: 14 breaths/min

Dental History

- Her last dental cleaning was more than a year ago.
- She had her wisdom teeth extracted many years ago
- She had some dental restorations in the past, however she does not remember having any restoration placed recently

Social History

Negative.

Extraoral and Intraoral Mucosal Examination

No cervical lymphadenopathy. No clicking or deviations noted in the temporomandibular joint area. Cheek biting

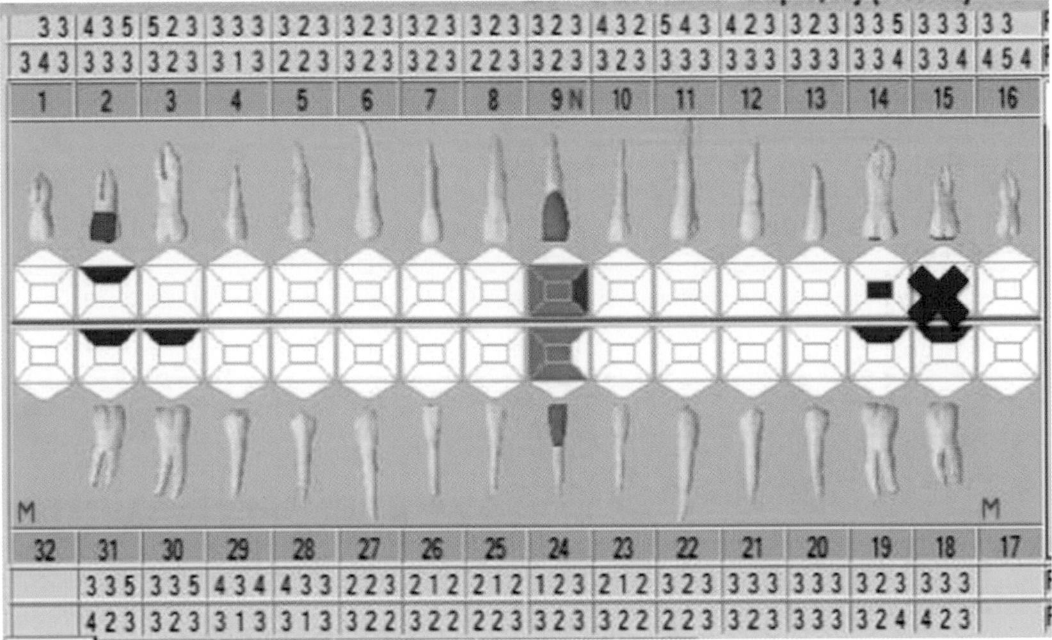

Figure 10.4.1: Clinical dental examination.

noted in the oral mucosa in the left side. Color of the gingiva and mucosa is within normal limits (WNL). Normal salivary flow.

Clinical Dental Examination

Mild to moderate gingival inflammation, especially in the interproximal of the posterior teeth where visible plaque is observed on the lingual and interproximal surfaces of lower posterior teeth (Figure 10.4.1).

No visible caries, multiple restorations.

Visible calculus on the lingual aspect of the mandibular teeth.

Radiographic Examination

Mild to moderate bone loss on the posterior teeth.

Dental restorations.

Broken tooth #15, which is not restorable.

Treatment Plan and Management

Dental Considerations

The patient will require:

- Periodontal evaluation
- Periodontal treatment
- Oral hygiene reinforcement

Medical Considerations

- Antibiotic prophylaxis for dental procedures that involve manipulation of gingival tissue, the periapical region of teeth or perforation of the oral mucosa that will include antibiotic prophylaxis for periodontal probing and the scaling and root planing visits (Wilson et al. 2007, 2008).
- Patient is allergic to penicillin. The choice for antibiotic prophylaxis in this case is clindamycin or azithromycin or clarithromycin. If clindamycin is prescribed, the patient should be instructed to take 600 mg 30 to 60 minutes before the dental appointment (Wilson et al. 2007, 2008).
- Assess bleeding risk due to the use of anticoagulant: request recent laboratory test International Ratio (INR) which should be taken 24–78 hours prior to treatment. Results should be less than 3.5 in order to safely perform the dental procedure and achieving hemostasis (Webster and Wilde 2000).
- Scaling and root planing. Expect more bleeding in the areas with inflammation.

Antibiotic Prophylaxis

Even though this case lacks dental complexity, there are a few important things to be taken into consideration. Antibiotic prophylaxis is still recommended by the AHA (Wilson et al. 2007, 2008) for a limited number of heart conditions that are still considered high risk for patients to develop bacterial endocarditis. As a result, the regimen for antibiotic prophylaxis is very important to remember.

The list of cardiac medical conditions that are considered high risk for developing infective endocarditis

Table 10.4.1: Cardiac prophylaxis.

Cardiac Prophylaxis

1. Prosthetic cardiac valve or prosthetic material used for cardiac valve repair
2. History of infective endocarditis
3. Cardiac transplant that develops cardiac valvulopathy
4. Congenital heart disease:
   a. Unrepaired cyanotic congenital heart disease including palliative shunts and conduits
   b. Completely repaired congenital heart defect with prosthetic material or device, whether placed by surgery or by catheter intervention, during the first six months after the procedure
   c. Repaired congenital heart defect with residual defect at the site or adjacent to the site of a prosthetic device (that inhibit endothelialization)

Except for the conditions listed above, antibiotic prophylaxis is no longer recommended for **ANY** other form of congenital heart disease

DENTAL PROCEDURES REQUIRING ANTIBIOTIC PROPHYLAXIS

All dental procedures that involve manipulation of gingival tissue, the periapical region of teeth or perforation of the oral mucosa.

EXCLUDES THE FOLLOWING:

1. Routine anesthetic injections through non-infected tissue
2. Taking dental radiographs
3. Placement or adjustment or removable prosthodontics or orthodontic appliances, placement or orthodontic brackets.
4. Shedding of primary teeth
5. Bleeding from trauma to the lips or oral mucosa

Source: Extracted and adapted from Wilson et al. (2008).

includes the history of a prosthetic valve. In addition, the following are the other conditions, recommended by the American Heart Association, that warrant antibiotic prophylaxis: a history of infective endocarditis, cardiac transplant that develops valvulopathy and congenital heart disease that includes unrepaired cyanotic congenital heart defects, including shunts and conduits, completely repaired congenital heart defects during the first six months after the procedure and repaired heart defects with residual defect at the site or adjacent to the site (see Table 10.4.1).

The taking of dental radiographs does not require antibiotic prophylaxis.

As a general rule, antibiotic prophylaxis should be administered in a single dose before the dental procedure (see Table 10.4.2). However, if the dosage is inadvertently not taken before the procedure, the antibiotic may be taken up to two hours after the procedure. This should be the exception but not the rule. In patients allergic to penicillin, like in this case, suitable drugs to prescribe are clindamycin, clarithromycin, or azithromycin. It is important to remember one of the side effects of these medications is gastrointestinal (GI) distress.

About the use of antithrombotic agents, this patient is taking two drugs that affect the patient's coagulation time. Questions on the patient's medical history should include a history of bleeding. Patients are usually aware of the medications they are taking. Asking simple questions about that is an important part of the medical interview. In this case the patient is taking Warfarin (Coumadin), the patient needs to be checked regularly for the coagulation status. The laboratory test needed to assess the coagulation status in patients using Warfarin is the INR. An acceptable INR for invasive dental procedures, where bleeding is expected, should be less than 3.5 (Webster and Wilde 2000).

This patient is also taking low-dose aspirin (the action is at the level of platelet aggregation; antiplatelet) (Schrör 1997). However, the impact of bleeding is not in a grade that will preclude us to stop dental treatment or to stop the medication (Nematullah et al. 2009). There is no test available to check platelet aggregation and its effect on bleeding time. As health-care providers, it is important to remember that we should not suggest to the patient they stop any of the antithrombotic agents. However, it may be beneficial to stop the antithrombotic agent especially if the INR is not at an acceptable level. In these situations close consultation with the physician or cardiologist is necessary. The physician / cardiologist would be the health-care provider who would manage how long the discontinuation of the antithrombotic medications is needed, which would be patient and procedure specific.

In case of procedures where bleeding is expected to be longer, we should be prepared to control the bleeding locally (Svensson et al. 2013).

Table 10.4.2: Antibiotic dosage.

Regimens for a Dental Procedure			
Administration/situation	**Antibiotic**	**Regimen single dose 30–60 minutes before procedure**	
		Adults	**Children**
Oral	Amoxicillin	2 g	50 mg kg^{-1}
Unable to take oral medication	Ampicillin Cefazolin or Ceftriaxone	2 g IM or IV 1 g IM or IV	50 mg kg^{-1} IM or IV
Allergic to penicillin or ampicillin- oral	Cephalexin[a] OR Clindamycin OR Azithromycin or Clarithromycin	2 g OR 600 mg OR 500 mg	50 mg kg^{-1} OR 20 mg kg^{-1} OR 15 mg kg^{-1}
Allergic to penicillin or ampicillin-unable to take oral medication	Cefazolin or Ceftriaxone[b] OR Clindamycin	1 g IM or IV OR 600 mg IM or IV	50 mg kg^{-1} IM or IV OR 20 mg kg^{-1} or IV

Source: Extracted and adapted from Wilson et al. (2008).
IM: Intramuscular IV intravenous
[a] Cephalosporin should not be used in a person with a history of anaphylaxis, angioedema, or urticaria with penicillin or ampicillins.
[b] First or second generation oral cephalosporin.

Table 10.4.3: Dental management.

Issue	Potential Problem	Management
Heart valve replacement	Infective endocarditis	Antibiotic prophylaxis for procedures with invasive procedures/ manipulate gingiva
Penicillin allergy	Anaphylactic shock	Use clindamycin or alternative antibiotic for prophylaxis
Antithrombotic agents	Increased bleeding	Assess the coagulation status. INR less than 3.5 only for invasive dental procedures. Be prepared to control bleeding. Local hemostatic agents. Atraumatic surgery – sutures and prepare adjuncts to promote hemostasis

Table 10.4.3 summarizes the suggested management.

Take-Home Hints

1. The administration of antibiotic prophylaxis is not risk free.
2. Only a few cardiac medical conditions require antibiotic prophylaxis before dental treatment.
3. Antithrombotic agents may alter the coagulation process. You need to identify the class and mechanism of action to request the appropriate test, if needed.
4. INR is needed for patients taking Warfarin (Coumadin) only, with the newer medications Novel Oral Anticoagulants (NOACs) such as dabigatran (Pradaxa), rivaroxaban (Xarelto), and apixaban (Eliquis) laboratory tests are not indicated but you should contact the medical provider in cases that prolonged bleeding is expected.
5. We do not suggest stopping any antithrombotic agent. This should be done by the physician or cardiologist if necessary. You should assess the risk and benefits and be able to control the bleeding locally prior to any procedure (Douketis et al. 2012). Look for signs and symptoms of potential bleeding problems (such as petechiae and ecchymosis).

Self-Study Questions

1. According to the American Heart Association, which medical conditions still require the use of antibiotic prophylaxis?
   A. Prosthetic cardiac valve or prosthetic material used for cardiac valve repair
   B. History of infective endocarditis
   C. Cardiac transplant that develops cardiac valvulopathy
   D. Congenital heart disease
   E. All of the above

2. For what dental procedures is antibiotic prophylaxis still recommended?
   A. Dental procedures that involve manipulation of gingival tissue, the periapical Region of teeth or perforation of the oral mucosa
   B. alginate impression
   C. X-rays
   D. Removal of sutures

3. Which of the following drug categories contains low-dose aspirin?
   A. Anticoagulant
   B. Antiplatelet
   C. Antibiotic
   D. Arthritic

4. For antibiotic prophylaxis, which of the following antibiotics can be prescribed to a patient who is allergic to amoxicillin?
   A. Clindamycin 600 mg
   B. Azithromycin 600 mg
   C. Clarithromycin 300 mg
   D. Penicillin 500 mg

5. If a patient is taking warfarin it should be discontinued before dental procedures.
   A. True
   B. False

References

Douketis, J.D., Spyropoulos, A.C., Spencer, F.A. et al. (2012). Perioperative Management of Antithrombotic Therapy: antithrombotic therapy and prevention of thrombosis, 9th Ed: American College of Chest Physicians Evidence-Based Clinical Practice Guidelines. *Chest* 141 (2 Suppl): e326S–e350S.

Nematullah, A., Alabousi, A., Blanas, N. et al. (2009). Dental surgery for patients on anticoagulant therapy with warfarin: a systematic review and meta-analysis. *J. Can. Dent. Assoc.* 75 (1): 41.

Schrör, K. (1997). Aspirin and platelets: the antiplatelet action of aspirin and its role in thrombosis treatment and prophylaxis. *Semin. Thromb. Hemost.* 23 (4): 349–356.

Svensson, R., Hallmer, F., Englesson, C.S. et al. (2013). Treatment with local hemostatic agents and primary closure after tooth extraction in warfarin treated patients. *Swed. Dent. J.* 37 (2): 71–77.

Webster, K. and Wilde, J. (2000). Management of anticoagulation in patients with prosthetic heart valves undergoing oral and maxillofacial operations. *Br. J. Oral Maxillofac. Surg.* 2000 38 (2): 124–126.

Wilson, W., Taubert, K.A., Gewitz, M. et al. (2007). Prevention of infective endocarditis. *Circulation* 116: 1736–1754.

Wilson, W., Taubert, K.A., Gewitz, M. et al. (2008). Prevention of infective endocarditis: guidelines from the American Heart Association. *J. Am. Dent. Assoc.* 139: S11–S24.

Answers to Self-Study Questions

1. E. Unrepaired cyanotic congenital heart disease including palliative shunts and conduits

- Completely repaired congenital heart defect with prosthetic material or device, whether placed by surgery or by catheter intervention, during the first six months after the procedure
- Repaired congenital heart defect with residual defect at the site or adjacent to the site of a prosthetic device (that inhibit endothelialization).

2. A. Dental procedures that involve manipulation of gingival tissue, the periapical region of teeth, or perforation of the oral mucosa.

3. B. Aspirin is an antiplatelet drug that inhibits the aggregation or clumping of platelets.

4. A. Clindamcyin 600 mg is the correct answer. Azithromycin and clarithromycin can be prescribed to a patient allergic to amoxicillin but it has an incorrect dosage. Amoxicillin is a type of penicillin.

5. B. Numerous articles have been published documenting that it is not necessary to discontinue Warfarin, an anticoagulant, before dental procedures.

Case 5

Patient with Kidney Disease

CASE STORY

The patient is a 35-year-old man with the chief concern "I want a complete denture." The patient states that he is on dialysis. He had a dental examination about six months prior to this visit and was told that he had many cavities that needed to be restored. The dentist was not comfortable treating him because of his medical issues.

PROBLEM-BASED LEARNING OBJECTIVES

As a result of studying this case the dental hygienist will be able to:

- Take a medical history of a patient with chronic kidney disease and renal dialysis to establish the patients' medical status and identify issues of concern prior to dental hygiene treatment
- Ask appropriate questions on a medical consultation for a patient on renal dialysis
- Interpret the patients laboratory findings in relationship to his dental treatment
- List oral mucosal and jawbone changes that may be associated with chronic kidney disease and renal dialysis
- List the dental hygiene management concerns for treating a patient with chronic kidney disease on renal dialysis

Medical History and Review of Systems

The patient has a long history of hypertension. As a result he developed end stage renal disease (ESRD). He receives hemodialysis every Monday, Wednesday, and Friday. He has an arterio-venous (AV) shunt in his left arm. He has an allergy to shellfish and no known drug allergies. See Table 10.5.1 for laboratory values.

- **Medications:**
  - Simvastatin 10 mg per day for high cholesterol
  - Calcium carbonate – Vitamin D 500 mg/5 mg to maintain serum calcium level
  - Calctinol 5 mg – Vitamin D to maintain serum calcium
  - Aspirin 85 mg per day to prevent platelet aggregation

Dental History

Until recently he had no caries or restorations. He brushes his teeth twice a day and never flosses. His last dental visit was six months ago for an examination, but no treatment. He was told he had many cavities.

Social and Family History

He denied alcohol and smoking. His mother and sister both have high blood pressure.

Table 10.5.1: Selected laboratory values.

Complete Blood Count	Patient's Results	Normal (Laboratory)
WBC	6.3	3.4–11.2 x 10^3 μl^{-1}
Hemoglobin	9.3 (Low)	13.3–17.7 g dl^{-1}
Hematocrit	27.4% (Low)	40.0–50.0%
Mean Corpuscular Volume (MCV)	106.4 fl (High)	81.0–100 fl
Mean Corpuscular Hemoglobin (MCHb)	36.1 (High)	27.0–34.0 pg
Red Blood Cell (RBC) count	2.57 (Low)	4.40–5.90 x 10^6 μl^{-1}
Blood Chemistry		
Serum Chloride	96 (Low)	101–111 mmol l^{-1}
Urea Nitrogen (BUN)	45 (High)	18–20 mg dl^{-1}
Serum Creatinine	6.0 (High)	0.64–1.27 mg dl^{-1}
Serum Calcium	6.0 (Low)	8.90–10.3 mg dl^{-1}

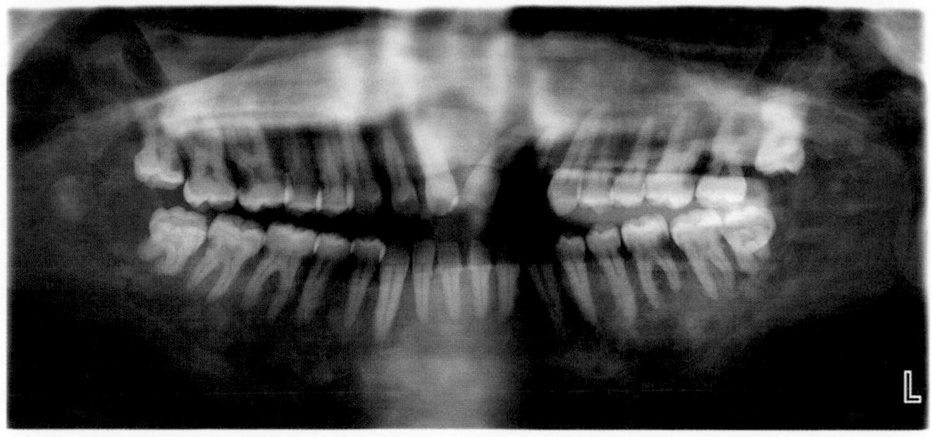

Figure 10.5.1: Panoramic radiograph showing "ground glass" appearance of trabeculae and loss of lamina dura.

Extraoral and Intraoral Examination

- No cervical lymphadenopathy
- Clicking noted over right temporomandibular joint area
- No intraoral mucosal abnormalities noted
- Missing left lateral incisor with resultant shifting of adjacent teeth
- Multiple extensive carious teeth

Panoramic Examination

- Diffuse bone changes consistent with renal osteodystrophy
- Generalized alveolar bone loss
- Multiple carious lesions
- Calculus visible on mandibular anterior teeth

Figure 10.5.1 shows a panoramic radiograph of the patient.

Problem List

- End-stage renal disease on dialysis
- High blood pressure
- Osteodystrophy
- Anemia
- Generalized caries and periodontal disease

Treatment Plan

- Medical consultation to confirm medical status: request prothrombin time/partial thromboplastin time (PT/PTT) and platelet count prior to dental hygiene appointments and oral surgery appointments. Need for antibiotic prophylaxis to prevent endarteritis in patients with AV shunt is controversial. Request medical consultation. Antibiotic prophylaxis is not required for peritoneal dialysis.
- Take blood pressure at each visit – use arm without AV shunt (usually right arm) to take blood pressure
- Avoid dialysis days for dental hygiene appointments
- Dental hygiene: scaling, root planing, and oral hygiene instructions
- Extraction of maxillary teeth and fabrication of full denture
- Selective extraction of nonrestorable mandibular teeth
- Treatment of restorable carious teeth
- Fabrication of mandibular partial denture

Discussion

End stage renal disease occurs when 50–70% of the kidneys' two million nephrons lose function. Once destroyed, the nephrons cannot be restored. End stage renal disease begins with an asymptomatic stage and progresses to severe disease. Hypertension, diabetes mellitus, and chronic glomerulonephritis are common causes. Chronic kidney disease is a serious consequence of systemic lupus erythematosus. In many cases of kidney failure the cause is unknown. As the disease progresses to severe disease, either kidney dialysis (artificial filtration of the blood) or kidney transplantation is required.

As a result of the destruction of nephrons, there is a failure of the kidneys to excrete waste products and multiorgan involvement. There is interference with endocrine and metabolic functions, and neuromuscular, cardiac, gastrointestinal, hematological, and dermatological manifestations. The resulting syndrome is called *uremia*. Patients develop anemia, bleeding problems including platelet deficiencies, hypertension, electrolyte and fluid imbalance, and altered metabolism of drugs. Laboratory abnormalities include decreased red blood cells and platelets, increased serum creatinine, and blood urea nitrogen (BUN) levels. An increased creatinine level is an important indicator of kidney disease. Dosages of medications that are metabolized by the kidney may need to be adjusted. With decreasing kidney function and decreased glomerular filtration there is an increase in serum phosphate. The excess phosphate tends to cause serum calcium to be deposited in bone resulting in decreased serum calcium. The parathyroid glands increase their secretion of parathormone (PTH) resulting in secondary hyperparathyroidism and bone disorders. The bone disorders in ESRD are referred to as renal osteodystrophy.

Oral manifestations of ESRD include xerostomia, uremic stomatitis (painful oral mucosal lesions), petechiae, and ecchymoses. Anemia results in mucosal pallor. Radiographically, the bone trabeculae develop a "ground glass" appearance and there is loss of the lamina dura (Figure 10.5.1). Well-defined unilocular and multilocular radiolucencies also occur. Histopathologically, these are identical to central giant cell granulomas. In these lesions the multinucleated giant cells are osteoclasts.

The medical management of ESRD involves renal dialysis in which the blood is artificially filtered. Renal dialysis results in improvement of the consequences of ESRD.

Hemodialysis is done through a permanent shunt: an AV shunt in the forearm. The arm with the shunt must not be used for measuring blood pressure. Dialysis is usually scheduled on alternate weekdays (i.e., Monday/Wednesday/Friday or Tuesday/Thursday/Saturday). Patients receive the short-acting anticoagulant, heparin, at the time of dialysis. For this reason, dental hygiene and dental treatment is best scheduled on weekdays alternate to dialysis. In addition, patients usually experience fatigue on dialysis days. There is no clear consensus on whether patients with hemodialysis shunts require antibiotic prophylaxis to prevent bacterial endarteritis. The guidelines from the AHA for prevention of infective endocarditis have been suggested, but there is no convincing evidence that patients with AV shunts are at risk of infection from transient bacteremia.

Prior to initiating dental hygiene and dental treatment a medical consultation should be obtained from the patient's medical-care provider. This should include information about the status of the patient's kidney disease, dialysis schedule, medical complications, and laboratory values including any bleeding abnormality and the schedule dialysis treatment. It is important that the medical provider be informed that dental hygiene treatment is invasive dental treatment.

Take-Home Hints

1. A medical consultation should be obtained prior to initiating dental hygiene/dental treatment.
2. For patients on renal dialysis, dental appointments should be scheduled on alternate days from dialysis.
3. For patients with kidney disease and renal dialysis, blood pressure should be taken and recorded at each dental hygiene/dental appointment.
4. The arm with the AV shunt must not be used for taking blood pressure
5. Bone changes due to kidney disease may include a "ground glass" appearance of trabeculae, loss of lamina dura, and unilocular and multilocular radiolucencies.
6. Dental hygiene treatment is important in eliminating sources of oral infection for patients with kidney disease and on renal dialysis.

Self-Study Questions

1. For patients on renal dialysis, dental hygiene appointments should be scheduled on:
- **A. Alternate days from dialysis**
- **B. The same day as dialysis**
- **C. Once a week**

2. Which of the following laboratory values is an important indicator of kidney disease?
- **A. Increased neutrophil count**
- **B. Cholesterol**
- **C. Creatine**
- **D. Glucose**

3. End state kidney disease occurs when ____ percent of the nephrons lose function.
- **A. 10%**
- **B. 20%**
- **C. 50–70%**
- **D. 90–100%**

4. Bone manifestations of ESRD include all of the following except one. Which one is the exception?
- **A. Loss of lamina dura**
- **B. Brown tumor (giant cell granuloma)**
- **C. "Ground glass" appearance of trabeculae**
- **D. Osteomas**

Additional Resources

Little, J.W., Miller, C.S., Rhodus, N.L., and Falace, D.A. (2013). *Dental Management of the Medically Complex Patient*, 8e. St. Louis: Mosby.

Patton, L.L. and Glick, M. (2016). *The ADA Practical Guide to Patients with Medical Conditions*. Hoboken NJ: Wiley Blackwell.

Rada, R.E. (January 2015). Oral effects of kidney disease. *Dimensions of Dental Hygiene* 13 (1): 24,26,28.

Tadakamadia, I., Kumar, S., and Mamatha, G.P. (2014). Comparative evaluation of oral health status of chronic kidney disease (CKD) patients in various stags ad healthy controls. *Spec. Care Dentist.* 34 (3): 122–126.

Answers to Self-Study Questions

1. A. Patients receive the short-acting anticoagulant, heparin, at the time of dialysis. For this reason, dental hygiene and dental treatment is best scheduled on weekdays alternate to dialysis.

2. C. Increased creatinine level is an important indicator of kidney disease.

3. C. End stage renal disease occurs when 50–70% of the kidneys two million nephrons lose function.

4. D. Secondary hyperparathyroidism results in bone changes including loss of lamina dura, "ground glass" appearance of trabeculae, brown tumor (central giant cell granuloma).

11

Professional Responsibility

Clinical Cases in Dental Hygiene, First Edition. Edited by Cheryl M. Westphal Theile, Mea A. Weinberg and Stuart L. Segelnick.

Case 1

Ethical Principles – Informed Consent

CASE STORY

A 49-year-old female presents with her 18-year-old daughter for comprehensive dental hygiene care. The mother has Limited English Proficiency (LEP). The daughter relates to the dental hygienist that her mother hasn't had any dental care in many years. She says her mother sometimes has discomfort when chewing, has bad breath, and complains of a funny taste in her mouth. She also informs the dental hygienist that she is there to interpret what is said and translate any papers her mother has to sign (Figure 11.1.1).

PROBLEM-BASED LEARNING GOALS AND OBJECTIVES

- Define the ethical obligation of providing autonomy for the patient
- State the legal responsibility of attaining a patient's informed consent
- Identify the ethical dilemma and steps to reach an ethical decision

Medical History

There are no significant issues in the medical history and the patient takes no prescribed or over-the-counter medications.

Dental History

There are no records or memory of the patient having been seen for dental care since she left her country 15 years previously. The chief complaint as related by her daughter appears to be halitosis and occasional discomfort when chewing and taste alteration. Patient nods yes to brushing every day but shakes her head no when shown floss and other interdental biofilm removal aids.

Gingival tissues are red in color, with generalized edematous tissue. The tissue readily bleeds on probing and probing depths in the posterior areas are generally 4 and 5 mm. There are moderate biofilm and calculus deposits. There appears to be occlusal decay on several molars in all four quadrants. Gingival recession is 2 mm and is generalized.

Social History

The daughter reports her mother does not smoke or drink but eats a diet high in carbohydrates, indicative of some cultural recipes she continues to prepare from her country. The family depends on her to make the best sweets for dessert that they enjoy throughout the day. Her diet is strongly influenced by culture. Although fresh foods are a part of daily consumption, so too are dishes and snacks with high concentrations of sugar.

Dental Hygiene Diagnosis

Problems	Related to Risks and Etiology
Periodontal disease	Inadequate biofilm control and preventive dental visits
Caries	Inadequate biofilm control and diet high in carbohydrates
Halitosis and foul taste	Periodontal infection
Discomfort chewing	Presence of carious lesions

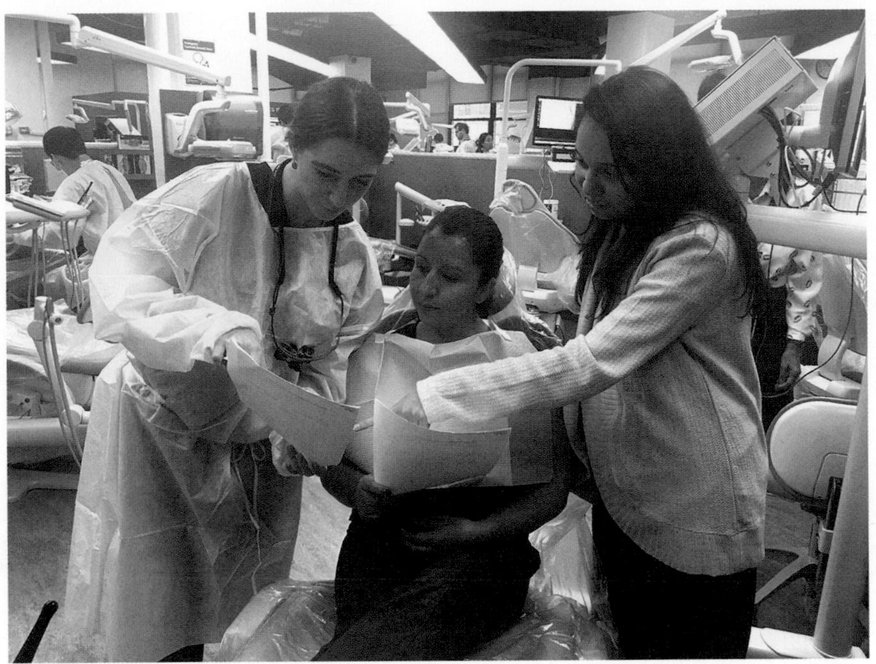

Figure 11.1.1: Staff members can be utilized as certified translators.

Planned Interventions

Clinical	Education/Counseling	Oral Hygiene Instruction
Full mouth series of radiographs	Needed for diagnosis	Explain the results of the series
Scaling and root planing by quadrant	Periodontal infection present	Etiology and progression of periodontal disease
Homecare instructions	Importance of home care	Modified Bass brushing, flossing, and fluoride rinse
Fluoride treatment	Needed for remineralization	Action of fluoride and home fluoride rinse
Nutritional advisement	Carbohydrates contribution in development of caries	Reduction in intake of carbohydrates
Arrange for a health care professional	Importance of understanding treatment plan and home care	Engage a professional interpreter to relay all interactions
Restorative appointment for fillings	As determined by diagnosis	Stress continued appointments until completion
Evaluate tissue response in 6 weeks	Document tissue response	Adjust instructions as needed
Periodontal maintenance every 4 months	Monitoring treatment, host response, and home care	Continue as instructed or adjust treatment as needed

Discussion

All health-care providers have an ethical obligation to treat the public applying defined principles of action. This is a result of the knowledge and skills achieved to be licensed to deliver care. The public respects this and seeks out this expertise. The public expects the highest levels of care and the health-care provider is obligated to meet these expectations.

Autonomy is an ethical principle that addresses the patient's right to make an informed decision about their care. Affording autonomy to a patient gives them the ability to be self-governing and in turn they can choose

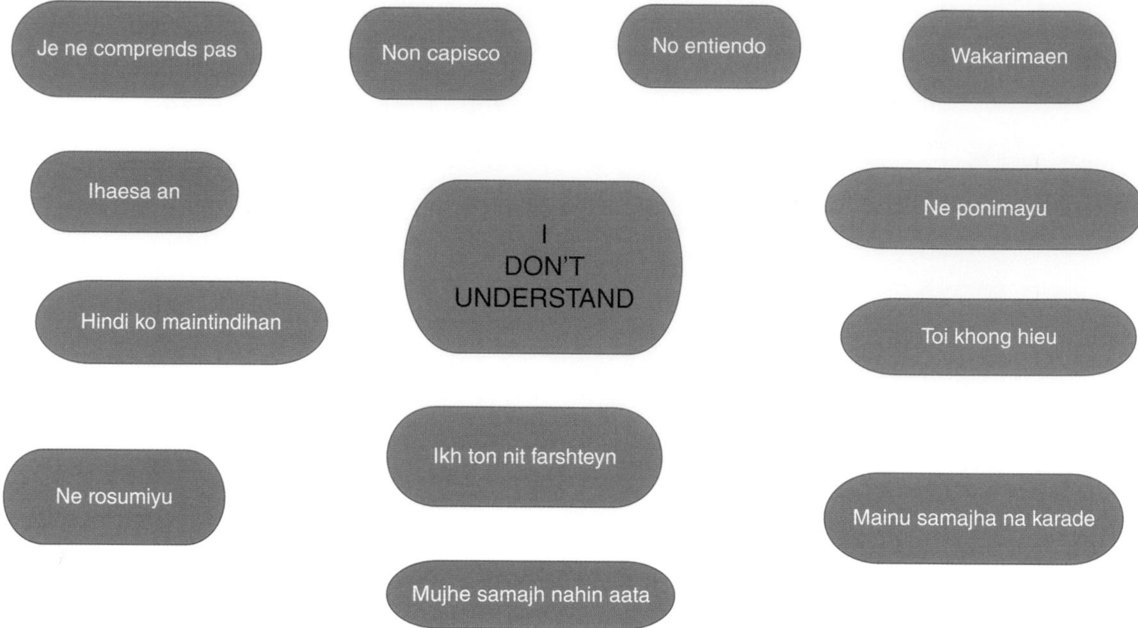

Figure 11.1.2: If you can't understand a patient's response then they can't understand you.

what is relevant to their needs. Autonomy gives individuals permission to make decisions regarding their health care. To do this they must be given explanations about treatment choices and consequences of those and the consequences of rejecting the treatment services (Beemsterboer 2010).

The American Dental Hygienists' Association (ADHA) lists autonomy, beneficence, nonmaleficence, justice, fairness, societal trust, veracity, and confidentiality as core values for practice. All these are the principles the dental hygienist incorporates into care (ADHA 2016a).

The dental hygienist is now faced with an ethical dilemma. A dilemma exists when two or more principles are in conflict. To ensure autonomy for the patient, the etiology of the infection needs to be explained and understood by the patient in order to accept the treatment plan (Figure 11.1.2).

The teenage daughter may not have understood the treatment plan sufficiently to relay it to the patient. In fact, the patient's LEP has probably contributed to her not seeking professional care.

Having a patient sign a consent form without her understanding the financial obligation, the benefits, the risks, the possible outcomes, and giving her a chance to ask questions can be considered Battery. (A dentist who does something without consent on a patient is considered to have committed Battery. In this example, although the patient signed the consent form, they did not give actual consent due to the patient not understanding the form. Any procedures carried out on this patient by the health-care professional would be considered Battery. Having them sign the form itself is not Battery.) In this case the clinician is practicing below the standard of care professionally and is violating legal protections and ethical principles (Figure 11.1.3).

The dilemma has two principles in conflict: the patient's autonomy and the responsibility of beneficence to do good. Doing good for the patient would involve taking actions to remove existing harm. A model for analyzing a dilemma follows the steps of gathering facts, identifying the ethical principles in conflict, listing alternatives, selecting, justifying the action, acting on the decision, and finally evaluating the decision. If the dental hygienist accepts the daughter as interpreter, the hygienist would not know whether everything was related to the patient in a satisfactory manner. The dental hygienist does not know if anything may have been omitted or misunderstood. The dental hygienist cannot be sure that the daughter has told her mother everything about her needs. If treatment proceeds with exposing x-rays and scaling there cannot be a certainty that this is what the patient understood or if her questions were answered correctly. The dental hygienist wants to afford beneficence by doing good for the patient with home care instructions, scaling, and recommending restorations.

Proceeding with any treatment without certainty that the patient understands is unethical and the patient's autonomy is denied. If the dental hygienist doesn't proceed the treatment could be delayed considerably

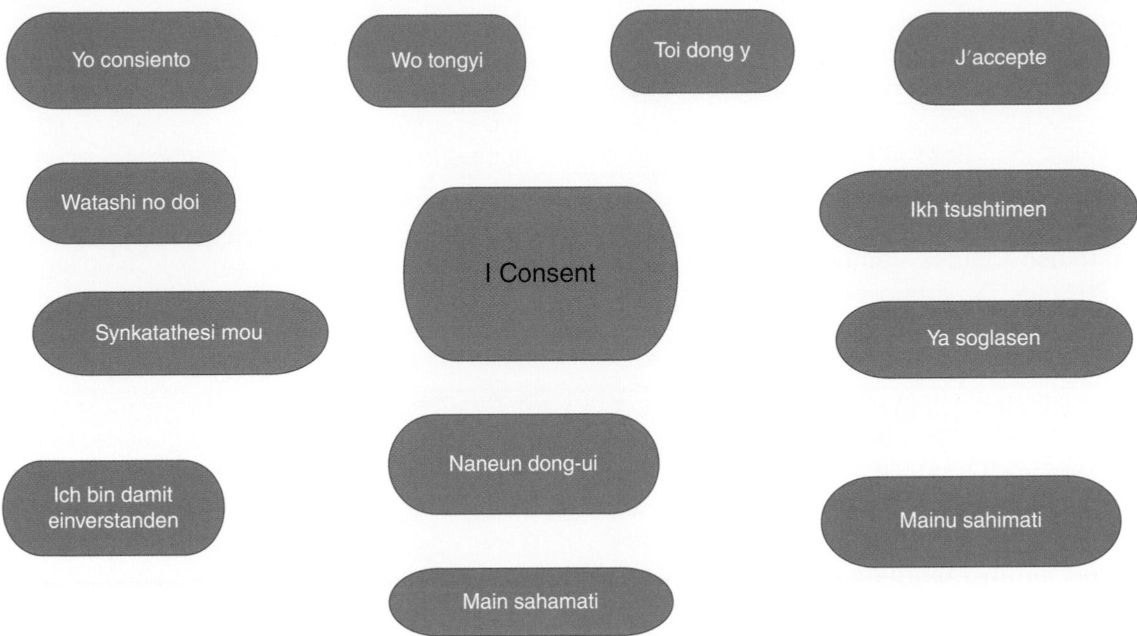

Figure 11.1.3: A patient cannot give informed consent unless they know the facts and can ask questions.

and the patient would also continue to experience discomfort.

An important obligation of all health-care providers is to act within the confines of law. Without informed consent the patient does not experience autonomy. Patients have not given permission for treatment and so the crime of Battery can be claimed. When analyzing a dilemma, the law takes precedence and the standard of care should be respected.

Lack of informed consent is noted in civil and criminal cases against providers in dentistry. Patients should understand treatment outcomes and all risks possible including having no treatment at all. The health-care provider must ensure the patient receives all pertinent information about planned care. Patients should have their questions answered truthfully without prejudice or exclusions. This is standard practice without exception (ADHA 2016b). It is also necessary to document this as a permanent part of the patient's record. Documentation is first of all data collected for the definitive diagnosis. The ADHA has published the document, *Standards for Dental Hygiene Clinical Practice.*

American Dental Hygienists' Association Standards for Clinical Dental Hygiene Practice 2

Standard 1 Assessment

The collection and analysis of systematic and oral health data in order to identify client needs.

Standard 2 Dental Hygiene Diagnosis

The identification of an individual's health behaviors, attitudes, and oral health care needs for which a dental hygienist is educationally qualified and licensed to provide. The dental hygiene diagnosis provides the basis for the dental hygiene care plan.

Standard 3 Planning

The establishment of realistic goals and the selection of dental hygiene interventions that can move the client closer to optimal oral health.

Standard 4 Implementation

The act of carrying out the dental hygiene plan of care. Care should be defined in a manner that minimizes risk, optimizes oral health, and recognizes issues related to patient comfort including pain, fear, and/or anxiety.

Standard 5 Evaluation

The measurement of the extent to which the client has achieved the goals specified in the dental hygiene care plan.

Standard 6 Documentation

The primary goals of good documentation are to maintain continuity of care, provide a means of communication between/among treating providers, and to minimize the risk of exposure to malpractice claims.

For the language barrier, there are two options in this case. The dental office could have a team member who can speak the language and relay this information or the clinician can use a call service, at no charge to the patient, which specializes in the practice of interpreting for health-care providers. Some of these services are available 24 hours a day. It is poor risk management to use a family member as an interpreter. (On May 13, 2016 the Department of Health and Human Services (DHHS) formally adopted final changes to section 1557 of the *Affordable Care Act ACA*. The new rules took effect on July 18, 2016 and will be codified as 45 CFR part 92. These changes are sweeping in scope as they apply to "every [federal] health program or activity, any part of which receives Federal financial assistance." **The final rule prohibits the use of adult family members and friends as medical interpreters**. However, the final regulations allow two exceptions to this general rule. First, adult family members and friends may be used as medical interpreters in an emergency involving an imminent threat to the safety or welfare of an individual or the public where there is no qualified interpreter is immediately available. (Note: since most leading national telephonic and video remote interpreting companies can make qualified interpreters available in hundreds of languages within seconds, this exception should be regarded as limited.) Second, adult family members and friends may be used as medical interpreters where the LEP person "specifically requests that the accompanying adult interpret or facilitate communication and the accompanying adult agrees to provide such assistance." However, the rule makes plain that providers are not relieved of their legal duty to provide a qualified medical interpreter where an LEP patient elects to use an adult family member or friend since even then, "reliance on that adult [family member or friend must be] appropriate under the circumstances." The treatment plan must not go forward until these qualifications are met. The patient must be allowed to understand and choose to accept or reject the plan. The dental hygienist should reschedule the patient until these are all satisfied.

There is a Code of Ethics for Dental Hygienists and a Code of Ethics for Dentists (ADA 2016; ADHA 2016a). Several of the concepts, core values, and principles are the same. They both include autonomy, beneficence, nonmaleficence, veracity, and justice. The American Dental Association's (ADA) code makes reference to auxiliaries for dentists. They are reminded that they are obliged to protect the health of their patients by only assigning to qualified auxiliaries those duties that can be legally delegated. The ADHA further includes the fundamental principle of Universality, which expects that if one individual judges an action to be right or wrong in a given situation, other people considering the same action in the same situation would make the same judgment. The principle of Complementarity "recognizes the existence of an obligation to justice and basic human rights. In all relationships, it requires considering the values and perspectives of others before making decisions or taking actions affecting them" (ADHA 2016a). ADHA's principle of Community is the concern for the bond between individuals, the community, and society in general. It leads to the preservation of natural resources and inspires a sense of concern for the global environment. Responsibility is the recognition that there are guidelines for making ethical choices and the acceptance of responsibility for knowing and applying them. Dental hygienists accept the consequences of their actions or the failure to act and are willing to make ethical choices and publicly affirm them. Ethics, in the code, are considered to be the general standards of right and wrong that guide behavior within society. As generally accepted actions, they can be judged by determining the extent to which they promote good and minimize harm. Ethics compel dental hygienists to engage in health promotion/disease prevention activities.

The ADHA lists as core values, individual autonomy, and respect for human beings, that is, people have the right to be treated with respect. They have the right to informed consent prior to treatment, and they have the right to full disclosure of all relevant information so that they can make informed choices about their care. Confidentiality, in respect of client information and relationships, is a demonstration of the value placed on individual autonomy. Dental hygienists acknowledge their obligation to justify any violation of a confidence. Societal Trust is the principle in which dental hygienists value client trust and understand that public trust in their profession is based on individual actions and behavior. Nonmaleficence states that dental hygienists accept their fundamental obligation to provide services in a manner that protects all clients and minimizes harm to them and others involved in their treatment. Beneficence declares that dental hygienists acknowledge they have a primary role in promoting the well-being of individuals and the public by engaging in health-promotion/disease-prevention activities. When referring to Justice and Fairness, dental hygienists value justice and support the fair and equitable distribution of health-care resources. They believe all people should have access to high-quality, affordable oral health care. The last core value for dental hygienists is Veracity, wherein dental hygienists accept their obligation to tell the truth and expect that others will do the same. They value self-knowledge and seek truth and honesty in all relationships.

Take-Home Hints

1. Autonomy is a right afforded to patients.
2. Dental hygienists must practice according to federal, state, and local statutes and regulations.
3. Dental hygienists have ethical responsibilities to all patients.
4. When faced with a dilemma: gather the facts, list the ethical principles in conflict, list the alternates, and act on this decision.

Self-Study Questions

1. For informed consent to be valid, the following are true except one. Which is the exception?
- **A. The patient understands how much the treatment will cost and how long it will take**
- **B. The patient understands the risks of accepting or not accepting the plan**
- **C. The patient is given the opportunity to ask questions and have them answered**
- **D. The patient gives consent as a courtesy, it is not a legal obligation**

2. As stated in the ADHA Code of Ethics autonomy is defined as:
- **A. being truthful and fair to the patient in all interactions**
- **B. doing only good for the patient and not causing harm**
- **C. the patient has a right to all relevant information so that they can make choices about their care**
- **D. treating all patients the same: justly and fairly**

3. The following is true for using family members as interpreters
- **A. is acceptable if the patient is comfortable with them**
- **B. the practitioner is at risk of breaching the law**
- **C. cannot be used until they are of legal age**
- **D. can explain the treatment plan the best**

4. Five steps in analyzing an ethical dilemma include all except:
- **A. identifying the principles in conflict**
- **B. listing the options**
- **C. obtaining informed consent**
- **D. selecting and justifying the action**

References

American Dental Association. 2016 Code of Professional Conduct, [Online]. Available at: http://www.ada.org/en/about-the-ada/principles-of-ethics-code-of-professional-conduct (May 23, 2018).

American Dental Hygienists' Association 2016a, Code of Ethics, [Online]. Available at: https://www.adha.org/resources-docs/7611_Bylaws_and_Code_of_Ethics.pdf (May 23, 2018).

American Dental Hygienists' Association 2016b, Standards for clinical dental hygiene practise, [Online]. Available at: http://www.adha.org/resources-docs/2016-Revised-Standards-for-Clinical-Dental-Hygiene-Practice.pdf (May 23, 2018).

Beemsterboer, P. (2010). *Ethics and Law in Dental Hygiene*. St. Louis: Saunders Elsevier.

Additional Resources

Diversity RX, Resources on cross-cultural healthcare including translation, interpretation and other issues, [Online]. Available at: www.diversityrx.org

Language Line Services, [Online]. Available at: www.languageline.com

National Council on Interpreting in Health Care, [Online]. Available at: www.ncihc.org

Answers to Self-Study Questions

1. D

2. C

3. B

4. C

Case 2

Regulatory Compliance

CASE STORY

The 53-year-old female patient lives on the same street as the dental hygienist. The dental hygienist has a casual yet cordial relationship with the patient. She comes to the office because of this relationship. During the last appointment the dental hygienist recalls the patient seemed edgy but attributed it to nervousness. Her home-care and oral health status is very good and she has maintained a preventive care visit every six months for the past four years that she has been a patient. The patient relays some major changes during her medical history update. These will have to be documented and reported to the dentist. The changes could have effects on her treatment plans and for patient management protocols.

PROBLEM-BASED LEARNING GOALS AND OBJECTIVES

- Identify practice laws and regulations in state issuing dental hygiene license(s)
- Define the purpose and scope of state Boards of Dentistry
- Identify the risks and consequences of violating statutes and regulations

Medical History

The patient's medical history update now includes a recent diagnosis of schizophrenia and she takes the prescription medication Risperdal (risperidone) daily. She states she wants preventive care as usual but is now too afraid of needles, pain, and all health professionals. Her physician also prescribes Xanax (alprazolam) three times a day for this condition. The dental hygienist's research into these drugs and side effects include increased lightheadedness and possible drying of oral tissues. The patient reports she has not experienced any negative side effects of the medications yet. There are no other significant findings in her health history.

Dental History

The patient's gingiva is a normal pink color. She has been compliant with good homecare and regular preventive care visits. There are no signs of gingival disease. Her chief complaint is her anxiety about the new health diagnosis and having to take medications to be "normal." She also states she only wants female health care providers to treat her. She is relieved to know the dentist will not be in today until the very end of her appointment. There is a chance she will forego routine care because of the diagnosis of schizophrenia coupled with her high anxiety level.

Social History

The patient does not report any social habits that would negatively affect her oral health. Her four cups a day of herbal tea contribute to generalized extrinsic staining. She is a married parent of two children and spends her days providing care for her family.

Dental Hygiene Diagnosis

Problems	Related to Risks and Etiology
Anxiety and fear of treatment and male providers	Medical diagnosis of schizophrenia
Lightheadedness and Generalized staining	Complication of medications and intake of 4 cups of herbal tea daily

Planned Interventions

Clinical	Education/counseling	Oral hygiene instruction
Prophylaxis and polishing	Staining effect from herbal teas	Consume less and use toothpaste with baking soda
Monitor saliva at each appointment	Discuss drying effect of medications	Sip water or use dry mouth rinse
Nitrous oxide analgesia	Less stressful appointments	No residual after effects

Discussion

The state laws where the dental hygienist practices allow the administration of nitrous oxide analgesia and the dental hygienist is certified to do so. This can only be practiced under the direct supervision of a dentist. The dental hygienist fears the patient will not return if not helped to relieve her anxiety as soon as possible. Even though it is taught that nitrous oxide analgesia is contraindicated for patients with severe personality disorders, the patient is a neighbor, and the dental hygienist wants to help her (Wilkins 2009). This consideration is a standard of practice by which dental hygienists are expected to practice. It would be illegal to administer nitrous oxide analgesia without the dentist present in that state yet administering it to someone with a personality disorder may be considered below the standards. The *Standards for Clinical Dental Hygiene Practice* are elements of a document that describe a competent level of dental hygiene care (ADHA 2016). It is provided as a guide for all practitioners to be aware of what dental hygienists are expected to perform and at what level. It is not a law. Yet, if the situation ever became a complaint with a subsequent law suit as a result of the patient experiencing unforeseen reactions, it is likely the dental hygienist would be cited for practicing below the standards of care in addition to administering nitrous oxide before the supervising dentist was on site. That is a legal issue which is practicing outside the scope of practice of the dental hygienist in the state and a violation of law. These violations can be considered civil, criminal, and in some case breaches or violations of both categories of violations (Figure 11.2.1).

Laws come under different categories. One is Civil Law and a breach is against an individual wherein the individual initiates the action. Under Civil Law there is tort and contract. Another category is Criminal Law and this is an act against society or the public and its interest. The government initiates this action. This may include: practicing without a license, and insurance fraud. It can result in being both civil and criminal. Consequences of these actions range from fines to loss of liberty.

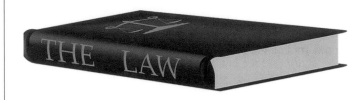

Figure 11.2.1: It is imperative that a dental hygienist is familiar with the laws governing practice.

Under civil law, contract law deals with a legally binding agreement as in services for payment. These agreements are expressed in signatures as obtained for treatment plans. For a breach to occur under contract law a patient's financial or privacy rights have to be violated, or services agreed to were not performed, or the services were delayed for an extended period of time. Under Contract Law a dental hygienist has the duty to be licensed, provide the services by the Standards of Care, obtain informed consent, keep skills current, treat within a reasonable time, refer when necessary, charge reasonable fees, treat within the scope of practice, and keep accurate records. Additional duties include achieving reasonable results, providing patient instruction, informing the patient of unexpected problems, maintaining confidentiality, not abandoning the patient, observing a fiduciary relationship that respects the confidence patients have in one who has superior knowledge and training, and exercise reasonable skill and judgment using evidence-based practice.

Also under Civil Law in addition to Contract Law there is Tort law. Breaches in Tort Law can be intentional or unintentional. They can be breaches in omission or commission. These include negligence (a form of malpractice), assault, battery, defamation (libel and slander) misrepresentation, and breach of privacy.

In the case of negligence, a person is harmed by a professional and it is considered malpractice. Malpractice can be defined as the failure to perform as a reasonably prudent professional would under the same circumstances and the patient is harmed as a result. A dental hygienist may be accused of negligence

Table 11.2.1: Top reasons dental hygienists are sued.

- Failure to update medical history
- Failure to detect oral pathology
- Failure to detect periodontal disease
- Injury to a patient

if harm comes to a patient by not maintaining skills necessary to perform treatment, by neglecting to apply the standards of care, by failure to refer, and other actions that may be considered misconduct. The dental hygienist should practice good risk management by accurate record keeping, documentation, and consents.

Assault is the part of Tort Law wherein a threat is made. Battery is the part of Tort Law wherein there is nonconsensual contact with intent to harm. And lastly, defamation is the part of Tort Law that is a false statement, made to a third person, which harms a person's reputation. It is libel when the statement is conveyed in writing. It is slander when the statement is conveyed orally. *The dental hygienist should remember that criticizing another professional's care can be considered defamation.*

There have been occasions that dental hygienists have been sued. Table 11.2.1 shows the most common reasons.

Laws and regulations exist that in essence define a profession's scope of practice. Every practitioner is responsible for not only knowing these and their limitations but strictly adhering to the parameters they define. There are strict penalties for infractions of scope of practice laws. One can be sued by a patient and/or have charges brought against him/her for practicing another profession without a license. Practicing without competence is also included. These can be considered both civil and criminal acts. A civil offense occurs if a dental hygienist injures a patient by violating the standards, the statutes, and the regulations. This is considered malpractice. When one fails to exercise the degree of care, skill, and learning expected by others acting in the same or similar circumstances, it further defines malpractice (Beemsterboer 2010).

Laws or statutes for health-care practitioners are enacted by both the federal government and the individual states. The regulations accompanying the laws of the state practice acts are defined by boards that oversee each licensed profession. In most states, the dental hygiene profession is under the auspices of a State Board for Dentistry. The members of these boards work to protect the consumer of dental care. The state boards of dentistry's responsibilities include assisting in the licensing rules for practice and for investigating any breaches of these rules. Many have the ability to

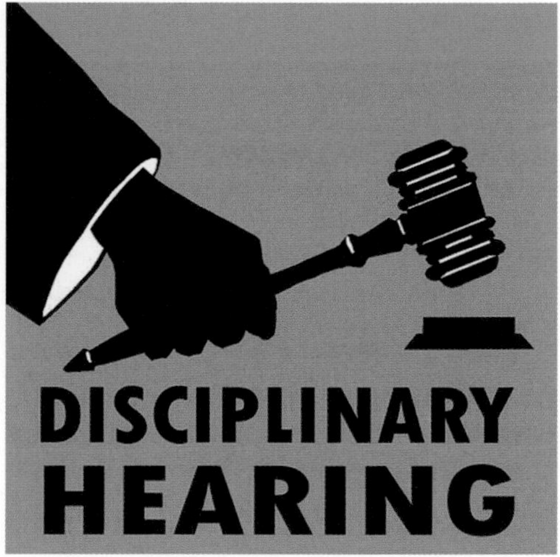

Figure 11.2.2: One way State Boards of Dentistry protect the public is by holding disciplinary hearings.

determine consequences for a licensed dental practitioner from license suspension, revocation, monetary fines, to mandatory remediation or rehabilitation. The regulatory bodies can receive reports from practitioners and the public. It is imperative that a dental hygienist becomes familiar with the laws governing practice. It is imperative to know how the system for reporting and investigations proceed and what consequences can be imposed for failure to comply (Figure 11.2.2).

The top four areas of potential liability and documented cases of dental hygienists being sued include: Failure to update medical history (Glasscoe Waterson 2013). The patient medical history should be updated every time the patient is seen. The dental hygienist should ask if there have been any changes since the last visit. If there are no changes, a note should be made that the patient stated that. On average a complete new medical history should be taken every three years.

Another area for legal action has been failure to detect oral pathology. It is the dental hygienist's responsibility to perform a thorough intraoral/extraoral assessment on every patient. This should not be omitted even in the interest of time.

Dental hygienists are not expected to be able to identify every oral pathology that exists, but hygienists are expected to know when something in the oral cavity is abnormal. If a lesion is detected in the course of an assessment, the hygienist has a responsibility to thoroughly describe the lesion in the patient narrative – color, size, texture, shape – and then to call any pathology to the attention of the dentist. If a persistent oral lesion is identified a referral for a biopsy should be made. Early detection may be key for the patient to get treatment to prevent any cancer from advancing. A patient with a lesion thought to be benign, who much later develops a malignancy and who is not adequately followed, will invariably claim failure to diagnose or delayed diagnosis.

A third reason dental hygienists are sued for is failure to detect periodontal disease. Generally speaking, one way dental hygienists detect periodontal disease is through periodontal probing. In many practice settings hygienists have this as a primary responsibility. The standard of care for periodontal charting is one full-mouth probing at least once per year for every adult patient.

The fourth but not last reason dental hygienists are sued is injury to a patient. Any time during patient care an injury may occur. Instruments have broken and have been aspirated, chemicals have been spilled on patients, and lacerations of soft tissue have occurred. If an accident occurs the patient should be made aware of it and it should be thoroughly documented.

These are some additional reasons that hygienists have been sued:

Not protecting patient privacy/divulging protected patient information;
Practicing outside the scope of legal duties;
Not adhering to standards of care;
Breaching infection control standards;
Failure to ask if the patient has premedicated;
Failure to record thorough documentation;
Failure to identify or take precautions with a medically compromised patient;
Upcoding or incorrectly coding procedures; and
Soliciting patients upon change of employment venue

Take-Home Hints

1. State Boards for Dentistry and Dental Hygiene exist to protect the public.
2. Dental hygienists are bound by the federal, state, and local statutes for practice.
3. Treatment planning must consider side effects and interactions of prescribed and over the counter drugs.
4. Dental hygienists are responsible for providing high levels of professional knowledge, skill, and judgment.

Self-Study Questions

1. Which of the following statements are true? In many states:

A. A State Board for Dentistry or Dental Hygiene exists to protect the public
B. The Standards of Care are part of the practice laws
C. The State Boards may revoke or suspend a license
D. All are true
E. A and C are true

2. Which of the following statements are true? When injury to a patient that should have been avoided occurs:

A. Only the dentist employer is responsible
B. This can be defined as malpractice
C. The dental hygienist is responsible for their actions
D. The State Boards for Dentistry and the legal system are involved
E. A and D are true
F. B, C, and D are true

3. If a dental hygienist performs treatment that is not in the legal limits of his or her jurisdiction, it can be considered:

A. A civil infraction
B. A criminal violation
C. Both a civil and criminal act
D. Neither a civil or criminal act

4. All of the following are true except one. Which one is the exception

A dental hygienist can protect oneself from legal and civil violations by:

A. Managing and maintaining professional competency
B. Being familiar with statutes and regulations in their state for practicing dental hygiene
C. Adhering to the standards of care and code of ethics
D. A and C are true
E. All are true

References

American Dental Hygienists' Association 2016, Standards for clinical dental hygiene practise, [Online]. Available at: http://www.adha.org/resources-docs/2016-Revised-Standards-for-Clinical-Dental-Hygiene-Practice.pdf (May 23, 2018).

Beemsterboer, P. (2010). *Ethics and Law in Dental Hygiene*. St. Louis: Saunders Elsevier.

Glasscoe Waterson, D 2013 Strategies for avoiding malpractice, [Online]. Available at: http://www.rdhmag.com/articles/print/volume-33/issue-11/features/top-reasons-hygienists-are-sued.html (May 23, 2018).

Wilkins, E. (2009). *Clinical Practice of the Dental Hygienist*. Baltimore: Lippincott Williams & Wilkins.

Additional Resources

Dental Hygiene Practice Act Overview: Permitted functions and Supervision Levels by State. Available at: http://www.adha.org/scope-of-practice

State Dental Boards – American Dental Association. Available at: http://www.ada.org/en/education-careers/licensure/licensure-dental-students/state-dental-boards

Answers to Self-Study Questions

1. E

2. F

3. C

4. E

Case 3

Patient and Professional Communication

CASE STORY

A dental hygienist had finally after many oral cancer screenings on all her patients discovered a suspicious lesion. Even the dentist employer agreed that the patient should be referred for a biopsy. There was a sense of pride and accomplishment. The dental hygienist envisioned being the one to save this patient's life by the thoroughness of the examination. It felt so good to apply the knowledge and experience in such a way that it could have a profound effect. An intraoral photograph was taken to show the patient its exact location, size, and color. The dental hygienist was so happy and just had to share with 500 closest and not-so-close friends. Many of these friends were present patients. Using a smartphone, the photo of the lesion was messaged to the group of dental hygiene friends. On a Facebook page the dental hygienist posted it for the rest of the people who were "friends." Both had the caption "last patient of the day made my day and I think I made his."

PROBLEM-BASED LEARNING GOALS AND OBJECTIVES

- Identify protected patient information
- Distinguish between social and professional communications
- Understand the role of incoming and outgoing communication
- Choose appropriate means for sharing professional experiences

Medical History

The patient is a 51-year-old male and has been diagnosed with hypertension and states he complies with medication regimen daily. He sees his physician twice a year and his blood pressure has been controlled through medication for the past six years.

Dental History

His dental visits have been less frequent. His last preventive visit was one year ago. He has posterior amalgam restorations on his maxillary first molars and composite restorations on both first and second molars in the mandible. There are generalized pocket depths of 3 mm and slight bleeding on probing. His biofilm control is fair, as he reports brushing twice a day but uses no aids to remove interproximal biofilm. No new carious lesions appear present.

Social History

The patient is also a recovered alcoholic who states that he has not consumed alcohol in two years since his divorce. He claims he is a light smoker, which for him is a few cigarettes a day. He has an active social life and uses social media to make and meet new friends.

Dental Hygiene Diagnosis

Problems	Related to Risks and Etiology
Generalized gingivitis	Inadequate home care no interproximal biofilm removal
Leukoplakia lesion on tongue	Prior alcoholism and smoking

Planned Interventions

Clinical	Education/Counseling	Oral Hygiene Instruction
Record blood pressure at every appointment	Continue physician recommended regimen	Consult with pharmacist when taking any over-the-counter remedies
Chairside home care demonstration	Biofilm role in gingival disease	Flossing for interproximal biofilm removal
Smoking cessation	Suggest aids and counseling	Explain deleterious effects of alcohol and smoking
Assess and document lesion. Record location, size, color	Importance of referral	Follow recommendation of oral surgeon
Consult with dentist for referral. Take intraoral photograph	Lesion related to social habits	
Document referral		Regularly do self inspections of oral cavity

Discussion

It is difficult to establish the oral effects of alcohol alone but as a mucosal irritant it can have etiologic importance. Persons who consume alcohol as a habit many times do so in conjunction with smoking. This trauma to the tissues can be extremely important in the etiology of oral cancer and the presence of leukoplakia. These habits are also associated with increased risk for other oral diseases such as caries and periodontitis. It is imperative for the dental hygienist to inform patients of this relationship and recommend cessation options. Professional communication with the patient must exhibit the principle of veracity. Veracity is communicating the truth and is expected between the patient and the health-care provider and anyone else the patient may deem privileged to their information.

The private information of any patient is protected by law. The dental hygienist must communicate to the patient that his social habits may be contributing and exacerbating factors for his oral health and now for the appearance of a suspicious lesion (Shafer et al. 1983).

Patients have privacy and confidentiality rights afforded to them by the Health Insurance Portability and Accountability Act of 1996 (HIPAA). Individually identifiable health information is information, including demographic data, that relates to: the individual's past, present, or future physical or mental health or condition, the provision of health care to the individual, or the past, present, or future payment for the provision of health care to the individual, and that identifies the individual or for which there is a reasonable basis to believe it can be used to identify the individual. Individually identifiable health information includes many common identifiers (e.g., name, address, birth date, Social Security Number) (USDHH 2016).

Confidentiality must be maintained by the health-care provider and no information can be released without the patient's consent or otherwise noted in public health laws. Information must be respected by the professional in both health-care and social settings (Figure 11.3.1). The American Dental Hygienists' Association states in its Code of Ethics that "we respect the confidentiality of client information and relationships as a demonstration of the value we place on individual autonomy" (ADHA 2016). Communication today has a wealth of options. Face-to-face communication has been lessened by technology. The telephone, email, text, Twitter, Instagram, and the use of social networking sites are common modalities of communication. These have become acceptable means of messaging. Friends and family, professionals, employers, employees, health providers, insurance carriers, and patients use these means on a daily basis. It is the patient's choice to post private and public information not the health-care provider's choice.

Health-care providers must respect the confidentiality of client information and relationships. Information that is shared from patients becomes part of their health record and cannot be shared with other parties not directly involved with their care.

Patients expect their medical and other health information to be private and should be protected. A breach of patient privacy and confidentiality of records was committed in this case story. The dental hygienist communicated possible identifiable protected information with patients and others via a social network. A social network is not a forum for professional communication. It is conceivable that one can determine who the male, last patient of the day, was. It is conceivable that the patient could be made aware of the post and see this breach. There are situations wherein a case may be presented and discussed in the professional community. Cases may be shared in a professional publication and as examples in educational presentations. Even then identifiable information should be anonymized.

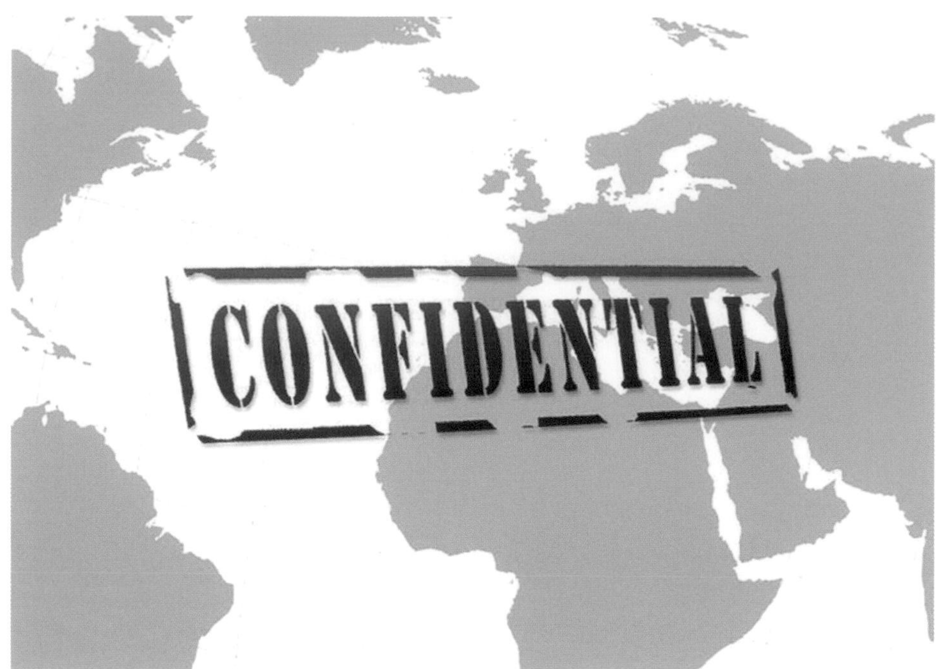

Figure 11.3.1: HIPAA protects patients' personal information from being shared to unauthorized entities.

To maintain professionalism, all professionals should strive to maintain the public's trust in the profession. All professionals act within certain boundaries. They are professional boundaries. There are rules and codes that help one to clarify what is acceptable professionally and what are social relationships. Yet the professional faces daily challenges to keep those boundaries. Social networking and other electronic media are means of communication that can present these challenges and threaten the ability to maintain those boundaries. As a result, there are more and more opportunities and instances of lapses in professional judgment. Professionals must become aware and concerned about the possible ramifications of sharing certain information. Communication is a means to transmit information. In dentistry, as in other professions, communication takes on different forms. Much information exists about verbal and nonverbal communication. Even listening can be a form of communication. The dental hygienist is also obligated to communicate in a manner that includes intercultural considerations. Nonverbal communication is complicated and inconsistent. It can be unintentional and easily misunderstood (Adams 2011).

Theories abound as to what a person is "saying" and feeling in body language. Even the ubiquitous smile, which can be universally understood to promote content, friendliness, and happiness, can be faked. Appearance is also a form of communication. The first impression one gets through personal and office appearance is usually a lasting one.

Dental hygienists treat diverse patients from nearly every cultural background in the world. This would make it impossible to know all verbal, nonverbal, and norms associated with each one. The dental hygienist is obliged to become aware that the cultural norms in one society may be completely different in another. They must learn to respect those differences, and treat and communicate in a nonjudgmental and respectful way. There is research to read, courses to take, and experience to gain in the realm of intercultural communication. Studying is a way to gain understanding. In the professional/patient scenario it is appropriate to ask a patient if there are cultural boundaries a dental hygienist may not be aware of. It is appropriate to ask about touching when one is used to handshaking. It is a mistake to assume everyone has the same rules and then judge others on the basis of that assumption (Adams 2011).

In verbal communication, the dental hygienist must keep in mind that patients will have different levels of literacy: literacy in language and/or health literacy. It is important to become familiar with plain language to accommodate a patient's lack of literacy in both. This is crucial especially when explaining a diagnosis and when giving instructions for patients to follow. Miscommunication can bring about untoward consequences and result in injury. Information and instructions can be communicated in writing or depicted in print or video. This is especially important when a patient has limited language proficiency in the hygienist's language choice.

In personal social media communication, dental hygienists should be aware that employers frequently visit social pages of potential and present employees. These ramifications can have dire consequences for their positions, working lives, and even their license to practice.

As an aide to help keep the boundaries, professionals should utilize options for privacy. The Facebook network offers its users options for privacy settings. Profiles that do not have privacy limits allow a "friend" to access personal photo albums that contain information about one's children, spouse, family, lifestyle, and other groups they may belong to. The privacy settings limit access to the user's profile. Open access to one's profiles is not typical of a health professional–patient relationship. Others can easily search a name and unintended information can be accessed into the future. Friends can easily copy a post or picture and forward it on and on out of the control of the person who posted the information. Other aides to keep professionalism in social media can be presented as a list of dos and don'ts. Do pause before posting and think of the ramifications of the post. Do use correct and appropriate language, spelling, and grammar. Be mindful of offensive or harassing words. Don't complain about current or past employers, current or past patients, or the trivia faced daily. Don't relate overly opinionated ideas. Share opinions tactfully especially issues about religion and politics. Don't post inappropriate images (Ruesink 2014).

In a positive way social networks can have a dental hygienist become familiar with the patient's family, and interests and this is being social but these are the types of "friends" that should not have access to all of a dental hygienist's information. So some information is taken not given. It is good practice to minimize risk of legal actions and putting a professional career in jeopardy. It is expected that the dental hygienist has concerns and be cognizant of who is "friended" or who they invite to be "friends." The dental hygienist should keep personal and professional relationships separate. One has to think first and be mindful of crossing any of the boundaries. There is no list available of what is acceptable information to share, yet professionals must determine what is acceptable and balance what is revealed to maintain the public's trust and to protect the public they serve. Even a single lapse in judgment by a dental hygienist to create unprofessional content online can reflect poorly on not only themselves but on the entire profession. Social media can be an opportunity to educate the public about oral health and the profession

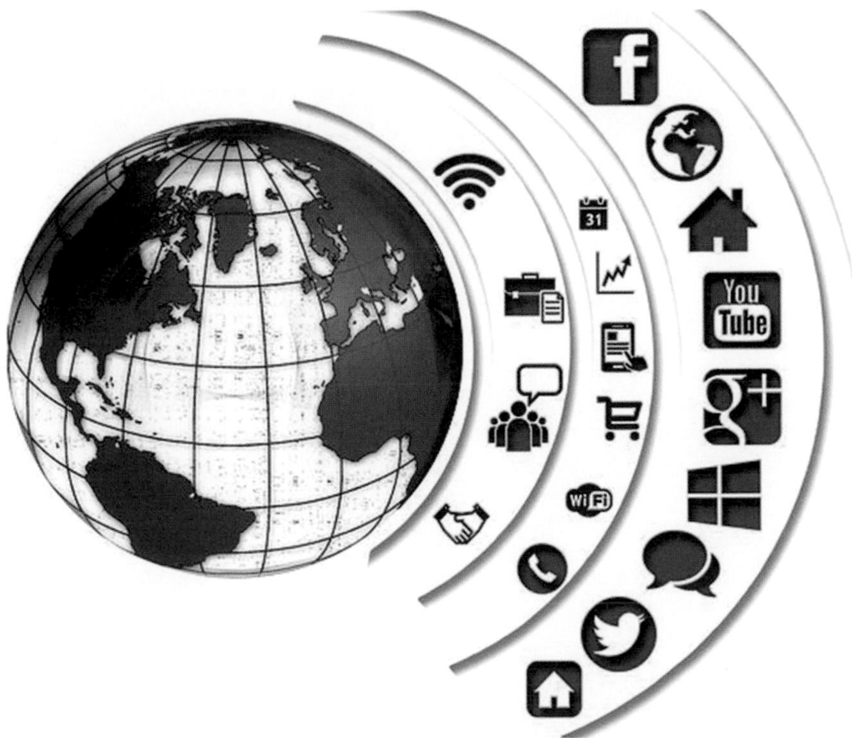

Figure 11.3.2: Dental hygienists must be aware of the pros and cons of all social media.

of dental hygiene. It can be a means to gain professional exposure and putting the professional in a good light. Many professionals use the network LinkedIn to expose themselves to others with the revelations of skills, experience, and expertise. All social media has a potential to raise the respect for oneself and one's profession. Encourage colleagues to become aware of the pros and cons of using social media (Figure 11.3.2).

Take-Home Hints

1. When counseling patients about smoking cessation use the ADHA's "ask, advise, refer" paradigm without personal judgment.
2. Record any atypical lesions for possible referral and follow up.
3. Confidentiality of patient information is to be respected as a demonstration of the value placed on individual autonomy.
4. Accept the obligation to tell the truth and expect others will do the same. Seek truth and honesty in all relationships.
5. Keep social and professional communications separate and abide by the legal requirements for confidentiality.
6. Become cognizant of different forms of communication, their positives and negatives in the context of cultural sensitivity.

Self-Study Questions

1. Which of the following statements is true?
- **A. The confidentiality of patient records is protected by law**
- **B. A patient can give consent to tell others on social media**
- **C. A health-care provider can share a case if the patient's name is not revealed**
- **D. Always using professional language with patients is the way to increase patient literacy**
- **E. A and B**
- **F. All are correct**

2. HIPAA and the ADHA Code of Ethics are in conflict with each other concerning veracity and confidentiality.
- **A. True**
- **B. False**

3. Which of the following demonstrates how the dental hygienist breached the patient's right to confidentiality?
- **A. She told her employer dentist**
- **B. She will communicate with the oral surgeon**
- **C. She posted information that may identify the patient**

References

Adams, T. (2011). *Dental Communication Brief Book Series*: Book 2, 3, 4. Rocklin, CA: Odontocomm Productions.

American Dental Hygienists' Association 2016, Code of Ethics, [Online]. Available at: https://www.adha.org/resources-docs/7611_Bylaws_and_Code_of_Ethics.pdf (May 23, 2018).

Ruesink, M 2014. Social Media Do's and Don'ts: 10 tips for keeping your profiles professional, [Online]. Available at: http://www.rasmussen.edu/student-life/blogs/main/guide-to-soc-media-dos-and-donts/ (May 23, 2018).

Shafer, W., Hine, M., and Levy, B. (1983). *A Textbook of Oral Pathology*, 94–98. Philadelphia, PA: Saunders.

US Department of Health and Human Services. 2016. HIPAA for professionals, [Online]. Available at: http://www.hhs.gov/hipaa/for-professionals (May 23, 2018).

Additional Resources

ADHA Smoking Initiative: www.askadviserefer.org
HIPAA enforcement: http://www.hhs.gov/ocr/hipaa
HIPAA and mental health: http://www.hhs.gov/ocr/privacy/hipaa/understanding/special/mhguidance.html
Health Privacy Project: www.healthprivacy.org
Makely, S. (2000). *The Health Care Worker's Primer on Professionalism*. Upper Saddle River, NJ: Brady/Prentiss Hall.

Answers to Self-Study Questions

1. E

2. B

3. C

12

Community and Oral Health Promotion

Clinical Cases in Dental Hygiene, First Edition. Edited by Cheryl M. Westphal Theile, Mea A. Weinberg and Stuart L. Segelnick.

Case 1

Participating in Community Programs

CASE STORY

The dental hygienists from the local component were contacted after Palomar Hospital was awarded a grant to assess the oral health needs and plan an education program for the senior population who regularly visit the health education center (see Figure 12.1.1A). The hospital has many different programs for health education and disease prevention that are targeted at the senior population. The health education director informed the dental hygienists that the patients would like to know more about oral health. It was assumed the needs of the target population would be more education in denture care. The dental hygienists conducted a needs assessment survey (see Figure 12.1.1B). They developed a questionnaire utilizing closed-ended questions with a Likert scale response with only two open-ended questions for a more in-depth discussion. To ensure collection of detailed information and a wide range of respondents that would represent the target population, it was decided to conduct the survey as a face-to-face interview (see Figure 12.1.1C). The results from the survey revealed a strong interest in information about the prevention of xerostomia and more education about implant care. The seniors also reported that holding small groups rather than a large lecture would be the preferred method in delivering the information on oral health promotion. The dental hygienists developed a plan to meet the needs of the targeted senior population.

(A)

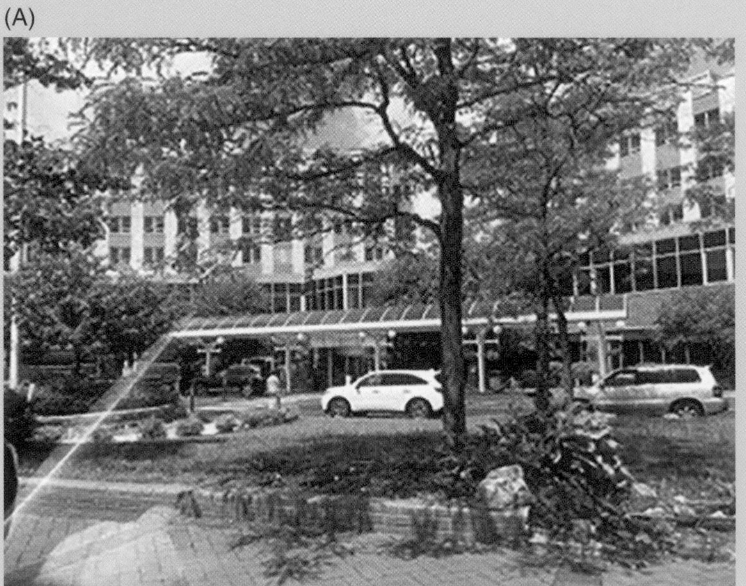

(B)

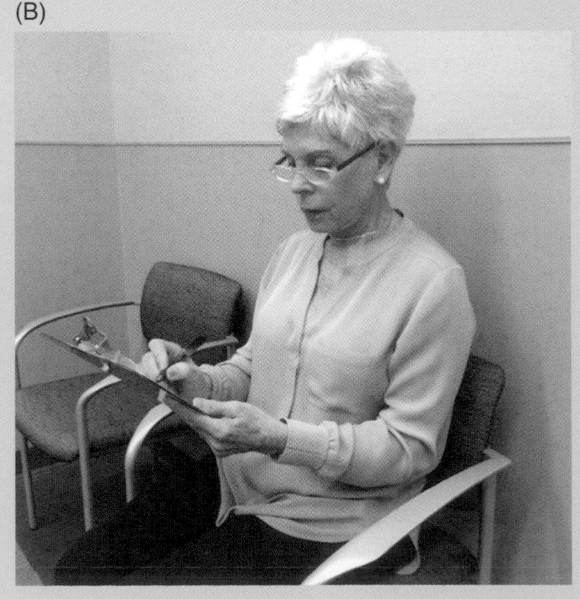

Figure 12.1.1: (A) Hospital setting. (B) Patient completing needs assessment. (C) Dental hygienist conducting face to face interview. (D) Dental hygiene process of care. (E) Dental hygiene program planning paradigm.

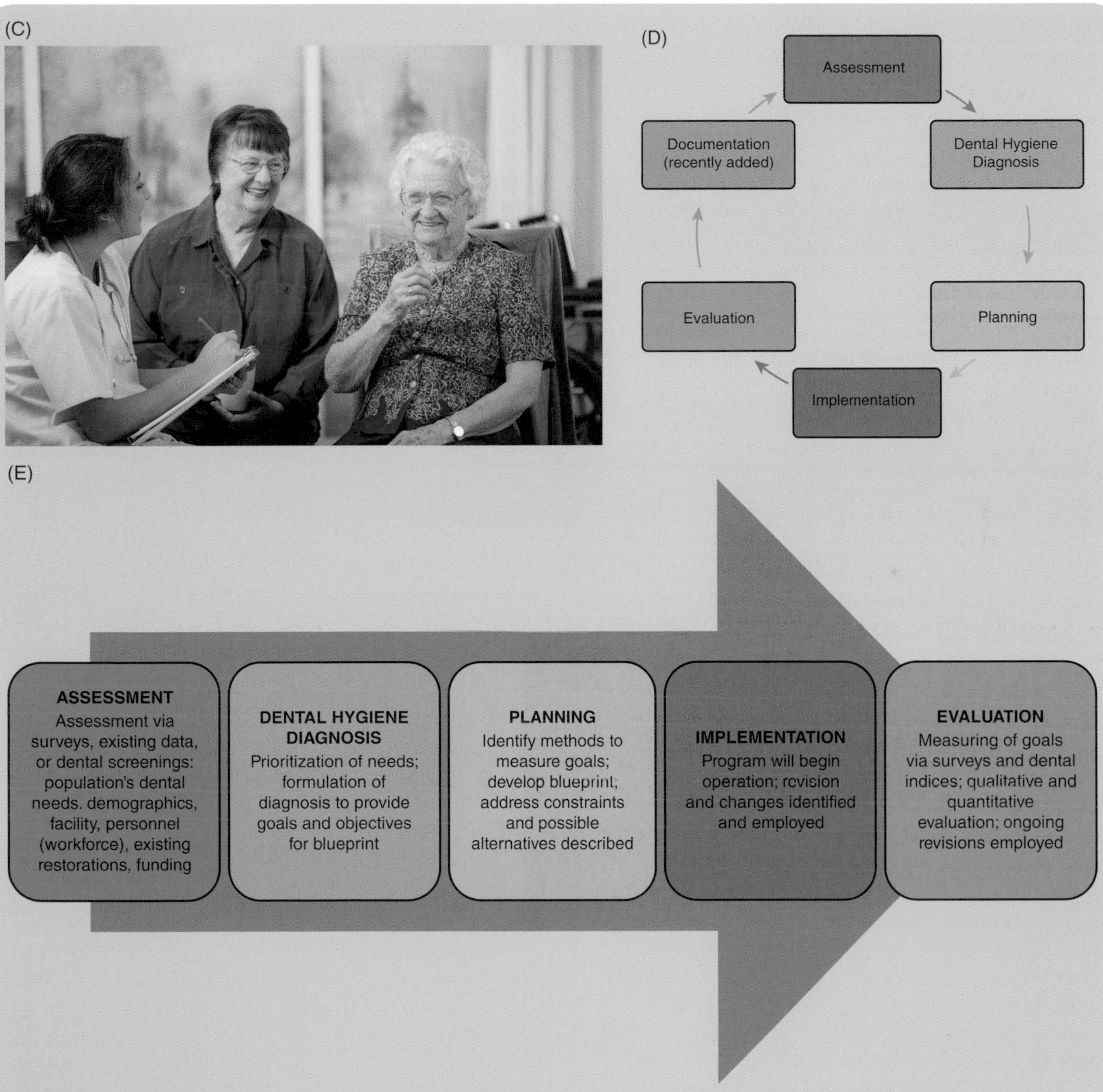

(C)

(D)

Assessment

Dental Hygiene Diagnosis

Planning

Implementation

Evaluation

Documentation (recently added)

(E)

ASSESSMENT
Assessment via surveys, existing data, or dental screenings: population's dental needs. demographics, facility, personnel (workforce), existing restorations, funding

DENTAL HYGIENE DIAGNOSIS
Prioritization of needs; formulation of diagnosis to provide goals and objectives for blueprint

PLANNING
Identify methods to measure goals; develop blueprint; address constraints and possible alternatives described

IMPLEMENTATION
Program will begin operation; revision and changes identified and employed

EVALUATION
Measuring of goals via surveys and dental indices; qualitative and quantitative evaluation; ongoing revisions employed

Figure 12.1.1: (Continued)

PROBLEM-BASED LEARNING GOALS AND OBJECTIVES

- Explain the structure and steps of the Dental Hygiene Program Paradigm
- Distinguish appropriate data collection survey methods in assessing community needs
- Differentiate between closed- and open-ended questions

Discussion

Note the dental hygiene process of care and dental hygiene program planning paradigm are similar in that they are both a structured process for dental hygienists to follow when caring for an individual or group. Both consist of steps that include: assessment of the situation, formulation of a dental hygiene diagnosis, planning the program, putting the plan into action, and evaluation (see Figure 12.1.1D and E, and Table 12.1.1).

Table 12.1.1: Patient care vs. community health programs.

Stage	Patient Care	Community Health Programs
Assessment	Conducts a health assessment and comprehensive oral examination of individual patient to identify oral and general health status based on patient problems, needs, and strengths	Conducts a needs assessment of target population to analyze needs, interests, abilities, and resources
Dental hygiene diagnosis	Formulate conclusions about the patient's dental hygiene needs based on all available assessment data and evidence in the literature	Formulate findings from assessment and prioritize needs
Planning	Develop a dental hygiene care plan with realistic goals and outcomes based on patient needs, expectations, values, and current scientific evidence to plan dental hygiene interventions Select appropriate interventions to implement plan	Develop a program based on the analysis of needs assessment data, priorities, and alternatives; community interaction; and resources available for which measureable assessment mechanisms are used Select appropriate resources to implement program
Implementation	Implement dental hygiene care plan while minimizing risk and optimizing oral health	Implement self-generated treatment plan effectively
Evaluation	Review and assess outcomes of dental hygiene care via dental, gingival, and periodontal evaluations, modifying plan when necessary	Review and assess program outcomes via index and community evaluations, modifying plan when necessary
Documentation	Document all collected data, interventions planned and provided, recommendations, and other information relevant to patient care and treatment	Document all data gathered throughout all stages

Source: Adapted from Darby and Walsh (2015); Nathe (2017).

Data collection is the gathering of information that the community can use to make decisions and set priorities. Different types of data are necessary to make certain that a complete assessment accurately describes the factors influencing the health of the community. Community health assessment efforts can evaluate determinants of health needs, assess needs, and assets, quantify disparities, and inequalities among population groups, measure preventable disease, injury, disability, and death (Geurink 2012, p. 64).

Assumptions should not be made of a population's needs. A need is a gap between what the current condition is and what it should be. It can be defined as a judgment based on professional knowledge, skill, and experience as to the amount and kind of health-care services required to attain or maintain health (Nathe 2017, p. 41). A needs assessment is required to provide the evidence that will guide the development of appropriate program planning. It provides a systematic method to determine needs, identify related cause(s), and priorities for future interventions. A needs assessment has the ability to identify health-care situations regarded as unwelcome or harmful and needing to be dealt with and overcome within the community. The assessment provides information not only about the issues but about the community (Geurink 2012). Assessment is a core public health function and dental hygienists involved in public health practice must be proficient in the various aspects of oral health assessment. This is an integral component of a community oral health improvement process. Information gained form a community assessment can be used to plan, implement, and evaluate oral health improvement strategies.

A survey is a method of collecting information to determine the views of the target group. The assessment survey to evaluate community needs may be conducted in a variety of forms, such as interviews, questionnaires, or indices. The method chosen depends on the scope of the intention and available resources. Methods include: face-to-face interviews, phone interviews, direct mailers, email questionnaire, focus groups, indices, and multiple methods of distribution. The appropriate data collection survey approach should be determined. Interviews and questionnaires provide measurement of knowledge, attitudes, and values related to health and disease (Nathe 2017, p. 200). Interviews involve direct verbal questioning of participants and questionnaires are simple to administer when a large amount of data is needed. Interviews may be more time consuming than questionnaires, but assures more adequate responses. A dental index is a standardized quantitative method for measuring, scoring, and analyzing oral conditions in individuals and groups (Nathe 2017, p. 166).

Closed-ended questions are those that may be answered with a single word or a short phrase, while open-ended questions are those that require more thought and a longer answer. Closed-ended questions may be dichotomous, multiple choice, or scaled questions. The Likert scale is the most widely used rating scale to measure responses and survey research. It is an ordered scale from which respondents choose one option that best aligns with their views. A typical scale might be "Strongly agree, Agree, Neutral, Disagree, Strongly disagree" (CDC 2012). Open-ended questions have no predefined options or categories.

After the needs assessment is completed and the data has been evaluated, the dental hygienists began the planning by determining the goals and objectives for the program. A plan for community-based interventions consists of strategies that will be implemented. Planning is an organized response to a community's established need to reduce or eliminate one or more problems. A course of action is developed from the diagnosis. Developing goals, objectives, and program activities is part of the planning process. During this stage, it is essential to have community involvement and participation by community leaders, stakeholders, health group representatives, foundation leaders, government agencies, and all dental hygiene and dental associations (Geurink 2012).

Implementation is the step defined as the process of putting the plan and activities into action (Beatty 2017). Personnel, equipment, resources, supplies, and preliminary progress toward program goals are monitored. Many community oral health programs commence on a smaller scale – short term. This is referred to as a pilot testing or a pilot program. This provides information and allows for future decisions to be made that would work in practice.

Evaluation is continuous and measurements of the program's intended outcomes determine if the population's needs were met or if revisions are needed. A successful program meets its goals and objectives. Evaluation is a mandatory phase of all types of community programs. Although it is the final step of the program or community health improvement plan, formal, and informal evaluation results are reported regularly as this phase is ongoing and involves constant feedback and interaction. Program evaluation is a systematic method for collecting, analyzing, and using information to answer questions about community health programs. During this stage of the process, the results of the program are measured against the goals and objectives developed during planning. This is summative evaluation (Beatty 2017). Formative evaluation or process evaluation takes place before or during a project's implementation with the goal of improving the project (Beatty 2017). This type of evaluation allows for better understanding of the process of change or continual improvement. The dental hygienist can improve future design and implementation.

Take-Home Hints

1. If you are unfamiliar with the target population, always begin with a needs assessment.
2. Closed-ended questions are time-efficient, but make sure to not ask for simplistic responses to a complex issue when an open-ended question is more appropriate.

Self-Study Questions

1. What would one of the first steps be in planning this community program?
- **A. Arranging a time for an in-service session with the community staff and health education director**
- **B. Planning an educational session for the older adults**
- **C. Arranging a meeting with the director and seniors involved to assess the needs and determine goals and objectives for the program**
- **D. Determine which seniors have dentures**

2. When collecting data, the advantage of using the interview technique over a questionnaire is that the interview technique:
- **A. Is less time consuming**
- **B. Can reach a broader population**
- **C. Is less expensive**
- **D. Assures more adequate responses**

3. If the dental hygienists had a limited amount of time to determine areas of interest and dental knowledge for the older adults, one efficient tool to evaluate the group's knowledge would be a(an):
- **A. Look at past activities**
- **B. Questionnaire**
- **C. Intraoral examination**
- **D. Interview**

4. After which step are the program goals and objectives formulated?
- **A. Analyzing assessment results**
- **B. Initial meeting with the health education director**
- **C. Program evaluation**
- **D. Creating the survey questions**

5. Some of the survey questions the dental hygienists asked involved responses such as strongly agree, agree, neutral, disagree, and strongly disagree. What type of question requires this type of response?
- **A. Open-ended question**
- **B. Closed-ended question**
- **C. Likert scale**
- **D. Interview**

6. The face-to-face interview is conducted in which phase of the program planning paradigm?
- **A. Assessment**
- **B. Diagnosis**
- **C. Planning**
- **D. Implementation**
- **E. Evaluation**

References

Beatty, C.F. (2017). *Community Oral Health Practice for the Dental Hygienist*, 4e. St. Louis, MO: Elsevier.

CDC (2012) *CDC coffee break: Using Likert scales in evaluation survey work*, [Online]. Available at: https://www.cdc.gov/dhdsp/pubs/docs/cb_february_14_2012.pdf (July 19, 2016).

Darby, M.L. and Walsh, M.M. (2015). *Dental Hygiene Theory and Practice*, 4e. St. Louis, MO: Saunders.

Geurink, K.V. (2012). *Community Oral Health Practice for the Dental Hygienist*, 3e. St. Louis, MO: Elsevier.

Nathe, C.N. (2005). *Dental Public Health & Research: Contemporary Practice for the Dental Hygienist*, 2e. Upper Saddle River, NJ: Prentice Hall.

Nathe, C.N. (2017). *Dental Public Health & Research: Contemporary Practice for the Dental Hygienist*, 4e. Boston: Pearson.

Additional Resources

Altarium Institute (2012) *Recommendations to promote health and well-being among aging populations: Prepared for trust for America's health*, [Online]. Available at: http://healthyamericans.org/assets/files/Prevention%20Recommendations%20for%20Aging%20Populations2.pdf (September 11, 2016).

National Council on Aging (n.d.) *Healthy aging fact sheet*, [Online]. Available at: https://www.ncoa.org/news/resources-for-reporters/get-the-facts/healthy-aging-facts (June 3, 2018).

Work Group for Community Health and Development at the University of Kansas (2016) *Community tool box*, [Online]. Available at: http://ctb.ku.edu/en/toolkits (July 19, 2016).

Answers to Self-Study Questions

1. C

2. D

3. B

4. A

5. C

6. A

Case 2

Promoting Health and Preventing Disease within Groups

CASE STORY

The dental hygienists that are members of a local component have been awarded funds by the regional dental society to conduct research with the purpose of determining and implementing the most effective and efficient caries prevention options to meet the needs of the children at New East Elementary School. There are 182 children ranging from first to sixth grade (see Figure 12.2.1A). The target elementary school is located in a nonfluoridated, rural community that has limited access to dental health care (see Figure 12.2.1B). However, there is a school nurse that is responsible for all students. The closest dental office is located 45 minutes away from New East Township and there is no public transportation available. The one local dentist volunteered on a limited basis to accompany the dental hygienists to the elementary school during this research. He informed the dental hygienists that members of this community often come to his dental office for restorative or emergency treatment, not for prevention. Water in the community contains less than 0.1 ppm natural fluoride. Five years ago, water fluoridation was sent to legislation, but it was defeated. After a conversation with the school nurse, the dental hygienists were told the referendum had failed due to the lack of education of the community on the benefits

(A)

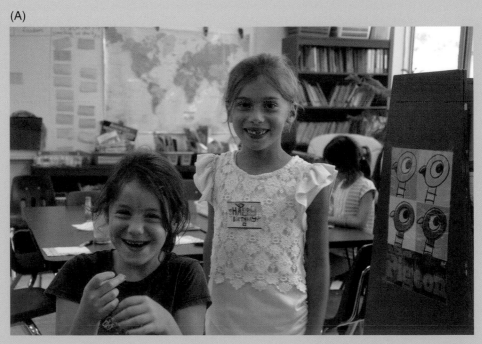

Figure 12.2.1: (A) Children in elementary school. (B) Elementary school setting. (C) Children with signs of demineralization. *Source:* Courtesy of Travis Nelson. (D) Variety of fluoride varnish products.

of fluoride and lack of awareness of other preventive modalities. A survey went home with each child to have the parents complete and give consent to an oral examination for initial assessment. The results of the survey showed a lack of knowledge in oral health and disease prevention. Of the parents, 98% provided consent for their children to participate in the screening. The dental hygienists conducted decayed/missing/filled teeth (DMFT)/dmft indices on the children to determine their current oral health status. This showed a high rate of decayed teeth on the older children and the dental hygienists noticed a prevalence of demineralized teeth on children of all ages (see Figure 12.2.1C). After compiling results of the assessment data, it was determined that a fluoride varnish program would be the most efficient and effective method of preventing decay, which was affordable by the program (see Figure 12.2.1D). The dental hygienists will also be placed on the agenda at the parent-teacher organization meeting in October for Children's Dental Health Month and in April for the school-wide health fair. The dental hygienists will train the school nurse to support teachers in the inclusion of classroom oral health education. At the conclusion of this program, 178 students were examined and varnish was placed as needed. A year later, the dental hygienists wanted to evaluate the effectiveness of the varnish and education program and the hygienists decided they would conduct another DMFT/dmft index. They found a decrease in decay rate by 26%, filled rate increased by 13%, and noticed a decrease in demineralization.

(B)

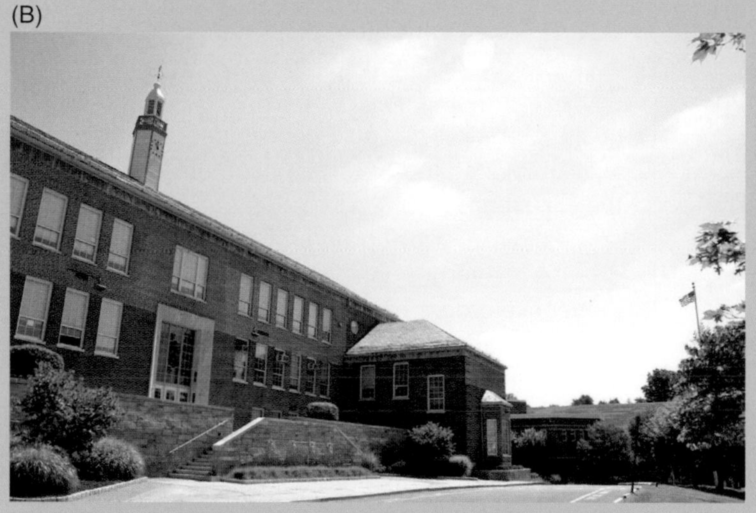

(C)

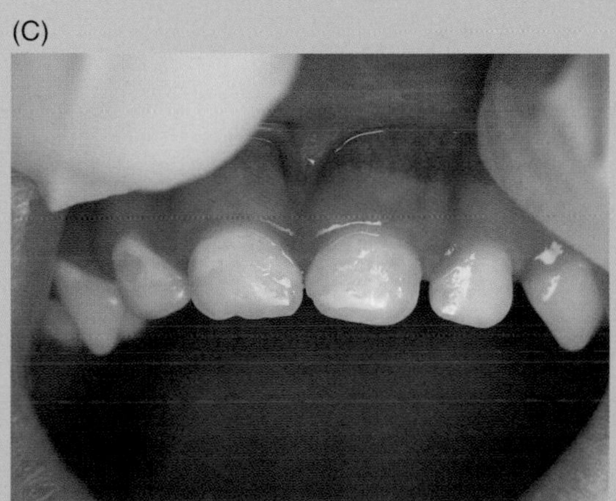

(D)

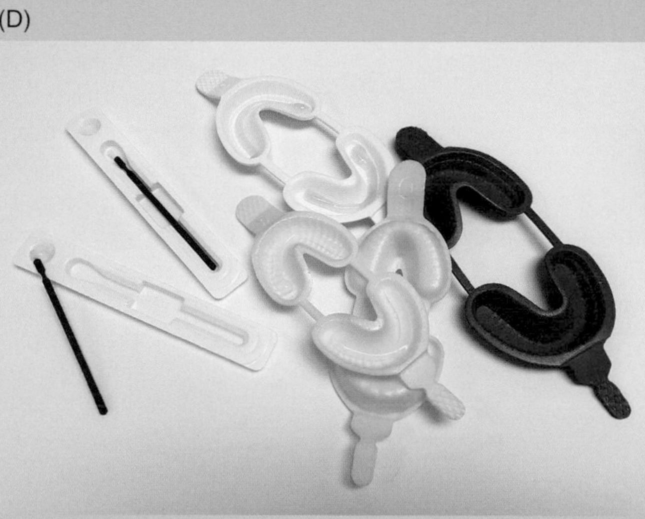

Figure 12.2.1: (Continued)

PROBLEM-BASED LEARNING GOALS AND OBJECTIVES

- Explain the three levels of disease prevention
- Identify possible barriers to dental health care
- Describe the evaluation of dental health programs in the dental hygiene program planning paradigm
- Differentiate between qualitative and quantitative methods and data
- Describe the use and purpose of indices in community programs

Discussion

Public health focuses on the prevention of disease. Three levels of disease prevention have been identified: primary, secondary, and tertiary (Mason 2010, p. 112). Primary prevention is the intervention in disease before it occurs. Examples of primary preventive interventions include community water fluoridation, fluoride varnish, pit and fissure sealants, and preventive education. Secondary prevention is the treatment or control of disease early in the process. Remineralization of early caries and periodontal debridement are examples of secondary prevention methods. Tertiary prevention involves strategies to replace lost tissues through rehabilitation to restore the functions of the oral cavity to as close to normal as possible. An example is the replacement of a missing tooth with an implant.

Preventive oral health services are essential in maintaining the dental health needs of the population. However, there are many barriers that should be considered when providing these services. Examples of major factors that prevent or deter the population from gaining access to care are the following (Darby and Walsh 2015; Nathe 2017):

1. Financial barriers – unaffordable costs, no spendable income, cannot afford time off if an hourly paying job.
2. Transportation – public transportation is often unreliable, unaffordable, nonexistent, and confusing. Homebound, hospitalized, or institutionalized clients frequently cannot be transported for care.
3. Psychological barriers – fear or inability to comprehend dental procedures, feelings of anxiety, low pain tolerance.
4. Special needs – needs to rely on others for transportation or care impact scheduling and compliance; sensory and physical impairments.
5. Geographic barriers – shortages of providers in rural areas, regional maldistribution of health-care personnel.
6. Physical facilities – nowhere to park safely, too many stairs, narrow doors, and entryways, bathrooms without grab bars, dimly lit hallways, and small signage, and inconvenient office hours.
7. Cultural diversity/influences – based on cultural, family, and individual beliefs patients will have different orientations toward health; language barriers.

School-based oral health programs are designed to improve access to dental care by reducing barriers. Barriers that may be reduced may include parents taking time off of work to take their child to the dentist during the day, children missing classroom time for dental visits, dealing with limited access to oral care in rural communities, and lack of reliable transportation (MCOH 2011). All children and often parents can benefit from children receiving oral health screenings in school, which is a familiar, nonthreatening environment. Services that are typically performed in this setting include dental education, oral screenings, fluoride applications, sealant placement, and referral for follow up treatment if needed (MCOH 2011). School-based health programs can also be included in the curriculum in all grades so teachers can incorporate oral health into the classroom.

Health preventive programs are created to prevent disease in a target population (Nathe 2005, p. 171). Preventive programs may occur in a wide range of settings in addition to schools, such as communities and health-care facilities. Dental health programs that involve dental hygienists have included oral health education programs to provide dental health tools to large populations, use of fluoride to prevent caries, dental sealants, athletic mouth guards, nutritional advising, and provision of other preventive services to large populations of need. Regardless of the preventive program designed, the program planning paradigm must be considered to be able to address the specific needs of the target population and available evidence-based resources.

The dental hygiene program planning paradigm is similar to the dental hygiene process of care consisting of the same steps: assessment of the situation, formulation of a dental hygiene diagnosis, planning the program, putting the plan into action, and evaluation. During the evaluation stage in the program planning paradigm, the results of the program are measured against the objectives developed during planning. Evaluation is ongoing throughout the program and upon its completion. The dental provider uses scientific techniques to discern the program effectiveness. A combination of quantitative and qualitative methods

Table 12.2.1: Indices and purposes.

Indices that measure *oral hygiene status* to determine daily oral care and monitor results of oral hygiene education programs.

Index	***Purpose***
Biofilm Index (also known as Pl I)	To assess the thickness of plaque biofilm at the gingival area.
Biofilm Control Record (also known as plaque control record)	To record the presence of plaque biofilm on individual tooth surfaces to permit the patient to visualize progress while learning biofilm control.
Biofilm-Free Score (also known as plaque-free score)	To determine the location, number, and percentage of biofilm-free surfaces for individual motivation and instruction. Interdental bleeding can also be documented.
Patient Hygiene Performance (PHP)	To assess the extent of plaque biofilm and debris over a tooth surface.
Simplified Oral Hygiene Index (OHI-S)	To assess oral cleanliness by estimating tooth surface covered with debris and/or calculus.

Indices that measure *gingival and periodontal health* to assess need for treatment, treatment success or treatment failure.

Index	***Purpose***
Community Periodontal Index (CPI)	To screen and monitor the periodontal status of populations. Later modified to form the PSR index for scoring individual patients.
Periodontal Screening and Recording (PSR)	To assess the state of periodontal health of an individual patient. Designed to indicate periodontal status in a rapid and effective manner and motivate the patient to seek necessary complete periodontal assessment and treatment. Used as a screening procedure to determine the need for comprehensive periodontal evaluation.
Sulcus Bleeding Index (SBI)	To locate areas of gingival sulcus bleeding and color changes in order to recognize and record the presence of early (initial) inflammatory gingival disease.
Gingival Bleeding Index	To record the presence or absence of gingival inflammation as determined by bleeding from interproximal gingival sulci.
Eastman Interdental Bleeding Index (EIBI)	To assess the presence of inflammation in the interdental area as indicated by the presence or absence of bleeding.
Gingival Index (GI)	To assess the severity of gingivitis based on color, consistency, and bleeding upon probing.

Indices that measure *dental caries* to determine number of persons in any age group who are affected by dental caries, the number of teeth that need treatment, or the portion of teeth that have been treated.

Index	***Purpose***
Permanent Dentition: Decayed, Missing, and Filled Teeth (DMFT) or Surfaces (DMFS)	To determine total dental caries experience, past, and present, by recording either the number of affected teeth or tooth surfaces.
Primary Dentition: Decayed, indicated for Extraction, and Filled (df and def)	To determine the dental caries experience for the primary teeth present in the oral cavity by evaluating teeth or surfaces.
Primary Dentition: Decayed, Missing, and Filled (dmf)	To determine caries experience for children. Only primary teeth are evaluated.
Early Childhood Caries (ECC and S-ECC)	To provide case definitions that determine dental caries experience of children aged five years of age or younger.
Root Caries Index (RCI)	To determine total root caries experience for individuals and groups and provide a direct, simple method for recording and making comparisons.

Indices that measure *dental fluorosis* to investigate the effects of fluoride concentration on dental enamel.

Index	***Purpose***
Dean's Fluorosis Index	To measure the prevalence and severity of dental fluorosis.
Tooth Surface Index of Fluorosis (TSIF)	To measure the prevalence and severity of dental fluorosis. More sensitive than Dean's Fluorosis Index in identifying mildest signs of fluorosis.

Indices that are *community oral health screenings* to monitor health status and determine population access to or need for oral health services.

Index	***Purpose***
WHO Basic Screening Survey (BSS)	To collect comprehensive data on oral health status and dental treatment needs of a population. Suitable for surveying both adults and children.
Association of State and Territorial Dental Directors (ASTDD) Basic Screening Survey (BSS)	To screen adult, school age, and/or preschool populations for a variety of categories (untreated caries, treated decay missing, sealants, treatment urgency, dentures, number of natural teeth, root fragments, need for periodontal care, suspicious soft tissue lesions).

Source: Adapted from Wilkins et al. (2017).

should be used to measure if objectives were met (Kaur 2016). Quantitative methods are based on numbers to claim objectivity; whereas, qualitative methods generate theories relying on subjectivity (Kaur 2016, p. 94). Quantitative data is precise and qualitative data is descriptive.

To aid in assessment and evaluation by providing quantitative data, indices are used by community programs to determine and record the oral health status of groups (see Table 12.2.1). They can assess the needs of a community, assist in planning community-based health promotion/disease prevention programs, and compare the effects or evaluate the results of community-based programs (Wilkins et al. 2017, p. 371). Indices provide a way to express clinical observations in the use of numbers.

Take-Home Hints

1. Although evaluation is listed as the last step in the program planning paradigm, the program must be evaluated continuously throughout each step.
2. If fluoride varnish is not an available option for a caries prevention program in a community that does not have a fluoridated public water supply, an alternative would be to investigate fluoridation of the school water supply.

Self-Study Questions

1. What would be the most effective method for caries prevention education at the elementary school?

A. Meet with each parent to discuss benefits of fluoride
B. Plan an oral health fair
C. Educate the nurse and teachers on caries prevention
D. Discuss with local politician to get the referendum passed

2. The decision to use fluoride varnish at New East Elementary as the method for preventing decay is which level of disease prevention?

A. Primary
B. Secondary
C. Tertiary

3. What may be the possible reason(s) for the community to have limited access to dental health care?

A. Dentist too far away with community members having limited transportation options
B. Limited hours of dental offices
C. Unaffordable costs
D. Fear of the dental health-care provider
E. All of the above

4. During which stage of the process of care is the evaluation method(s) considered?

A. Treatment planning
B. Diagnosis
C. Evaluation
D. Examination
E. Assessment

5. Quantitative methods inform the dental hygienists how many children in the New School received fluoride varnish. Quantitative methods inform the dental hygienists what the students, teachers, and parents liked or did not like about the product or process.

A. First statement is true; second statement false
B. First statement is false; second statement is true
C. Both statements are true
D. Both statements are false

6. Which of the following indices will determine total dental caries experience by recording the number of affected teeth for mixed dentition?

A. DMFT
B. Combined DMFT/dmft
C. dmft
D. ECC

References

Darby, M.L. and Walsh, M.M. (2015). *Dental Hygiene Theory and Practice*, 4e. St. Louis, MO: Saunders.

Gladwin, M. and Bagby, M. (2012). *Clinical Aspects of Dental Materials*, 4e. Philadelphia, PA: Lippincott Williams & Wilkins.

Kaur, M. (2016). Application of mixed method approach in public health research. *Indian Journal of Community Medicine* 41 (2): 93–97.

Mason, J. (2010). *Concepts in Dental Public Health*, 2e. Philadelphia, PA: Lippincott Williams & Wilkins.

Massachusetts Coalition for Oral Health (MCOH) (2011) Reaching new heights in health with school-based oral health programs, *White Paper*, [Online]. Available at: http://www.masscoalitionfororalhealth.org/files/2009/06/9134_White-Paper_r5aPROOF.pdf (September 11, 2016).

Velan, E. & Nelson T. (2014) Evaluating Caries Risk, *Dimensions of Dental Hygiene,* [Online], Available at: http://www.dimensionsofdentalhygiene.com/2014/02_February/Features/Evaluating_Caries_Risk.aspx (September 6, 2016).

Wilkins, E., Wyche, C., and Boyd, L. (2017). *Clinical Practice of the Dental Hygienist*, 12e. Philadelphia, PA: Lippincott Williams & Wilkins.

Additional Resources

American Dental Association Council on Scientific Affairs (2006). Professionally applied topical fluoride: evidenced-based clinical recommendations. *Journal of American Dental Association* 137 (8): 1151–1159.

Marinho, V., Worthington, H., Walsh, T., and Clarkson, J. (2013). Fluoride varnishes for preventing dental caries in children and adolescents. *Cochran Database of Systematic Reviews* (6): –CD002280.

National Network for Oral Health Access (NNOHA) (2014) *Survey of school-based oral health program operated by health centers: Descriptive findings*, [Online]. Available at: http://www.nnoha.org/nnoha-content/uploads/2014/07/SBHC-Report-FINAL_2014-07-28.pdf (September 11, 2016).

Answers to Self-Study Questions

1. C

2. A

3. E

4. C

5. C

6. B

INDEX

Clinical Cases in Dental Hygiene, First Edition. Edited by Cheryl M. Westphal Theile, Mea A. Weinberg and Stuart L. Segelnick.